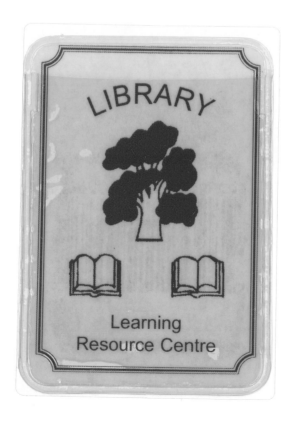

Conceptual Foundations of Occupational Therapy Practice

EDITION

4

Conceptual Foundations of Occupational Therapy Practice

Gary Kielhofner, DrPH, OTR/L, FAOTA
Professor and Wade-Meyer Chair
Department of Occupational Therapy,
College of Applied Health Sciences
University of Illinois at Chicago

EDITION

4

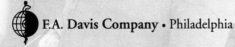 F.A. Davis Company • Philadelphia

F. A. Davis Company
1915 Arch Street
Philadelphia, PA 19103
www.fadavis.com

Printed in the United States of America

Last digit indicates print number: 10 9 8 7 6 5

Publisher: Margaret Biblis
Manager, Creative Development: George W. Lang
Senior Acquisitions Editor: Christa A. Fratantoro
Senior Developmental Editor: Jennifer A. Pine
Manager, Art and Design: Carolyn O'Brien

As new scientific information becomes available through basic and clinical research, recommended treatments and drug therapies undergo changes. The author(s) and publisher have done everything possible to make this book accurate, up to date, and in accord with accepted standards at the time of publication. The author(s), editors, and publisher are not responsible for errors or omissions or for consequences from application of the book, and make no warranty, expressed or implied, in regard to the contents of the book. Any practice described in this book should be applied by the reader in accordance with professional standards of care used in regard to the unique circumstances that may apply in each situation. The reader is advised always to check product information (package inserts) for changes and new information regarding dose and contraindications before administering any drug. Caution is especially urged when using new or infrequently ordered drugs.

Library of Congress Cataloging-in-Publication Data

Kielhofner, Gary, 1949-
  Conceptual foundations of occupational therapy practice / Gary Kielhofner. — 4th ed.
      p. ; cm.
  Rev. ed. of: Conceptual foundations of occupational therapy. 3rd. ed. c2004.
  Includes bibliographical references.
  ISBN-13: 978-0-8036-2070-4
  ISBN-10: 0-8036-2070-5
  1. Occupational therapy. I. Kielhofner, Gary, 1949- Conceptual foundations of occupational therapy. II. Title.
  [DNLM: 1. Occupational Therapy. WB 555 K47ca 2009]
  RM735.K54 2009
  615.8'515—dc22

                                                                            2008050043

For Amber, Halfie, Jane, Lorna, & Pookey
You guys are the best!

The first edition of *Conceptual Foundations* came about as an attempt to characterize the range of knowledge within occupational therapy. It appeared at a time when the field was in the midst of debate over what should be its central identity or focus. This book espoused the view that occupation was the central idea that led to the field's emergence and remained its best hope as a central theme in the field. I have been heartened over the years by the field's realization that we cannot neglect the "occupation" in occupational therapy.

This current volume was inspired by my increasing concern that the pendulum has swung too far in the other direction. It was greatly influenced by a concern that the field, in its eagerness to develop a science of occupation, may be leaving behind or forgetting the "therapy" in occupational therapy.

Thus, the fourth edition of *Conceptual Foundations* has been designed to restore some balance between the field's commitment to the occupational and everyday work of practitioners who serve the needs of their clients. The central theme of this text is that the conceptual foundations of occupational therapy must be in the service of practice. Occupational therapy is, above all, a practice profession. Thus, the knowledge that we should celebrate, support, and develop is that which advances practice.

With this in mind, I've revised the title to emphasize the centrality of practice to occupational therapy and its conceptual foundations. Further, the entire book is organized to reflect the everyday work and perspectives of a group of outstanding practitioners.

Gary Kielhofner

Yvette Hachtel, JD, MEd, OTR/L
Professor
School of Occupational Therapy
Belmont University
Nashville, Tennesee

Jane Painter, EdD, OTR/L
Associate Professor
Occupational Therapy Department
East Carolina University
Greenville, North Carolina

Neil Penny, EdD, MS, OTR/L
Assistant Professor
Occupational Therapy Department
Alvernia College
Reading, Pennsylvania

Linda Russ, PhD, OTR
Assistant Professor
Rehabilitation Science Department
University at Buffalo
Buffalo, New York

William Sisco, MA, MS, OTR
Assistant Professor
Occupational Therapy Department
Grand Valley State University
Grand Rapids, Michigan

Sheree Talkington, MA, OTR
Occupational Therapy Assistant Program
Director
Allied Health Department
Amarillo College
Amarillo, Texas

ACKNOWLEDGMENTS

The contents of this book have been in the making for some time. Along the way, more people than I can recall have influenced the four volumes of this text. I am grateful to them all. Nonetheless, my thanks here are oriented to those who had a direct impact on this fourth volume.

Over the years this text has been inspired by writers and leaders in the field. With this edition, I decided on a major reorganization. A key change was to build the book around the work of several practicing therapists. I owe a great debt of gratitude to Heidi Fischer, MS, OTR/L, Clinical Research Coordinator, Sensory Motor Performance Program, Rehabilitation Institute of Chicago; Andrea Girardi, BA(OT), Occupational Therapist and Program Coordinator, Fundación Senderos; Alice Moody, BSc(hons)OT, Clinical Specialist Occupational Therapist, Mental Health Services for Older People, Gloucester Community Team, 2gether NHS Foundation Trust, and Gloucestershire and Herefordshire Pain Management Team, Gloucestershire Hospitals NHS Foundation Trust; Bacon Fung Leung Ng, MSc(OT), SROT, ROT(HK), OTR, Senior Occupational Therapist, Castle Peak Hospital; Hiroyuki Notoh, BA, OTR, Rehabilitation Section Occupational Therapist, Tokoha Rehabilitation Hospital; Karen Roberts, Occupational Therapy Senior Clinician, Caulfield General Medical Centre; Stacey Szklut, MS, OTR/L, Executive Director, South Shore Therapies, Inc.; and Maya Tuchner, OT, MSc, School of Occupational Therapy, Faculty of Medicine, Hadassah and Hebrew University of Jerusalem, and Occupational Therapist, Rehabilitation Department, Hadassah University Hospital, who opened their practices to me and to the readers of this text. They were all generous in responding to my many inquiries and requests and inspirational in the responses and examples they provided!

My research assistant, Abigail Tamm-Seitz, was exactly what every author needs. She gave constant helpful feedback, caught my mistakes, made editorial suggestions, composed materials, chose photographs for the text, and completed other innumerable tasks all with good cheer and amazing speed. It was a genuine pleasure to have her support through the writing of this text. I am also indebted to Emily Ashpole, Annie Ploszaj, and Jessica Kramer, who provided support to this text as research assistants.

F.A. Davis staff have always believed in and supported this volume and its predecessor, *Health Through Occupation*. Since the first edition, F.A. Davis has always provided the kind of editors who make producing this volume a pleasure. My current editor, Christa Fratantoro, is no exception. Her guidance, encouragement, and friendship are much appreciated. Jennifer Pine, my developmental editor, provided thoughtful and thorough assistance throughout the process of this edition coming together.

Special thanks to Carmen Gloria de las Heras for her input, feedback, and support of case material in this book, to Elizabeth Walker Peterson for her feedback on the biomechanical chapter, to Yvette Hachtel and Noomi Katz for feedback on the cognitive model chapter, to Susan Cahill for case materials, and to Renee Taylor for sharing materials on cognitive behavioral therapy and for her feedback on many aspects of this text. Mary Alicia Barnes was so kind as to review the chapter on the functional group model and to provide a case example; many thanks to her and Sharon Schwartzberg who kindly assisted with material on the new version of this model. Thanks also to Libby Asselin, Katie Fortier, Jane O'Brien, and Rebecca Schatz for providing case materials and photos.

The staff and clients at the University of Illinois Medical Center at Chicago contributed countless hours in order to provide meaningful images of occupational therapy. Thanks to Lisa Castle, Cathleen Jensen, Tunde Koncz, Mike Littleton, Erica Mauldin, Stephanie McCammon, Sarah Skinner, Kathy Preissner, and Supriya Sen.

In addition, the book is graced with photos were collected from around the world. Thanks are also owing to Cathleen Burden, Adina Hartman-Maeir, Kayo Itoh, Rita Lefkovitz, Hitomi Matsumoto, Takeshi Muraoka, David Wilson-Brown, and Sarah Wyer who took photographs or provided pictures for this text.

I would also like to express gratitude to members of the Senderos Foundation team: Ana María Aguirre, Josefina Becerra, Rocio Carmona, Susana Infante, and Mercedes Vial, and to participants in the Senderos Foundation: Gabriel Lopez, Beltrán Molina, Marisol Salosny, and Pablo Vial, for their support. Thanks are also due to the El Valor cooking group who graciously agreed to be photographed.

CONTENTS

SECTION

Related Knowledge 229

SECTION 4

Using the Conceptual Foundations in Practice 267

An Overview of Occupational Therapy's Conceptual Foundations

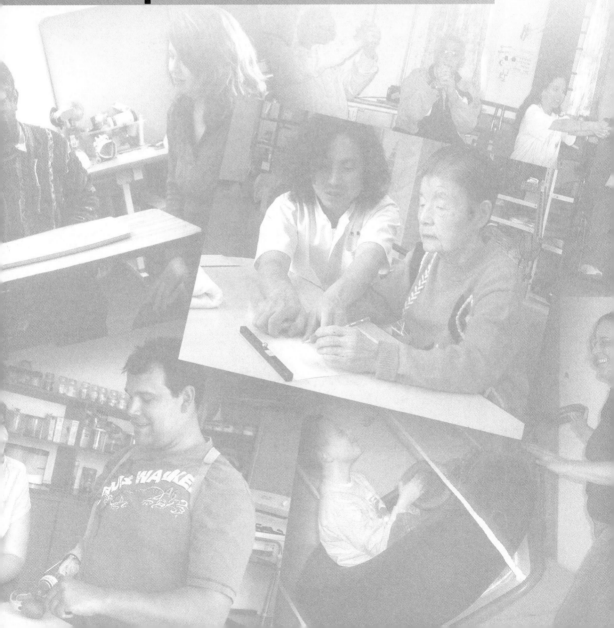

CHAPTER 1

From Practical Discovery to Conceptual Understanding

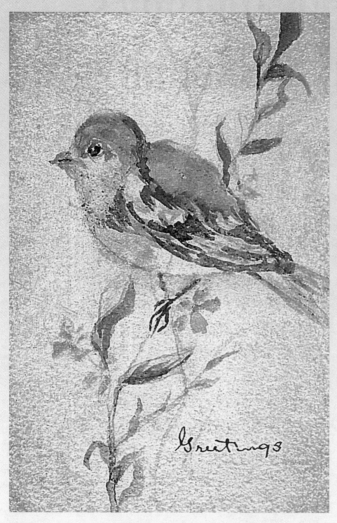

Early in the last century, Susan Tracy, one of the founders of occupational therapy in North America, sent a greeting card to another occupational therapist, Jennie K. Allen. The front of the card bore a finely executed watercolor of a bluebird perched on a blooming tree branch. On the reverse side of the card, Tracy wrote, "Done without help by a patient sent from the [psychiatrist] tagged 'not able to concentrate *at all*!' " Since she offered no further elaboration, Tracy apparently expected Allen straightaway to grasp the significance of the story she was relating.

Anyone who has practiced occupational therapy will have other versions of this story. For example, Chin-Kai Lin, a therapist from Taiwan, told of a client who had a severe head injury. Her face, distorted through facial nerve palsy and the weight of her dark future, seemed fixed in a permanent frown. One day Chin-Kai convinced the client to join in with a traditional Chinese choir. As she began to sing an ancient sacred poem her face slowly lifted, transforming into a cheerful smile.

Luc Vercruysse from Belgium shared the story of a client admitted to a psychiatric facility who was very withdrawn and despondent over his psychiatric illness and hospitalization. With a great deal of effort, Luc persuaded the client to join an occupational therapy group in which clients were busy drawing, painting, sewing, and doing other crafts. At the end of the group the client, surprised at himself, noted: "I made a candle myself. Maybe it sounds stupid, but it felt good. It showed me that I didn't need to lose heart and could go on with my life."

Patricia Laverdure, a therapist from Virginia who works for Fairfax County Public Schools, told of a second-grade girl with cerebral palsy with whom she had worked on self-care and learning to write with a pencil. One day, the little girl quietly asked if her therapist could help her learn to change her doll's clothes. The therapist put everything else aside and they worked together to figure out how the little girl could dress and undress her doll. The next week, the little girl's mother told, amidst a flurry of tears, how her daughter had gotten up the courage for the first time to invite some classmates to her house where they played with dolls all afternoon.

Such stories remain alive in occupational therapy across time and culture because they reveal the essence of the field's practice. They demonstrate how supporting clients to engage in occupations can evoke new thoughts, feelings, and actions and can result in positive changes in their lives. The observation that engagement in

an occupation had the potential to transform people is what brought the field into existence. It remains at the core of occupational therapy and is now supported by a substantial body of knowledge.

For example, contemporary occupational therapy theory states that when someone engages in an occupation, that person's unique characteristics interact with the specific occupation being done, creating a dynamic that leads people to think, feel, and behave in ways that they would not otherwise (Bass-Haugen, Mathiowetz, & Flinn, 2008; Christiansen, Baum, & Bass-Haugen, 2005; Kielhofner, 2008; Toglia, 2005). Supporting this idea, studies have shown that the kind of occupation in which a person engages can change how persons move their bodies, how effectively they can plan and attend to what they do, how much effort they use, and what they experience (Eastridge & Rice, 2004; LaMore & Nelson, 1993; Toglia, 2005; Wu, Trombly, & Lin, 1994; Yoder, Nelson, & Smith, 1989). There are assessment procedures and tools that examine how the occupations that clients do affect their cognition, motivation, and motor performance (Bass-Haugen et al., 2008; de las Heras, Geist, Kielhofner, & Li, 2002; Toglia, 2005). Finally, there are intervention protocols that provide guidance in how to select and modify the occupations to enhance what people do, think, and feel (Bass-Haugen et al., 2008; de las Heras, Llerena, & Kielhofner, 2003; Toglia, 2005).

The journey from basic observations or stories about practice to a conceptual understanding of the occupational therapy process is an important one. Everyday practice involves addressing problems such as a client's confusion, despondency, or difficulty with some aspect of performance. Practitioners often find solutions to such problems through trial and error, creative problem-solving, and application of accumulated experience. Practice-based problems and solutions eventually lead to more systematic attempts to explain what is going on and to develop even more resources for solving such problems. This

> **The observation that engagement in an occupation had the potential to transform people is what brought the field into existence.**

pathway from practical discovery to formal theory and research results in knowledge that strengthens and improves occupational therapy. All the knowledge generated from such efforts constitutes the field's conceptual foundations.

The Relationship of Occupational Therapy's Conceptual Foundations to Practice

Perhaps the best way to see why the conceptual foundations of occupational therapy are important for practice is to reflect upon what practitioners do. In what follows, we will consider four occupational therapists.

Karen Roberts works in an amputee unit of a hospital in Melbourne, Australia. Her clients are generally young men who have had traumatic amputations following worksite or motor vehicle accidents. Their amputations were sudden and unexpected, changing their lives in an instant. Many are not only experiencing a physical loss but are also grieving the loss of their future plans and dreams. When Karen introduces herself to a new client, she typically says something like the following: "I am interested in all of the things that you have to do or want to do within your life and how we are going to work together on helping you get on with your life. I am also interested in all of the things that are important to you and how you might be able to continue

doing those things in the future. When you get a prosthesis, I will be the person who will be teaching you how to operate that prosthesis and, over time, we will work together to integrate it into your daily life."

Andrea Girardi works in a community integration program at Senderos Foundation in Santiago, Chile. Her clients are young adults with mental illnesses. Overall, their histories are marked by frustrated goals and multiple failures in life roles. These young people all have in common a history of disappointments coupled with the experience of social misunderstanding and prejudice. They all feel dispirited since their previous mental health services have had limited benefits.

Andrea's clients typically behave as if they have few capacities, no personal control, and little possibility of continuing their lives in a positive direction. Most have substantial difficulties making friends or belonging to a group. These negative convictions interfere with their participation and success in life.

In working with these clients, Andrea begins with activities that facilitate their recovery of some meaning of life and then progresses toward facilitating their mastery of their own lives. Along the way, Andrea expresses her understanding of their struggles and her faith in their abilities. She views her occupational therapy process as one of helping clients slowly build a new foundation of belief in their own capacities and hope for their futures.

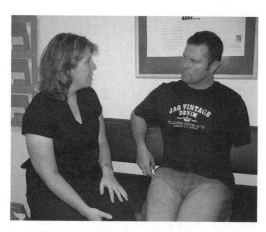

Karen discusses plans for therapy with a client who was born with limb deficiencies.

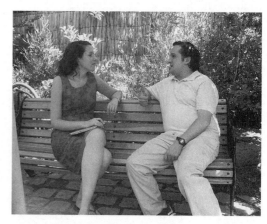

Andrea and a client discuss his progress in a community integration program.

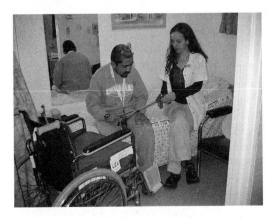

Maya shows a client who experienced a traumatic brain injury as a result of a car accident how to use a reacher to increase his independence.

Maya Tuchner works in a hospital-based rehabilitation department in Jerusalem. Many of her clients have brain damage due to strokes, traumatic accidents, or surgeries to remove brain tumors. In addition to physical problems, these clients often experience cognitive impairments that limit their ability to plan, problem-solve, and recognize errors in their own performance. Maya's clients come from a variety of backgrounds; they include, for instance, secular Jews, very religious Jews, Israeli Arabs, Palestinian Arabs, and immigrants from Russia and Ethiopia. Some of her clients were injured in terrorist bombings. With such heterogeneous clients, her largest challenge is to give all clients the best services according to their personal histories, cultures, and lifestyles.

Stacey Szklut owns and runs South Shore Therapies, a private pediatric clinic serving

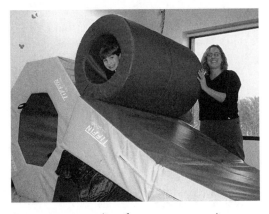

Stacey prepares a client for a sensory experience.

clients who have difficulties processing and organizing sensations that affect their motor development and ability to learn new skills. Her clients, along with their families, often struggle with the simple tasks of everyday living. The prospect of getting dressed, eating a meal, or going to the grocery store can cause anxiety and discomfort for some young clients who are hypersensitive to taste, touch, smell, and sound. Other clients, who have poor awareness of their bodies, struggle with such basic things as putting on their clothes and manipulating their fasteners or using a spoon to eat. These children often experience frustration and poor self-esteem and, therefore, exhibit difficult emotions and behaviors that affect family life and create difficulties as the children attempt to participate in the wider community.

Stacey views the therapy process as having three components: (1) enhancing the young clients' abilities to process sensations more effectively; (2) helping these children understand how their bodies work and how best to use them to do things; and (3) working with and teaching the families to adjust and adapt activities so these children can more successfully participate in family and community life. Stacey aims to make a difference in activities that are meaningful to the children and their families.

Each of these occupational therapists provides services to persons whose impairments interfere with satisfying participation in their everyday occupations. On any given day, Karen may help a client with an amputated arm relearn how to do his job using a prosthesis. Andrea may support a client to engage in an old interest and find renewed belief that she can enjoy life and do something worthwhile. Maya may help a client become aware of his tendency to forget steps in familiar tasks and use memory aids and other strategies to be able to dress and groom himself. Stacey may help a child with sensory sensitivities to try new foods or a child with poor balance to learn how to ride a bicycle.

In order to do what they do, these occupational therapists must have specialized knowledge. For instance, they must know how to:

• Augment limited ability using specialized equipment and environmental modifications that maximize the ability to do activities

• Enable clients to complete necessary tasks despite complex impairments
• Create appropriate activities that allow clients to develop new skills and participate in daily life routines
• Identify and use activities that are best suited to help a given client achieve success and rebuild the self-confidence for and interest in doing things
• Help families of clients understand their member's impairments and how those impairments affect the client's emotions, behavior, self-esteem, performance, and development

Clearly, Karen, Andrea, Maya, and Stacey each have specific knowledge and abilities that they bring to bear on the unique problems experienced by their clients. Their knowledge and abilities come, in large measure, from their field's conceptual foundations.

Karen, Andrea, Maya, and Stacey also have in common a conviction that being meaningfully occupied is fundamental to well-being. They share an understanding of the nature and purpose of their profession. They share a philosophical orientation that emphasizes respect for the unique desires and abilities of the individual. These perspectives also come from occupational therapy's conceptual foundations.

Conclusion

This book will introduce the reader to the various perspectives and knowledge that underlie

Karen's, Maya's, Andrea's, and Stacey's practices. It will discuss how their field came about and how it has changed over the years. It will present the kinds of theories and resources that they use in making sense of their clients' problems and what to do about them.

This chapter began with a story about a client with a serious impairment who was able to create a beautiful watercolor. The story was shared between two occupational therapists because it was an illustration of the potential of occupation to serve as a therapeutic tool. There is also another lesson to be taken from this story. The field of occupational therapy exists because its practitioners provide services that make a difference in the lives of their clients. This has always been and will always remain the central purpose and value of this profession.

Consequently, while this is a book about conceptual foundations, it is also a book about practice. It presents ideas, concepts, evidence, and resources that allow practitioners to support clients in achieving greater participation in the occupations they want and need to do. Said another way, this book will tell what occupational therapists have collectively learned about how to practice in the near century since Tracy sent a postcard telling her story of occupational therapy.

REFERENCES

Bass-Haugen, J., Mathiowetz, V., & Flinn, N. (2008). Optimizing motor behavior using the occupational therapy task-oriented approach. In M. Radomski & C. Trombly Latham (Eds.), *Occupational therapy for physical dysfunction* (5th ed., pp. 599–617). Philadelphia: Lippincott Williams & Wilkins.

Christiansen, C., Baum, C., & Bass-Haugen, J. (Eds.). (2005). *Occupational therapy: Performance, participation and well-being* (3rd ed.). Thorofare, NJ: Slack.

de las Heras, C.G., Geist, R., Kielhofner, G., & Li, Y. (2002). *The volitional questionnaire (VQ)* (version 4.0). Chicago: Department of Occupational Therapy, University of Illinois at Chicago.

de las Heras, C.G., Llerena, V., & Kielhofner, G. (2003). *Remotivation process: Progressive intervention for individuals with severe volitional challenges* (version 1.0). Chicago: Department of Occupational Therapy, University of Illinois at Chicago.

Eastridge, K.M., & Rice, M.S. (2004). The effect of task goal on cross-transfer in a supination and pronation task. *Scandinavian Journal of Occupational Therapy, 11,* 128–135.

Kielhofner, G. (2008). *Model of human occupation: Theory and application* (4th ed.). Baltimore: Lippincott Williams & Wilkins.

LaMore, K.L., & Nelson, D.L. (1993). The effects of options on performance of an art project in adults with mental disabilities. *American Journal of Occupational Therapy, 47,* 397–401.

Toglia, J.P. (2005). A dynamic interactional approach to cognitive rehabilitation. In N. Katz (Ed.), *Cognition and occupation across the life span: Models of intervention in occupational therapy* (2nd ed., pp. 29–72). Bethesda, MD: American Occupational Therapy Association Press.

Wu, C.Y., Trombly, C., & Lin, K.C. (1994). The relationship between occupational form and occupational performance: A kinematic perspective. *American Journal of Occupational Therapy, 48,* 679–687.

Yoder, R.M., Nelson, D.L., & Smith, D.A. (1989). Added purpose versus rote exercise in female nursing home residents. *American Journal of Occupational Therapy, 43,* 581–586.

CHAPTER 2

The Kind of Knowledge Needed to Support Practice

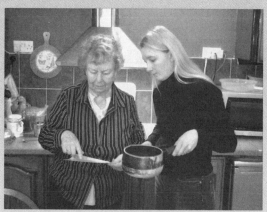

Alice and a client work on sequencing and kitchen safety.

Alice Moody works in community mental health and as part of a multidisciplinary pain management team in England. In her first role, she works with clients who have cognitive and other impairments related to severe mental illness. Her aim is to enable these clients to maintain their chosen lifestyles and goals. Part of her responsibility is conducting careful evaluations to make sure clients will be safe given their impairments and environmental contexts.

In her second role, Alice works with clients who have chronic pain. The aim of her interventions with these clients is to minimize the extent to which the pain interferes with their everyday lives and their quality of life. Among other things, Alice teaches clients how to pace what they do and how to physically undertake activities in ways that do not worsen their pain. This may involve helping one client to dress herself and another to manage his pain within a full-time job.

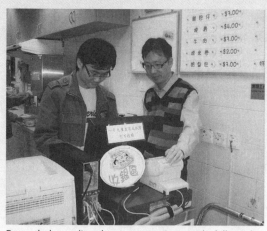

Bacon helps a client learn appropriate work skills and habits by teaching him how to operate a cash register.

Bacon Fung Leung Ng works in the largest psychiatric hospital in Hong Kong. He provides services to adult clients with severe mental illness who need work assessment and rehabilitation. Since most of his clients have severe motivational problems, he makes careful use of the therapeutic relationship to help his clients discover their own strengths and to work with them toward co-creating their futures and leading fulfilling and worthy lives.

Bacon also supervises the occupational therapy services provided to psychiatric clients with intellectual disabilities and to children and adolescents with psychiatric illness. His third professional responsibility is as a clinical educator supervising occupational therapy students during their fieldwork. In this role, he is active in demonstrating and sharing the various concepts he uses to guide his practice.

Heidi Fischer is a practitioner who has recently taken on an additional role as a clinical research coordinator in a neuro-muscular hand rehabilitation lab at a rehabilitation hospital in Chicago. She sees clients with impairments of one side of the body following stroke (hemiplegia). Part of her role is to assist with experiments that aim to improve problems with using the affected hand following stroke. Heidi uses her skills as an occupational therapist to work with the engineers to understand the barriers and supports to successful occupational performance in her clients in a number of ways. She assists in the fabrication and development of robotic devices to help clients with their hand function and to help them improve functioning in their daily lives. She designs therapy programs (that involve robotic devices or use virtual environments) to incorporate meaningful activities and help clients improve their performance in everyday activities. Her work helps assure that the interdisciplinary research of which she is a part ultimately improves the quality of life of stroke survivors.

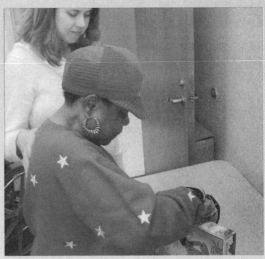

Heidi provides support to a client as she pours cereal using her hemiplegic arm.

Hiroyuki Notoh provides rehabilitation services to elderly clients in a long-term care unit. On a given day, he may see the following clients: a carpenter who broke his hip in a traffic accident and has not been able to walk, an elderly farmer who was diagnosed with dementia and has not been able to care for his orange orchard, and a grandmother who, following a stroke while shopping with friends, has lost movement on one side of her body. Each of these clients is experiencing not only a particular illness or injury but also a threat to being able to do things that really matter to them. Hiroyuki's job is to understand the nature of each client's medical and social problems, assess how the problems are affecting the client's ability to engage in life, and then involve each client in doing things in therapy that will help restore them to doing things they want to do.

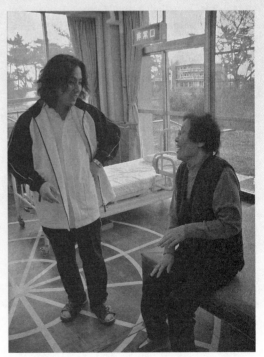

Hiroyuki discusses goals for therapy with a client who experienced a brain infarction and a hip fracture.

The Need for Different Types of Knowledge

Like all occupational therapists, Alice, Bacon, Heidi, and Hiroyuki must have a solid understanding of their unique professional roles. They must, for instance, explain what they do to clients, family members, students, and other professionals with whom they work. They must have a sense of the basic nature of their work so that they can function as occupational therapists in different practice settings, in different roles, or with very different types of clients. In short, these occupational therapists must all have a professional identity.

While important, having a professional identity is not enough for practice. These therapists must also have competence; that is, they must have knowledge and skills to understand the nature of their clients' problems and to know what types of services to provide them. The knowledge and skills that each of these therapists uses come primarily from within occupational therapy. Nonetheless, each therapist also uses some knowledge that comes from other fields such as medicine or psychology.

Thus, the conceptual foundations that guide these occupational therapists in their everyday work include three types of knowledge:

- Knowledge that defines the nature, purpose, scope, and value of occupational therapy practice
- Knowledge that enables them to understand the problems their clients are having and to know how to work with their clients to overcome those problems
- Knowledge borrowed from other fields that also informs what they do in their practice

These three types of knowledge will be referred to as the paradigm, conceptual practice models, and related knowledge. As shown in Figure 2.1, the paradigm can be thought of as the field's innermost core of knowledge in that it directly addresses the identity of occupational therapy. Surrounding the paradigm are several conceptual practice models that provide the unique concepts, evidence, and resources that occupational therapists use in their practice. The final layer, related knowledge, is a collection of concepts,

facts, and techniques from other fields that practitioners use to supplement unique occupational therapy knowledge (i.e., the paradigm and models). Table 2.1 summarizes the characteristics of these three layers of knowledge. The following sections discuss each layer in more detail.

The Paradigm

The concept of paradigm grew from the observation of how members of any discipline share a common vision (i.e., a collection of perspectives, ideas, and values that together constitute their unique perspective) (Kuhn, 1970). A paradigm defines the profession's practice for its members and presents ideals about how to practice (Tornebohm, 1985, 1986). It shapes how practitioners justify and define the services they provide to clients.

The paradigm also functions as a professional culture with common beliefs and values that make sense of and guide professional action (Macintyre, 1980). Thus, it allows therapists to understand, in a very broad way, what they are doing when they practice. That is, it defines the most basic nature of their work, its primary concerns and methods, and its values. The profession's paradigm shapes occupational therapists' understanding of the nature of the service that they provide and their particular professional perspective (how they view their clients' needs and what they hold as important).

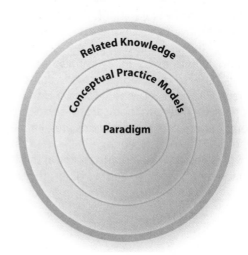

FIGURE 2.1 Concentric layers of knowledge in the conceptual foundations.

Box 2.1   A Scholarship of Practice

Scholarship (the development of theory and conduct of research) is important to occupational therapy practice. However, the relationship of theory, research, and practice is a matter of some debate. Authors in many fields have criticized scholarship for producing theory and research of questionable practical value (Barnett, 1997; Higgs & Titchen, 2001; MacKinnon, 1991; Maxwell, 1992; Schon, 1983). This problem has also been recognized in occupational therapy. In response, authors have proposed that the field needs a scholarship of practice (Hammel, Finlayson, Kielhofner, Helfrich, & Peterson, 2002; Kielhofner, 2002) in which researchers and theorists in the field work with practitioners to generate the field's theory and research and to advance practice. The scholarship of practice envisions an interaction between generating theory and research on the one hand and developing practice on the other (see figure, this box).

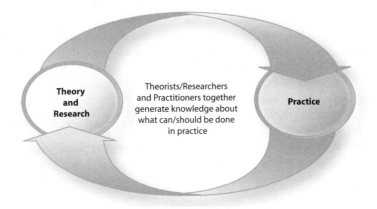

A scholarship of practice.

Theory and research provide necessary knowledge for practice. Practice points to what needs to be known and, by applying theory to real life, enriches the understanding and development of theory.

Table 2.1   Characteristics of the Layers of Knowledge

Layer	Content	Purpose
Paradigm	Broad assumptions and perspectives	• Unify the field • Define the nature and purpose of occupational therapy
Conceptual Practice Models	Diverse concepts organized into unique occupational therapy theory	• Develop theory • Provide rationale for and guide practice
Related Knowledge	Concepts, facts, and techniques borrowed from other disciplines	• Supplement unique knowledge of the field • Applied in practice

For instance, Alice, Heidi, Hiroyuki, and Bacon all see their professional roles as centered on helping clients do the everyday occupations that matter to them. They seek to achieve this aim by engaging clients in meaningful activities during therapy. These shared perspectives are all a function of a paradigm that Alice, Heidi, Hiroyuki, and Bacon share with other members of their profession.

Elements of the Profession's Paradigm

As shown in Figure 2.2, a paradigm is made up of core constructs, a focal viewpoint, and values. The core constructs define the nature of the field's service. They provide an understanding of why the service is needed, the kinds of problems that the service addresses, and how it solves those problems. The focal viewpoint directs practitioners' attention to certain things in practice and offers a way of seeing those things. Finally, because occupational therapists are engaged in practical action, they require ideas about the good they serve and about proper ways of going about what they do. Hence, values identify why

practice matters and what ought to be done in practice. The core constructs, focal viewpoint, and values together determine how occupational therapists, individually and collectively, make sense of their profession and its practice.

Paradigm Development

Chapters 3 through 5 will discuss how occupational therapy's paradigms have developed since the emergence of the field early in the last century. Those chapters will focus on how the paradigm is represented in the literature of the field. Of course, what matters most is the paradigm's influence on how individual occupational therapists make sense of what they do. After discussing the history of paradigm development, we will examine how it is reflected in the perspectives of four of the therapists introduced in Chapters 1 and 2.

Conceptual Practice Models

Although the paradigm provides a common understanding of what occupational therapy is, it does not provide specific details for how to

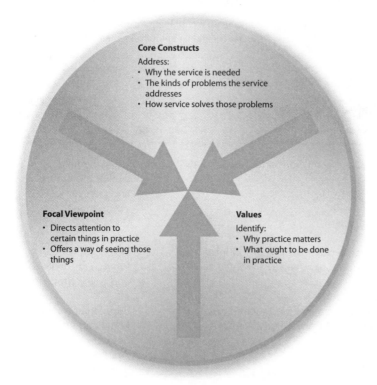

FIGURE 2.2   Elements of the paradigm.

engage in practice. The conceptual practice models provide this more detailed knowledge.

A conceptual practice model is an interrelated body of theory, research, and practice resources that is used by occupational therapists. Some models are organized around phenomena that are addressed in practice, such as problems of motion or cognitive difficulties that interfere with occupational performance. Other models address an aspect of practice such as the relationship of therapists with their clients or groups that are used in practice. All conceptual practice models provide theory, evidence, and resources that directly support practice. Because each model has a specific focus, a therapist usually employs a combination of models and uses them in the way that best addresses each client's situation.

Components of a Conceptual Practice Model

Models can be thought of as having the following components:

- Theory that explains some phenomena important to practice
- Practice resources (e.g., assessment protocols, instruments, and therapeutic methods)
- Research and evidence base that test the theory and demonstrate how the model works in practice

As shown in Figure 2.3, these components are parts of a dynamic and ongoing process of knowledge development.

One of the unique features of conceptual practice models is that they have their origins in some practice challenge. This challenge may be a particular type of problem that is often seen in clients or a process that needs to take place in therapy. The theory in each model gives logic and coherence to the practice applications that the model provides.

As a model develops, its practice resources are expanded and refined. Theorists and practitioners working within the model create assessments, accumulate case examples, write guidelines or protocols for application, and develop

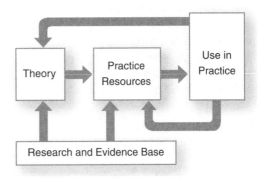

FIGURE 2.3 The dynamic and ongoing process of knowledge development in a conceptual practice model.

programs based on the model. Dissemination of these practice resources in journals, textbooks, and presentations make the model more useful in practice. Similarly, problems and insights encountered in practice may lead to changes in the model.

Research and evidence base allow for empirical scrutiny of the practice model. Studies test the accuracy of the theoretical arguments as they relate to the phenomena they seek to explain. Research also produces descriptive data helpful in elaborating the theory. Further, research tests the effectiveness of the technology for application based on the theory.

Each conceptual practice model represents a dynamic process in which knowledge is developed and used through theorizing, application, empirical scrutiny, and revision. The theory of the model provides explanations of phenomena with which it is concerned; these explanations can be verified, falsified, or refined through research. The theory also explains and directs practical application. Basic and applied research provide feedback to the model, allowing theory to be corrected and elaborated as scientific evidence is accumulated. Similarly, applications in practice can provide critical feedback leading to changes and elaborations of the theory. The conceptual practice models are part of the know-how of members of the field. When therapists use the field's knowledge,

> **Conceptual practice models provide special professional lenses through which the therapist sees the client and the therapy process, develops plans, and solves problems.**

they engage in an active process of reasoning using conceptual practice models. Conceptual practice models provide special professional lenses through which the therapist sees the client and the therapy process, develops plans, and solves problems.

Related Knowledge

Practice may require the use of some concepts and skills not unique to occupational therapy and not contained in occupational therapy's conceptual practice models. Related knowledge may include information that belongs to another profession that is also useful and necessary to occupational therapy practice. For example, medicine's knowledge of disease processes is critical to most areas of occupational therapy practice. Cognitive behavioral concepts and techniques from the field of psychology are sometimes used in occupational therapy practice. In these instances, occupational therapists use related knowledge to supplement the knowledge

that defines and guides the main elements of occupational therapy practice.

Conclusion

This chapter examined the types of knowledge that are required for practice and make up the field's conceptual foundations. We saw that practitioners use three types of knowledge in their everyday work. The first is knowledge reflected in the field's paradigm that provides therapists with a sense of professional identity, defining their service, their perspectives, and their values. The second is the knowledge of conceptual practice models that provide specific theory, resources, and evidence used to undertake the therapy process. Finally, therapists use related knowledge that originates in other fields but is used along with the unique occupational therapy paradigm and conceptual practice models. The remainder of this book will examine each of these three types of knowledge in detail and consider how therapists use them in practice.

REFERENCES

Barnett, R. (1997). *Higher occupational education: A critical business. The society for research into higher education.* United Kingdom: Open University Press.

Hammel, J., Finlayson, M., Kielhofner, G., Helfrich, C., & Peterson, E. (2002). Educating scholars of practice: An approach to preparing tomorrow's researchers. *Occupational Therapy in Health Care, 15*(1/2), 157–176.

Higgs, J., & Titchen, A. (Eds.). (2001). *Practice knowledge and expertise in the health professions.* London: Butterworth Heinemann.

Kielhofner, G. (2002). Knowledge development in occupational therapy: Directions for the new millennium. Keynote address at the World Federation of Occupational Therapy Conference, Stockholm, Sweden.

Kuhn, T. (1970). *The structure of scientific revolutions* (2nd ed.). Chicago: University of Chicago Press.

Macintyre, A. (1980). Epistemological crises, dramatic narrative, and the philosophy science.

In G. Gutting (Ed.), *Paradigms and revolutions; appraisals and applications of Thomas Kuhn's philosophy of science* (pp. 54–74). South Bend, IN: University of Notre Dame Press.

MacKinnon, C. (1991). From practice to theory, or what is a white woman anyway? *Yale Journal of Law and Feminism, 4*(13), 13–22.

Maxwell, N. (1992). What kind of inquiry can best help us create a good world? *Science, Technology, and Human Values, 17,* 205–227.

Schon, D.A. (1983). *The reflective practitioner: How professionals think in action.* New York: Basic Books.

Tornebohm, H. (1985). *Reflections on practice oriented research.* Goteborg, Sweden: University of Goteborg.

Tornebohm, H. (1986). *Caring, knowing and paradigms.* Goteborg, Sweden: University of Goteborg.

CHAPTER 3

The Early Development of Occupational Therapy Practice: The Preparadigm and Occupation Paradigm Period

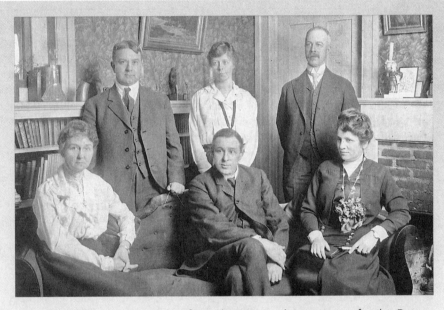

In 1917, a small group of individuals gathered to form the National Association for the Promotion of Occupational Therapy. This event is generally viewed as the formal beginning of occupational therapy in North America. In fact, this meeting was preceded by other significant accomplishments. Occupational therapy services were being offered in hospitals and other settings. Training of occupational therapists had already begun. Several books and numerous articles about occupational therapy had been published. This development of formal knowledge about practice earmarked the emergence of the profession's first paradigm. A single unifying idea brought together people from diverse professional backgrounds who were the first occupational therapists. This idea was articulated in many ways in the field's early literature and expressed in its practice. A 1915 book titled *The Work of Our Hands* neatly set forth this vision as follows:

When [the client] gets down to honest work with her hands she makes discoveries. She finds her way along new pathways. She learns something of the dignity and satisfaction of work and gets an altogether simpler and more wholesome notion of living. This in itself is good, but better still, the open mind is apt to see new visions, new hope and faith. There is something about simple, effective work with the hands that makes [humans] . . . creators in a very real sense, makes them kin with the great creative forces of the world. From such a basis of dignity and simplicity anything is possible. Many a poor starved nature becomes rich and full. All this is aside from the actual physical gains that may come from new muscular activities. (Hall & Buck, 1915, pp. 57–58)

As the quote illustrates, occupational therapy was predicated on the idea that engaging clients in occupations helped them achieve positive changes in their lives. This idea reflected a new and unique way of viewing and dealing

Herbert James Hall

Born in 1870, Herbert James Hall graduated from Harvard Medical School in 1895. He began a private general practice but soon developed an interest in the problems of persons with various forms of mental illness. In 1904, Hall and craftswoman Jessie Luther began a sanatorium called Handcraft Shops.

In 1905, Hall obtained a grant from Harvard to study the therapeutic use of occupation (Peloquin, 1990; Presidents of the AOTA, 1967). This grant built on Hall's work with persons who had neurasthenia, which Hall believed resulted in part from improper or misguided habits related to the overstrain of modern life (Creighton, 1993; Hall & Buck, 1915; Quiroga, 1995). Through his research, Hall intended to demonstrate that physical, mental, and moral health could be restored and maintained through occupation (i.e., involvement in a healthy pattern of activity) (Quiroga, 1995).

In 1912, Hall moved his sanatorium to Devereux Mansion at Marblehead, Massachusetts, where he used arts and crafts as the primary therapeutic approach. Hall considered crafts to present the just-right level of physical and mental stimulation to engage patients, allowing them to avoid idleness and isolation while preventing discouragement (Quiroga, 1995). He used progressively demanding occupations to eventually achieve a routine of alternating periods of work, play, and rest (Creighton, 1993; Hall & Buck, 1916; Quiroga, 1995). He developed a classification system for the crafts, grading them based on the demands of the task. Patients were advanced as they demonstrated improvements in attention span, coordination, and mastery of the craft (Creighton, 1993). This use of progressive and graded manual occupation allowed patients to improve their mental conditions gradually without becoming frustrated or bored in the process. Hall also espoused the idea that occupation was a useful tool in diverting a patient's thoughts away from illness. He also proposed that patients experienced the success of creation through crafts that eventually replaced their sense of failure (Quiroga, 1995).

Hall published three occupational therapy books, two with coauthor and teacher-craftswoman Mertice M.C. Buck. He created the editorial department of occupational therapy and rehabilitation in the journal *Modern Hospital* as a vehicle for promoting the profession (Presidents of the AOTA, 1967). Hall organized the Boston School of Occupational Therapy in 1918 (Hall & Buck, 1915; Hall & Buck, 1916; Presidents of the AOTA, 1967; Quiroga, 1995).

In 1921 Hall was elected to serve as the president of the National Society for the Promotion of Occupational Therapy, which was renamed during his term as the American Occupational Therapy Association (AOTA) (Quiroga, 1995). In addition to his tireless advancement of occupational therapy, Hall contributed greatly to the field's first paradigm.

with the problems of persons whose capacities were impaired. It was central to the field's first paradigm. This chapter will discuss that first paradigm, its origins, and how it defined and shaped occupational therapy practice.

The Moral Treatment Preparadigm

In the 18th and 19th centuries there arose, first in Europe and then in North America, an approach to the care of mentally ill persons referred to as moral treatment. The idea that engaging people in occupation could be used as therapy had its roots in moral treatment. For occupational therapy, moral treatment represents what is called a preparadigm—that is, a set of ideas that precedes and eventually leads to a paradigm (Kuhn, 1970). Early occupational therapists derived their fundamental concepts from the moral treatment writings, and the early practice of occupational therapy reflected its therapeutic concepts and practices (Bing, 1981; Bockoven, 1972; Dunton, 1915; Licht, 1948).

Moral treatment was inspired by the humanitarian philosophy of the Enlightenment (Magaro, Gripp, & McDowell, 1978). A central premise of moral treatment was that participation in the various tasks and events of everyday life could restore persons to more healthy and satisfying functioning. Proponents of moral treatment believed that people became mentally ill because they succumbed to external pressures by adopting faulty habits of living, becoming disengaged from the mainstream of life. Moreover, they believed that society had an obligation to help those with mental illness return to a satisfying life pattern.

The treatment approach was predicated on the assumptions that the mentally ill person retained a measure of self-command and that improvement depended largely on the person's own conduct. Thus, "employment in various occupations was expected as a way for the patient to maintain control over his or her disorder" (Bing, 1981, p. 504). In moral treatment,

> A central premise of moral treatment was that participation in the various tasks and events of everyday life could restore persons to more healthy and satisfying functioning.

the physical, temporal, and social aspects of the hospital environment were arranged to correct the person's faulty habits of living, which were believed to be a central factor in mental illness. Participation in such occupations as education, daily living tasks, work, and play was used to restore persons to healthy habits of living (Bockoven, 1972).

In the mid-19th century, converging forces led to the end of moral treatment in the United States. Rapid population growth due to large waves of immigration led to overcrowding in state hospitals. Social Darwinism and its "survival of the fittest" outlook, coupled with prejudice toward those in mental hospitals, eroded the social commitment to treat mentally ill persons. As state hospitals became congested and underfunded, moral treatment gave way to a custodial model in which people were primarily warehoused (Bockoven, 1972; Magaro et al., 1978). Although the reasons were somewhat different in Europe, moral treatment also came to an end there around this same time.

The Paradigm of Occupation

At the beginning of the 20th century, a diverse group of people in North America (e.g., physicians, nurses, architects, and craftspeople) began to reapply principles of moral treatment in several areas of caring for ill and disabled persons. Their approach came to be known as occupational therapy. As these early leaders developed and described the principles of using occupation to influence recovery from illness and adjustment to disability, they generated the core constructs, focal viewpoint, and values that made up the first paradigm.

Core Constructs

In the inaugural issue of the field's formal journal, *Archives of Occupational Therapy*, Meyer (1922) wrote:

> *Our conception of man is that of an organism that maintains and balances itself in the world of reality and actuality by being in*

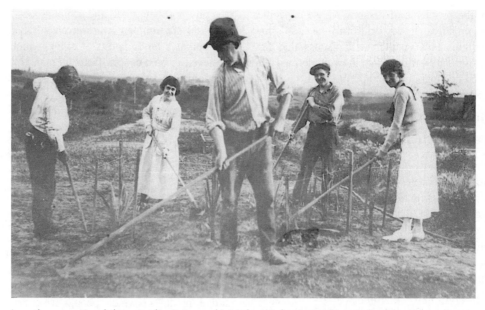

In early occupational therapy, clients in psychiatric hospitals engaged in productive outdoor occupations such as gardening and foresting.

active life and active use, i.e., using and living and acting its time in harmony with its own nature and the nature about it. It is the use that we make of ourselves that gives the ultimate stamp to our every organ. (p. 5)

Meyer identified humans as occupational beings who shaped their minds and bodies through the things they did. Meyer and William Rush Dunton, Jr., another physician and early leader of the profession, articulated a second construct that asserted that occupation consisted of an alternation between modes of existing, thinking, and acting (Dunton, 1919; Meyer,

1922). Early leaders postulated that a balance between creativity, leisurely diversion, aesthetic interests, celebration, and serious work was central to health (Dunton, 1919; Kidner, 1930; Meyer, 1922). Consequently, healthy living was seen to depend on and to be reflected in the habits that organized the everyday use of time (Meyer, 1922). Habits controlled the basic rhythm and balance of life. These habits were, in turn, maintained through ongoing engagement in everyday occupations.

A third construct asserted that the mind and body were inextricably linked. The concept of

Adolf Meyer

Adolf Meyer was a critical figure in the development of American psychiatry and occupational therapy. He received an M.D. in his native Switzerland, focusing in the area of neurology. After emigrating to Chicago in 1892, he began working as a pathologist. Influenced by his mother's mental illness, Meyer developed a growing interest in psychiatric problems (Lidz, 1985). He went on to work in New England and later at Johns Hopkins University, where he became director of its Henry Phipps Psychiatric Clinic and collaborated with Eleanor Clarke Slagle to develop occupational therapy services (Quen & Carlson, 1978). Meyer emphasized the connections of mind and body and of thinking to action along with the importance of cultivating a healthy pattern of living (Lidz, 1985).

Meyer also emphasized the role of the environment and stressed that a person's feelings could affect the body just as much as the body affected feelings. Meyer saw psychiatric disorders as patterns of behavior, action, and feeling that depended on a person's constitution and life experiences (Meyer, 1931). Rather than focusing on psychopathology, Meyer emphasized what could be changed in the client, such as habit patterns, problem-solving, and negative patterns of thinking (Lidz, 1985). Meyer also emphasized the importance of each client's unique life story and how it reflected personal attitudes, behavior, and life situation (Winters, 1951). Meyer argued that a large component of mental illness had to do with the development of faulty habits; he emphasized assisting clients by helping them recognize and change these habits (Kielhofner & Burke, 1977). He argued that an important part of the care of a person with mental illness was to "support development of a regime of work, rest, play, and socialization" (Meyer, 1931, p. 170). Meyer also emphasized that clients need to do work that is meaningful to them (Winters, 1952). Meyer's ideas significantly shaped the first paradigm of occupational therapy.

mind-body unity was interwoven with the observation that occupation was a powerful force in maintaining well-being; that is, while individuals employed their bodies in occupations, their attention was also directed to the creative and practical dimensions of the task at hand. Thus, both the body's capacities and the mind's morale and will were maintained by engagement in occupations (Dunton, 1919; Meyer, 1922). Morale, a concept borrowed from the moral treatment era, referred to the ability to see the present and future with a sense of interest and commitment. The concept of will referred to the ability to make decisions based on a clear sense of value and desire (Barton, 1919; Training of Teachers of Occupational Therapy, 1918).

A fourth construct concerned what occurred when participation in occupation was interrupted. Because occupation maintains mind and body, "enforced idleness ... [could] do damage to the mind and to the body of the ill person" (Slagle & Robeson, 1941, p. 18). Idleness (or lack of occupation) resulted in demoralization, breakdown of habits, and physical deterioration with the concomitant loss of ability to perform daily life occupations (Hass, 1944; Weiss, 1969). The following statement exemplifies this view:

> *In every functional disturbance, in addition to disorders of the central nervous system, there is a mental reaction. Pain, anemia, impairment of circulation, and sense impressions and emotions, such as anxiety and*

William Rush Dunton, Jr.

William Rush Dunton, Jr., was born in 1868 in Philadelphia (Licht, 1967). After earning a degree in medicine, he began working in Maryland at Sheppard Asylum, a private hospital for the mentally ill (Bing, 1967). Dunton's extensive reading in psychiatry led him to the work of Tuke, the moral treatment writer and founder of the York Retreat in England, as well as to the writings of his ancestor Benjamin Rush, the father of American psychiatry and early proponent of moral treatment. Exposure to moral treatment principles provided Dunton a foundation for leading the development of early occupational therapy. In 1912, he was appointed the director of occupation at the Sheppard Asylum and thereafter devoted a major portion of his time and energy to understanding occupation as a therapeutic agent.

(box continues on page 20)

In 1915, Dunton published *Occupational Therapy: A Manual for Nurses* and in 1919 a second book, *Reconstruction Therapy*, which outlined basic principles of occupational therapy. Dunton was the first to conceive of and originally use the term "occupational therapy" (Bing, 1967). He became one of the original founders of the National Society for the Promotion of Occupational Therapy in 1917 and a year later was elected president (Licht, 1967).

Dunton later opened a small private hospital, Harlem Lodge, where he developed occupational therapy as a key element of treatment. In 1939, he left clinical work to concentrate more on editing *Occupational Therapy and Rehabilitation,* the profession's first journal. In 1950, he collaborated with Sidney Licht to publish *Occupational Therapy: Principles and Practice*, which reintroduced many moral treatment writings to the field (Dunton & Licht, 1950).

In sum, Dunton was an important influence in the early development of the field. He was a founder and leader of the national association. He also introduced moral treatment principles that served as an important basis for the first paradigm.

depression, are all communicated to the brain . . . In ennui the tonicity of the muscles is affected so that they actually contract less strongly and develop less force. In melancholia the general physique, and especially the heart, is acted on . . . Morbid introspection produces a particularly vicious cycle of thinking, since continued attention focused on any particular part of the body may actually increase its morbid condition. (Training of Teachers for Occupational Therapy, 1918, p. 35)

As the statement illustrates, the negative effects of idleness were thought to infiltrate both body and mind, each magnifying the problem in the other.

A final construct asserted that, since occupation maintained the body and mind, it was particularly suited as a therapeutic tool for regenerating lost function. Occupation was recognized as a successful organizing force because it required an exercise of function in which mind and body were united (Dunton, 1919; Kidner, 1930; Training of Teachers for Occupational Therapy, 1918).

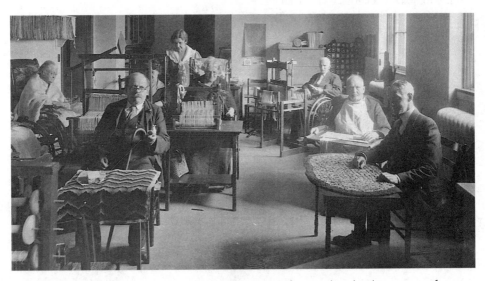

The therapeutic occupations of weaving and sewing were often used to develop a sense of competence and productivity.

Occupation was thought to provide a diversion from physical and psychic pain that encouraged the individual to use his or her mental and physical capacities. The following statement by Slagle and Robeson (1941) illustrates this view:

> Let our minds be engaged with the spirit of fun and competitive play and leave our

muscles, nerves and organs to carry on their functions without conscious thought—then our physical exercise will be correspondingly more beneficial and we can readily picture the effect exerted on the mood of the sullen, morose patient by the genial glow which suffuses the body following active exercise. (p. 53)

Eleanor Clarke Slagle

Eleanor Clarke Slagle was born circa 1871 in New York. There she attended a private academy and high school, where she studied music. Her interest in disability-related services likely grew from her experiences as a family caregiver to her father who returned from the Civil War impaired from a gunshot wound, her brother who had tuberculosis and problems with substance abuse, and her nephew who contracted polio and later experienced emotional problems (Quiroga, 1995).

In 1911, Slagle enrolled at Hull House in the Chicago School of Civics and Philanthropy in a course of amusements and occupation. Slagle deplored the prevailing negative social attitudes toward those with disabilities and took an active interest in how state institutions treated persons with mental illness. After completing her Hull House training, Slagle began organizing similar training programs in Michigan and New York mental health facilities, later returning to Chicago's Hull House as a faculty member (Schultz & Hast, 2001).

Next, Slagle joined Adolf Meyer at Johns Hopkins Hospital in Baltimore, where she created and directed a department of occupational therapy. In 1915, she returned to Chicago and served as director of the Henry B. Favill School of Occupations at Hull House and as director of Occupational Therapy for Illinois state mental hospitals (Schultz & Hast, 2001).

Building on Meyer's idea that disorganized habits characterized mental illness, Slagle developed programs of habit training. These programs, which were designed for patients with chronic and severe mental illness, included a 24-hour regimen of self-care, occupational classes, walks, meals in small groups, recreational activity, and physical exercise (Loomis, 1992). Slagle was later appointed by the governor of Illinois to be general superintendent of occupational therapy for the Illinois Department of Public Welfare. In this role, she supervised occupational therapy services throughout state institutions (Schultz & Hast, 2001). In 1922, Slagle became director of occupational therapy for the New York State Department of Mental Hygiene, where she continued promoting habit training in education. She held this position until her death in 1942.

At the outbreak of World War I, Slagle was asked by the Chicago Red Cross chapter to direct a six-week training course for volunteers in occupational therapy (reconstruction aides) to meet the urgent demands of returning injured and battle-fatigued soldiers. Slagle, along with William Rush Dunton, Jr., approached the American Armed Services with their evidence on occupational therapy's positive effect on rehabilitation of soldiers. Eventually, the U.S. Surgeon General appointed Slagle a consultant to the U.S. Army for the training of reconstruction aides. In six months, Slagle toured up to 20 military hospitals and directed the training of 4,000 therapists (Schultz & Hast, 2001).

(box continues on page 22)

In 1917, Slagle joined other early leaders in Clifton Springs, New York, to form the National Society for the Promotion of Occupational Therapy. Slagle was elected the Society's first vice-president and served in this post in 1919. She became president in 1920 (Schultz & Hast, 2001). As Executive Secretary for the American Occupational Therapy Association (formerly the National Society for the Promotion of Occupational Therapy), Slagle was instrumental in forming the Association's theoretical underpinnings and designing standards for occupational therapy educational and treatment programs. In 1933, she published the *Syllabus for Training of Nurses in Occupational Therapy*, and in the mid-1930s she worked with the American Medical Association to develop guidelines for the accreditation of occupational therapy programs as well as a system for registering trained practitioners.

In sum, Slagle's influence on occupational therapy was at multiple levels. She helped shape the concepts of the first paradigm. She developed new approaches to practice, especially habit training. She tirelessly promoted occupational therapy in state institutions and the military. Finally, she was one of the most influential leaders in developing the professional association and mechanisms for ensuring quality education and credentialing of occupational therapists.

Focal Viewpoint

The focal viewpoint of early occupational therapy centered on three phenomena and their interrelationships: mind, body, and environment. The mind was the pivotal area of concern. Motivating the person, influencing attitudes and morale, and eliciting physical activity through mental engagement were primary themes. In her explanation of how to motivate people, Tracy (1912) typifies discussions of the time:

> *It is easier to find something that he can do than to find something he will do. One needs to be resourceful, with a large variety of appeals, for it goes without saying that even in health what appeals to one person will not to another. The difference is even more marked*

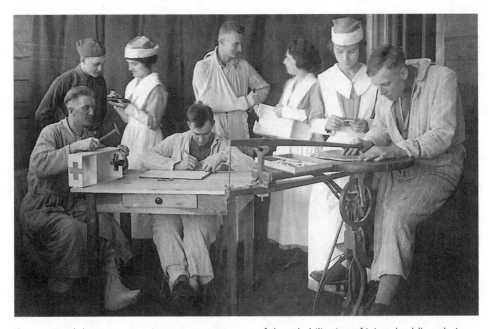

Occupational therapy was an important component of the rehabilitation of injured soldiers during World War I, supporting recovery from psychological and physical trauma.

among the insane. Appeals may be made through praise, competition, rewards; to the sense of the beautiful or to the useful; through affection for relatives, home needs, gifts to friends, or more diffuse altruism, as helping other patients, making preparations for special entertainments, such as Christmas gifts and decorations, or work for children . . . (pp. 157–158)

To early occupational therapists, motivation was seen not only as a problem of how to engage the person in therapeutic occupations but also as a necessary component of recovery. For example, there was the caveat, "Remember that restoration of physical capacity without the will to do is a futile thing. Good medical practice demands healing of the mind as well as of body or organ. . . " (Slagle & Robeson, 1941, p. 29). Therefore, the aim of therapy was to

    . . . create a wholesome interest in something outside the patient's morbid interest in himself and his symptoms . . . [and] to prepare his mental attitude so that he may adjust himself to normal demands and environment after

the hospital discharge. (Training of Teachers for Occupational Therapy, 1918, p. 50)

The human body was viewed as a dynamic entity, integrated into the larger pattern of everyday occupation:

    Our body is not merely so many pounds of flesh and bone figuring as a machine, with an abstract mind or soul added to it. It is throughout a live organism pulsating with its rhythm of rest and activity. . . . (Meyer, 1922, p. 10)

Consequently, practitioners tried to understand not only how the body was used in various tasks but also how it required regular rhythms of work, rest, recreation, and sleep. When the body was compromised through illness or injury, the immediate concern was to prevent further degeneration by engaging the body in occupations in whatever way possible.

Engaging clients in occupations required creativity. Tasks had to be adapted so that the person could use remaining capacities to perform. Kidner (1930) outlined the principle that

Susan Elizabeth Tracy

Susan Elizabeth Tracy was born in Massachusetts. She studied nursing at Massachusetts Homeopathic Hospital, graduating in 1898. There she observed that patients who engaged in activity during hospitalization fared better than those who were idle (Licht, 1967). Consequently, when Tracy went to work as a private nurse, she began using occupation in treatment (Parsons, 1917).

After studying hospital economics and manual arts in 1905, she became administrator of the training school for nurses at the Adams Nervine Asylum in Jamaica Plain, Massachusetts (Barrows, 1917; Licht, 1967). Tracy originally held occupation classes for patients in her own home. After construction of a new facility with specialized occupational therapy space, she began including student nurses in the occupation classes. Soon the nursing course in occupation extended to be year-round (Barrows, 1917).

In 1912, Tracy decided to devote her life to occupational therapy (Cameron, 1917). She began her own Experiment Station for the Study of Invalid Occupations in Jamaica Plain. There she instructed patients and public health and graduate nurses (Quiroga, 1995).

Although invited, Tracy was unable to join the 1917 meeting in which founders gathered to sign the certificate of incorporation of the National Society for Promotion of Occupational Therapy. Nonetheless, Tracy was listed as an incorporator and elected as an officer to the Board of Management (Barrows, 1917).

(box continues on page 24)

Tracy's first book, *Studies in Invalid Occupation,* was published in 1910, becoming the first American book on occupational therapy (Licht, 1967; Tracy, 1912). It was used widely as a textbook in the field until around 1940 (Quiroga, 1995). Tracy emphasized the importance of engaging patients properly in occupations by correctly matching activities to interests and by grading occupations to capacities. She emphasized that therapeutic occupation needed to "possess a certain dignity" (Tracy, 1912, p. 14) and hold meaning for the patient.

In sum, Tracy contributed to the founding of occupational therapy and development of the professional association. She developed some of the first education of practitioners. She contributed to the development of concepts and practice.

tasks had to be graded according to individuals' capacities throughout the course of therapy.

Like the proponents of moral treatment, early occupational therapists believed that the environment was an important element of the therapeutic process. They recognized that the environment included (1) social attitudes concerning involvement in occupations (e.g., the ideas of craftsmanship and sportsmanship; the value of work); and (2) occupations in which persons participated in ordinary life. Occupational therapy was viewed as a carefully structured environment in which people could explore potentials and learn about effective and satisfying ways to participate in everyday life. To this end, the social and task environments were carefully managed.

Therapists sought to provide a facilitating environment in the hospital. Natural rhythms of time use were seen as essential to the regeneration of habits in persons (Meyer, 1922; Slagle, 1922; Slagle & Robeson, 1941). Moreover, the occupational therapy environment, in order to be therapeutic, required the presence of creative and challenging opportunities and of persons (usually therapists) who demonstrated interest and a high level of competency in these occupations:

> *Much importance was placed on the occupation room, wherein opportunity was provided for various forms of interesting and useful work. Weaving rugs and finer fabrics, basket work, book binding and clay modeling were employed at the start. Fortunately there was*

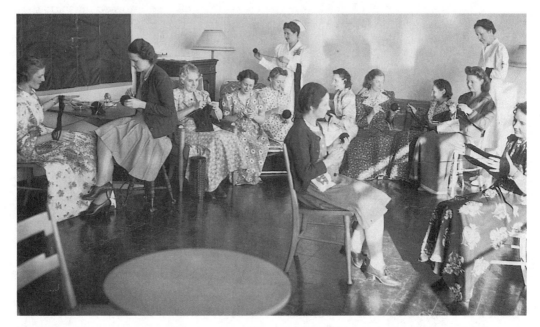

Occupational therapy groups provide an opportunity to socialize while engaging in creative occupations.

Thomas B. Kidner

Born in England, Thomas Bessell Kidner studied architecture and building construction at the Merchant Venturer's College in Bristol and London. He specialized in designing hospitals and other rehabilitation institutions. In 1900, he moved to Canada, going on to hold several positions; in 1915, he was appointed Vocational Secretary of the Canadian Military Hospitals Commission. Because of his experience in developing vocational rehabilitation for Canadian soldiers, in 1918 the Canadian government lent Kidner to the United States to become a special advisor to the Surgeon General of the Army on the vocational rehabilitation of disabled veterans (Obituary, 1932). In the following years, until his death in 1932, Kidner held various governmental and private positions in the United States as a consultant on planning, building, and organizing hospitals and other rehabilitation institutions for persons with tuberculosis and various other disabilities. He was on the staff of the Surgeon General, worked with the Public Health Service and the Veteran Bureau, and served from 1919 to 1926 as the Secretary of the National Tuberculosis Association. He played a major role in the early development of occupational therapy as a profession and a field of therapeutic practice.

Kidner's relationship with occupational therapy in the United States began in March 1917, when George E. Barton invited him to serve as one of the founders of the National Society for the Promotion of Occupational Therapy. At Consolation House, he became one of the six incorporators of the association and was elected a member of the Association Board; he later served as President of the American Occupational Therapy Association (AOTA) from 1922 to 1928 (Licht, 1967; Quiroga, 1995).

In his 1930 book, Kidner outlined his vision for the scope and structure of occupational therapy in various inpatient and outpatient settings, including mental hospitals, general hospitals, orthopedic cases, pediatrics, long convalescence, and community-based curative workshops. He wrote numerous publications that discussed the therapeutic nature of occupations and the structure and methods of occupational therapy in rehabilitation. In one he notes

> Occupational Therapy provides a means of conserving and bringing into play whatever remains to the sick and injured of capacity for healthy functioning. The patient is aided in mobilizing his physical, mental and spiritual resources for overcoming his disability. The tedium and consequent depression occasioned by the enforced idleness of illness are relieved, suffering is diminished, the care and management of the patient present fewer difficulties, convalescence is hastened, and the danger of relapses, invalidism and dependency is reduced. (Kidner, 1930, p. 40)

For this reason, he argued that engagement in occupations played a central role in rehabilitation (Kidner, 1922).

Kidner also discussed the methods for engaging patients in curative occupations and emphasized the overriding principle of gradualism (grading tasks in terms of the level of participation they require and their physical demands). Kidner suggested that occupational therapists begin with bedside habit training, progress patients to participation in simple occupations for diversion in the ward (e.g., reading or crafts), and then introduce them to the curative occupational therapy workshop (Kidner, 1930). In sum, Kidner played a major role in shaping occupational therapy's paradigm and its practice.

secured an excellent leader, trained in teaching, conversant with the work taken up and interested in it. The room was open at definite hours each day, but at other times those who wished could work without the presence of the teacher if their condition permitted. . . The atmosphere of interested activity prevailed. The work became the source of new purposes, of changed avenues of thought and of stimulated ambitions. (Fuller, 1912, p. 7)

In some cases the environment was highly regulated in an effort to develop healthy habits. Such habit-training programs for severely mentally ill persons employed highly organized schedules of everyday occupation.

The environment was also seen as a context for meeting a variety of needs. Simple games, music, and a colorful atmosphere were used to stimulate the senses of regressed individuals. As persons progressed, therapists directed them toward more demanding occupations that emphasized sportsmanship and craftsmanship (Dunton, 1922; Hass, 1944). Industrial therapy, the final phase of therapy, prepared people for the world of work (Bryan, 1936; Marsh, 1932). Individuals worked in various hospital industries (e.g., laundry, building and grounds maintenance, kitchen), engaging in real-life tasks under conditions that mirrored work outside the institution.

In sum, therapists saw the individual as a whole person (body and mind) in interaction with life tasks in the environment. Although the therapists realized that physical capacity was necessary to function, they put less emphasis on the detailed workings of the body than on environmental and mental matters. This is not to suggest that therapists did not consider how occupation could be used to achieve specific motor improvement. Rather, the therapists' fundamental vision was of occupation as the dynamic force that, by employing body and mind in interaction with the environment, maintained the ability to function. This focal viewpoint was both holistic and dynamic.

Values

Early occupational therapy inherited from moral treatment a belief in the essential worth of individuals and in their right to humane care. Interwoven with this belief were the convictions that:

• The individual achieved dignity in the performance of everyday occupations
• Meaning was realized in productive achievements and in creative and aesthetic pursuits

Thus, occupation was valued for its role in human life. Early therapists saw the importance of meaningful occupation as opposed to mere activity.

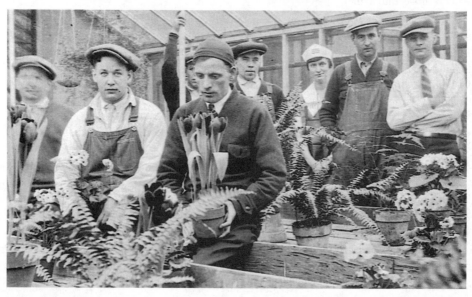

Occupational therapy clients developed a sense of responsibility and utility while working in a greenhouse caring for plants.

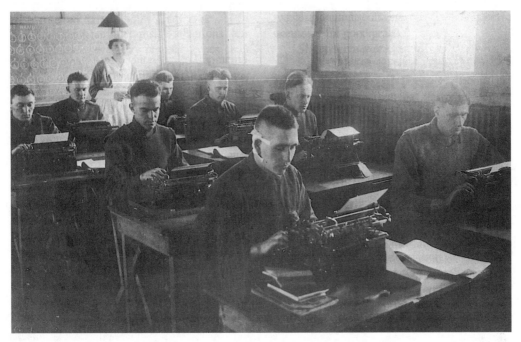

Soldiers injured in World War I learn new skills of shorthand and typing as part of a vocational rehabilitation program.

Crafts, sports, recreation, and work were all valued because they embodied something important about the human spirit as reflected in the workmanship, sportsmanship, and craftsmanship. Because humans were by nature doers and creators, they were seen as having a right to engage in occupations. Finally, therapists valued holism, recognizing the connection between mind and body and seeing the person as connected to the environment through participation in occupations (Hall & Buck, 1915; Slagle & Robeson, 1941).

> As a result of this early paradigm, occupational therapy identified itself as a field that appreciated the importance of occupation in human life, addressed problems of occupational disengagement, and used occupation as a therapeutic measure.

Summary

Occupational therapy's early paradigm focused on occupation, its role in human life and in health, and its potential as a therapeutic tool. The core constructs, focal viewpoint, and values of this paradigm (as shown in Table 3.1) shaped early occupational therapy practice. This practice approached people largely in terms of their motivation, emphasizing the importance of occupations as therapeutic media (e.g., crafts, dance, music, games, sports, and work activities). As a result of this early paradigm, occupational therapy identified itself as a field that appreciated the importance of occupation in human life, addressed problems of occupational disengagement, and used occupation as a therapeutic measure.

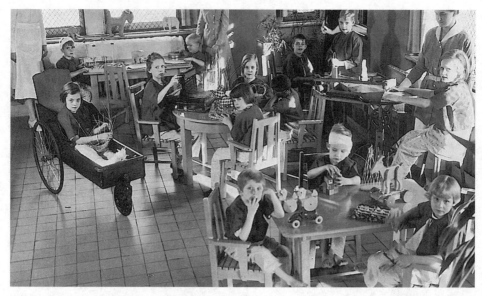

Play and crafts provide opportunities for children with physical impairments to develop a sense of enjoyment and mastery while developing their capacities.

Table 3.1 **The Paradigm of Occupation**

Core Constructs	• Occupation consists of alternation between modes of existing, thinking, and acting and requires a balance of these in daily life. • Mind and body are inextricably linked. • Idleness (lack of occupation) can result in damage to body and mind. • Occupation can be used to regenerate lost function.
Focal Viewpoint	• Environment, mind, and body, with a focus on motivation and environmental factors in performance. • Human dignity as realized in performance.
Integrated Values	• Importance of occupation for health. • Holistic viewpoint.

REFERENCES

Barrows, M. (1917). Susan E. Tracy, R.N. *Maryland Psychiatric Quarterly, 6*, 53–62.

Barton, G. (1919). *Teaching the sick: A manual of occupational therapy and re-education.* Philadelphia: W.B. Saunders.

Bing, R. (1981). Occupational therapy revisited: A paraphrastic journey. *American Journal of Occupational Therapy, 35*, 499–518.

Bing, R.K. (1967). William Rush Dunton, Jr.: American psychiatrist and occupational therapist 1868–1966. *American Journal of Occupational Therapy, 21*, 172–175.

Bockoven, J.S. (1972). *Moral treatment in community mental health.* New York: Springer.

Bryan, W. (1936). *Administrative psychiatry.* New York: W.W. Norton.

Cameron, R.G. (1917). An interview with Miss Susan Tracy. *Maryland Psychiatric Quarterly, 6*, 65–66.

Creighton, C. (1993). Graded activity: Legacy of the sanatorium. *American Journal of Occupational Therapy, 47*, 745–748.

Dunton, W.R. (1915). *Occupational therapy: A manual for nurses.* Philadelphia: W.B. Saunders.

Dunton, W.R. (1919). *Reconstruction therapy.* Philadelphia: W.B. Saunders.

Dunton, W.R. (1922). The educational possibilities of occupational therapy in state hospitals. *Archives of Occupational Therapy, 1,* 403–409.

Dunton, W.R., & Licht, S. (Eds.). (1950). *Occupational therapy: Principles and practice.* Springfield, IL: C.C. Thomas.

Fuller, D. (1912). Introduction: The need of instruction for nurses in occupations for the sick. In S. Tracy (Ed.), *Studies in invalid occupation.* Boston: Whitcomb & Barrows.

Hall, H.J., & Buck, M.M. (1916). *Handicrafts for the handicapped.* New York: Moffat, Yard & Company.

Hall, H.J., & Buck, M.M.C. (1915). *The work of our hands: A study of occupations for invalids.* New York: Moffat, Yard & Company.

Hass, L. (1944). *Practical occupational therapy.* Milwaukee, WI: Bruce.

Kidner, T.B. (1922). Work for the tuberculous during and after the cure. *Archives of Occupational Therapy, 1*(5), 363–375.

Kidner, T.B. (1930). *Occupational therapy: The science of prescribed work for invalids.* Stuttgart, Germany: W. Kohlhammer.

Kielhofner, G., & Burke, J.P. (1977). Occupational therapy after 60 years: An account of changing identity and knowledge. *American Journal of Occupational Therapy, 31,* 675–689.

Kuhn, T. (1970). *The structure of scientific revolutions* (2nd ed.). Chicago: University of Chicago Press.

Licht, S. (1948). *Occupational therapy sourcebook.* Baltimore: Williams & Wilkins.

Licht, D. (1967). The founding and founders of AOTA. *American Journal of Occupational Therapy, 21,* 269–277.

Lidz, T. (1985). Adolf Meyer and the development of American psychiatry. *Occupational Therapy in Mental Health, 5*(3), 33–53.

Loomis, B. (1992). The Henry B. Favill school of occupations and Eleanor Clarke Slagle. *American Journal of Occupational Therapy, 46,* 34–37.

Magaro, P., Gripp, R., & McDowell, D. (1978). *The mental health industry: A cultural phenomenon.* New York: John Wiley & Sons.

Marsh, C. (1932). Borzoi: Suggestions for a new rallying of occupational therapy. *Archives of Occupational Therapy, 11,* 169–183.

Meyer, A. (1922). The philosophy of occupational therapy. *Archives of Occupational Therapy, 1,* 1–10.

Meyer, A. (1931). *Psychobiology: A science of man.* Springfield, IL: Charles C. Thomas.

Obituary. (1932). *Occupational Therapy and Rehabilitation, 11,* 321–323.

Parsons, S.E. (1917). Miss Tracy's work in general hospitals. *Maryland Psychiatric Quarterly, 6,* 63–64.

Peloquin, S.M. (1990). Occupational therapy service: Individual and collective understandings of the founders, part 2. *American Journal of Occupational Therapy, 45,* 733–743.

Presidents of the American Occupational Therapy Association: 1917–1967. (1967). *American Journal of Occupational Therapy, 21,* 290–298.

Quen, J.M., & Carlson, E.T. (1978). *American psychoanalysis: Origins and development.* New York: Brunner/Mazel.

Quiroga, V.A. (1995). *Occupational therapy: The first 30 years 1900–1930.* Bethesda, MD: American Occupational Therapy Association.

Schultz, R.L., & Hast, A. (Eds.). (2001). *Women building Chicago 1790–1990: A biographical dictionary.* Bloomington, IN: Indiana University Press.

Slagle, E.C. (1922). Training aides for mental patients. *Archives of Occupational Therapy, 1,* 11–17.

Slagle, E.C., & Robeson, H. (1941). *Syllabus for training of nurses in occupational therapy* (2nd ed.). Utica, NY: State Hospitals Press.

Tracy, S. (1912). *Studies in invalid occupation.* Boston: Whitcomb & Barrows.

Training of teachers for occupational therapy for the rehabilitation of disabled soldiers and sailors. (1918). Federal Board for Vocational Education, Washington, DC: Government Printing Office.

Weiss, P. (1969). Living nature and the knowledge gap. *Saturday Review, 56,* 19–22.

Winters, E. (Ed.). (1951). *The collected papers of Adolf Meyer: Volume II: Psychiatry.* Baltimore: Johns Hopkins Press.

Winters, E. (Ed.). (1952). *The collected papers of Adolf Meyer: Volume IV: Mental hygiene.* Baltimore: Johns Hopkins Press.

CHAPTER 4

The Development of Occupational Therapy Practice in Mid-Century: A New Paradigm of Inner Mechanisms

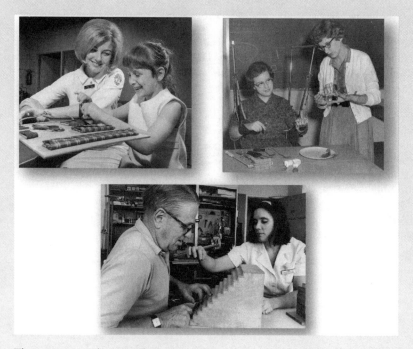

The previous chapter described the emergence and formation of the field's first paradigm. Paradigms can change, but the change is neither gradual nor incremental. Paradigm change results in such deep transformation of a profession that it is referred to as a revolution (Kuhn, 1970). This chapter presents the field's second paradigm, discussing why it came into existence and how it transformed occupational therapy practice.

The Call for a New Paradigm

In the late 1940s and the 1950s, occupational therapy came under pressure from medicine to establish a new theoretical rationale for its practice. The following typifies the kind of criticism that physicians leveled at the field:

> No one who has seen a good occupational therapy program in action can doubt that it seems to result in great help for some patients, and some help for many. There appears, however, to be no rigorous and comprehensive theory which will explain who is helped, how, by what, or why. . . (Meyerson, 1957, p. 131)

Medicine's critique of occupational therapy was grounded in its own particular viewpoint. In the 20th century, medicine increasingly sought to understand health and illness through careful identification and analysis of the inner workings of the human psyche and body (Riley, 1977). Medical intervention in such a framework aimed at identifying and repairing problems with these inner workings through such means as surgery, chemotherapy, and psychotherapy (Buhler, 1962). These medical perspectives and interventions were quite different from occupational therapy's perspectives and practice, which were grounded in the philosophy of moral treatment.

Along with physicians who criticized occupational therapy as insufficiently grounded in theory and research, many occupational therapists came to see their paradigm as unsuitable to explain and justify the field's practice. Moreover, physicians and occupational therapy leaders recommended replacing the paradigm with new concepts derived from medicine. For example, it was proposed that psychodynamic concepts used by psychiatrists were more important to mental health practice than concepts of occupation:

> According to our point of view occupation is neither the aim nor the mechanism operating in this field [and]. . . is undefinable if the framework within which it seeks theoretical clarification is psychodynamics. (Azima & Azima, 1959, p. 216)

The psychoanalytic perspective proposed that the only value of the client's engagement in occupation was that it served as a vehicle for expressing unconscious emotion. Similarly, critics writing from the physical disabilities practice area called for a refocusing to a neuromuscular perspective:

> A commonly accepted justification of the use of crafts and games as therapeutic media is the emotional value to the patient of an interesting and creative experience. The reasoning is accepted as a basic and important assumption empirically but not scientifically demonstrated. While the interest and pleasure of a creative activity are important, they do not provide the most fundamental and vital concept underlying occupational therapy of physical disabilities... Realization of the importance of neurophysiological mechanisms in the treatment of the motor system is increasing. A study of them increases understanding of how the neuromuscular system operates in terms of purposeful function. (Ayres, 1958, p. 300)

Forging a closer alliance with medicine, the field began to explain its practice increasingly in terms of medicine's perspectives (Rerek, 1971). Leading occupational therapists proposed a new view of the therapeutic process in terms of underlying neurological, anatomical, and intrapsychic mechanisms (Ayres, 1963; Fidler, 1958; Rood, 1958). They also argued that the value of occupational therapy depended on its ability to influence these inner mechanisms and thereby reduce clients' neurological, biomechanical, and psychodynamic impairments.

The Mechanistic Paradigm

Proponents of the new paradigm prevailed. Occupational therapists came to believe it would bring occupational therapy recognition as an efficacious medical service and increase its scientific respectability. Although the transition to a focus on inner mechanisms was gradual and subtle, by the end of the 1950s it dramatically changed how occupational therapists saw their practice and the kinds of services they delivered. One writer envisioned a new paradigm in the following words:

> As we talk of techniques let us think of underlying principles and build procedure on scientific fact. The clues lie in the basic concepts of psychology, physiology and anatomy. (McNary, 1958, p. 203)

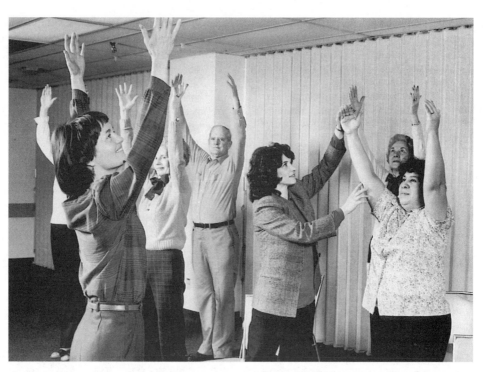

Clients engage in a range of motion dance exercise while the therapist helps them position their hands and arms properly to maximize the therapeutic value of the exercise.

Importantly, the adoption of this new paradigm meant that occupational therapists reformulated their focal viewpoint, core constructs, and values.

Focal Viewpoint

The focal viewpoint of the new paradigm centered on the internal intrapsychic, neurological, and biomechanical mechanisms as illustrated by the following quote:

> Much of the time both the sensory and the psychotherapeutic situation are dealing with semi- or non-conscious experiences. The psychotherapist thinks in terms of subconscious psychological complexes and dynamics; the sensory integrative therapist includes many subcortical integrative mechanisms in his thinking and treatment planning. While one therapist is considering the Oedipus complex, the other is considering brain stem integrating processes. In both cases the underlying mechanisms are recognized, their effect

> on behavior analyzed, and methods of dealing with them contemplated. (Ayres, 1972, p. 266)

This shift in the focal viewpoint meant that therapists were no longer focused on the broad benefits of occupation and the related, holistic themes of mind-body and person-environment interaction. The new focus was on understanding and addressing impairments related to the musculoskeletal, neuromotor, and intrapsychic systems. The focus of practice shifted, then, to looking within the person at those mechanisms that were disrupted and in need of repair.

The new focus was on understanding and addressing impairments related to the musculoskeletal, neuromotor, and intrapsychic systems.

Core Constructs

The orientation provided by this new paradigm is characterized in the following core constructs:

- All ability to perform is directly determined by the degree of integrity of the neuromotor, musculoskeletal, and intrapsychic functions
- Dysfunction or impairment can be traced to damage or abnormal development in the

A. Jean Ayres

A. Jean Ayres was born in 1920 and died in 1988 in California. At the University of Southern California she received bachelor's and master's degrees in occupational therapy and a Ph.D. in educational psychology. She did postdoctoral training in child development and neuroscience.

As a therapist, Ayres worked with children. Her observations of learning-disabled children sparked an interest in exploring perceptual and motor contributions to learning. She devoted her career to developing a theory explaining relationships among neural functioning, sensorimotor behavior, and early academic learning. She identified specific subtypes or patterns of sensorimotor dysfunction and developed specific intervention strategies for them. She was the first to identify and describe sensory integration dysfunction, previously thought to be a broad spectrum of unrelated and unexplained cognitive and perceptual-motor problems. She developed standardized tests to better understand children's problems. Ayres developed a rigorous research program to validate her tests and to test her theoretical arguments and clinical approaches.

In 1976, she founded the Ayres Clinic, which served as her private practice and as a training context for educating therapists in sensory integration principles and therapy. Her theory building and research always aimed to improve direct service. Ayres wrote numerous books and articles addressing her theory and techniques for clinical application. Her most definitive works on sensory integration theory include two books, titled *Sensory Integration and Learning Disorders* (1972) and *Sensory Integration and the Child* (1979).

In sum, Ayres devoted her career to the development of a specific applied theory. With her focus on the mechanisms underlying function and dysfunction, Ayres influenced development of the field's second paradigm. Her work exemplifies how knowledge should be generated for practice. She combined theory, research, and practice, developing tools to apply her theory in practice and conducting research to test the theory and its application. Her development of sensory integration was the first well-developed example of what is termed in this text a conceptual practice model.

neuromotor, musculoskeletal, or intrapsychic functions
• Performance can be improved by addressing neuromotor, musculoskeletal, or intrapsychic impairments

The Role of Inner Mechanisms in Performance

The first construct focused attention on how inner mechanisms affected performance. For instance, therapists recognized that performance requires coordinated movement and emphasized that neurological and musculoskeletal impairments that influenced movement should be directly and systematically addressed in practice (Smith, 1978). Detailed analysis of the neuromuscular features of task performance was emphasized, as in the following example:

> Synergistic muscles may be used to prevent an unwanted movement, thus assisting in the performance of a task. Forcefully gripping a tool is used to illustrate this concept; the long finger flexors cross more than one joint and have the potential to act on each joint they cross. Forceful gripping of a tool would cause the wrist to flex if the wrist extensors did not contract synergistically to prevent this unwanted motion.
> (Smith, 1978, p. 86)

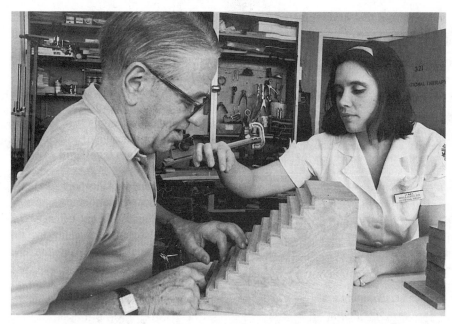

A client engages in a tabletop activity designed to provide appropriate exercise for his fingers.

The psychodynamic perspective stressed the relationship of unconscious processes to performance and the development of this relationship in the course of psychosexual maturation (Azima & Azima, 1959; Fidler & Fidler, 1958; Fidler & Fidler, 1963). From this point of view adequate performance required a normal process of psychosexual maturation.

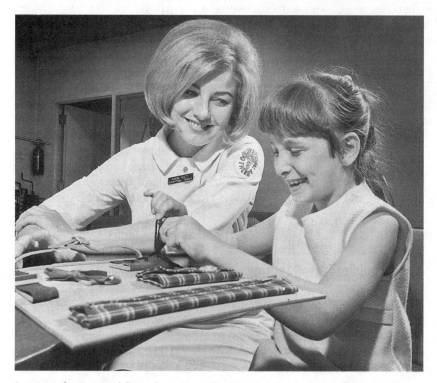

Practicing fine motor skills, a client manipulates zippers, buttons, and ties on a fastener board.

Understanding Impairment Related to the Neuromotor, Musculoskeletal, or Intrapsychic Functions

Therapists became increasingly concerned with understanding the nature of musculoskeletal, neurological, and intrapsychic impairments and how they were involved in a given performance problem. For example, therapists sought to understand how deficits in movement capacity were related to disease or trauma that affected muscles and joints. Therapists analyzed activities to determine the particular movements they required so that they could identify and bridge any gaps between a person's movement capacity and those demands.

From the psychodynamic perspective, dysfunctional behavior was seen as a result of internal tension (i.e., anxiety) or of early blocked needs that prevented maturation of the ego (Azima & Azima, 1959; Fidler & Fidler, 1958; West, 1959). Therapists sought to determine the underlying conflicts or unfulfilled needs that interfered with functioning because these were the mechanisms to be altered in therapy. Often, the therapists used activities to diagnose the person's hidden feelings and unconscious motives by interpreting the unconscious meaning of colors, themes, and other characteristics of a person's creations (Llorens & Young, 1960; West, 1959).

Addressing Neuromotor, Musculoskeletal, or Intrapsychic Impairments

In this new paradigm, therapy sought to identify the specific cause or problem underlying the inability to perform and to change and/or compensate for it. In cases of neurological disorders, new treatment methods stressed identification of abnormal movement patterns and techniques to inhibit them and facilitate normal movement (Bobath & Bobath, 1964; Rood, 1958; Stockmeyer, 1972). Other approaches used activities and specialized equipment to stimulate the

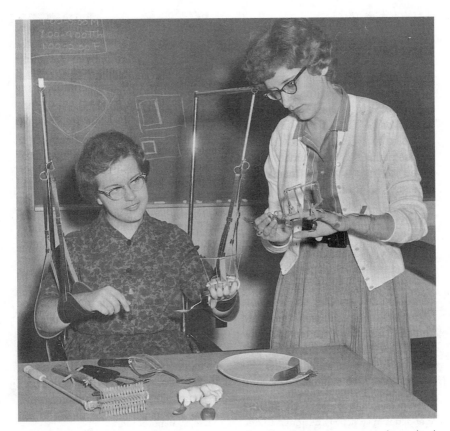

A client practices use of adaptive equipment designed to enable her to eat independently.

malfunctioning nervous system in order to elicit normal responses (Ayres, 1972, 1974). Therapists tried to provide a therapeutic rationale for every activity used in therapy, and the rationale had to be in terms of the impact on underlying mechanisms (i.e., reducing impairments). For example:

> *Sensory stimulus is developed through adapted cutaneous contact with tools, the beater of the loom, or the handle of a sander.... Gross motor reaching and throwing activities stimulate proprioception and kinesthetic awareness.... Use of a skateboard attached to the forearm for directed range of motion activities stimulates upper arm active movements. (Spencer, 1978, p. 355)*

Under the new paradigm, therapists also developed new treatment methods for musculoskeletal dysfunction, including such things as splinting and positioning limbs for optimal performance and providing exercises to restore muscle strength. Therapists analyzed activities to determine the movements needed for crafts and other activities. They made or prescribed adaptive devices to bridge the gap between persons' limited motion and the tasks they had to perform. Therapists also taught people compensatory techniques that allowed them to perform in spite of ongoing impairments.

Occupational therapy in psychiatry was predicated on the belief that if a person could learn to satisfy blocked childhood needs, the intrapsychic conflict could be removed, and the person would return to healthy functioning (Fidler, 1969; Llorens & Young, 1960; West, 1959). Thus, it was common to determine the psychosexual stage of development where needs had not been met and to provide activities as occasions for corresponding need fulfillment:

> *Occupational therapy can offer opportunities for the expression and satisfaction of*

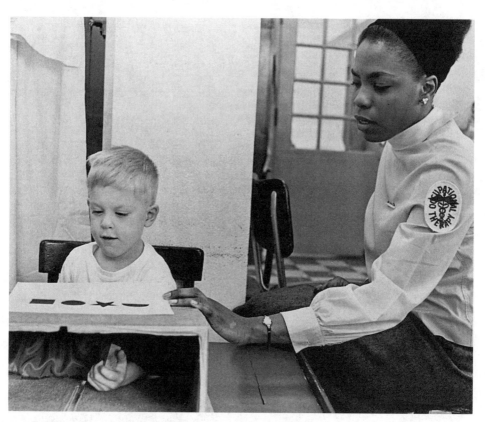

A client engages in an activity designed to develop perceptual motor skills.

*unconscious oral and anal needs in an actual
or symbolic way through activities which involve sucking, drinking, eating, chewing, blowing and those which use excretory substitutes
such as smearing or building with clay, paints,
or soil. (Fidler, 1958, p. 10)*

Overall, psychiatric occupational therapists conceptualized treatment as a means to
act out or sublimate feelings (Fidler & Fidler,
1963). In another approach, therapists used
activities to establish a therapeutic relationship that would permit the person to develop
healthy means of resolving intrapsychic conflict and fulfilling needs. As indicated in the
following quote, activities themselves were
less important than the therapist's therapeutic
use of self:

*The effective therapeutic approach in
occupational therapy today and in the future
is one in which the therapist utilized the tools
of his trade as an avenue of introduction.*

*From then on his personality takes over.
(Conte, 1960, p. 3)*

Across the three mechanistic approaches to
treatment (intrapsychic, neurological, and kine-
siological), therapists attempted to isolate particular effects that the activity was meant to have on
the neuromotor, musculoskeletal, or psychodynamic functions. By so doing, they sought to
achieve more specificity in the intended effects
of therapy.

Values

The values of the new paradigm reflected its
focus on scientific precision. Therapists came to
emphasize objectivity and exactness in problem
identification and measurement. Therapists also
changed their value orientation toward the activities in which clients engaged during therapy.
Therapists previously valued occupation as a
natural human need that was also therapeutic.
Now, therapists began to focus on the value of

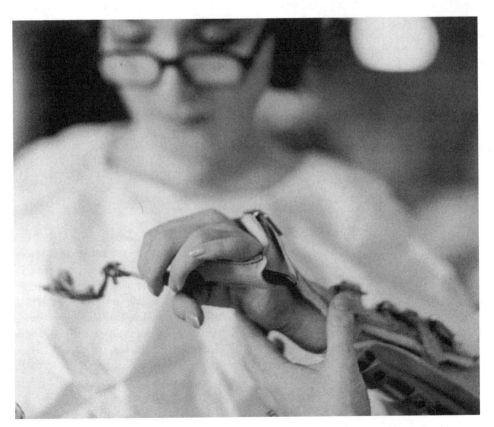

A client practices using an adaptive hand splint and an adapted utensil to eat independently.

Gail Fidler

Born in 1916, Gail Fidler spent her early childhood in South Dakota. She later moved to Pennsylvania, where she attended Lebanon Valley College, earning a bachelor's degree in education and psychology. Fidler worked briefly as a high school history teacher before securing a job as a hospital attendant at Wernersville State Hospital (Miller & Walker, 1993). There, Fidler encountered occupational therapy and was impressed with its impact on patients. She subsequently enrolled at the University of Pennsylvania and earned a certificate in occupational therapy. Later, Fidler once more returned to school, attending the William Alanson White Institute of Psychiatry and Psychology in New York. There, she studied and was influenced by interpersonal theory, in particular theories surrounding ego development, self-esteem, and competence (Miller & Walker, 1993).

In a career of more than 60 years, Fidler served as an occupational therapy practitioner, administrator, educator, and theorist. She also served as associate executive director and briefly as Interim Executive Director of the American Occupational Therapy Association (Miller & Walker, 1993).

Although Fidler made important contributions throughout her career, her early work rooted in psychodynamic theory was the most influential on the field's paradigm development. Fidler's early writing envisioned the occupational therapist as an integral part of the psychodynamic process.

The 1963 text *Occupational Therapy: A Communication Process in Psychiatry,* coauthored with her psychiatrist husband Jay Fidler, discusses how activity can be used to express thoughts and feelings nonverbally (Fidler & Fidler, 1963). The Fidlers asserted that communication that emerges through activity is more likely to reveal unconscious emotions (Miller & Walker, 1993).

A consistent theme in Fidler's work was activity analysis. She proposed that, through the analysis of activity, the occupational therapist can glean information on the specific needs, interests, and abilities of the client and use this information to design action-oriented experiences to benefit the client. Fidler's early work on activity analysis focused on the psychodynamic elements of activities. Over the years she expanded this idea to include motor, sensory integrative, psychological, cognitive, sociocultural, and interpersonal skills (Miller & Walker, 1993).

activity as a means for strengthening muscles, influencing the nervous system, and expressing unconscious desires.

Summary

By the 1960s occupational therapy's paradigm had radically changed. This meant that the field had adopted the new focal viewpoint, core constructs, and values that are summarized in Table 4.1. This mechanistic paradigm resulted in important advances in the field. The new paradigm resulted in a substantially increased technology for remediating impairments. The paradigm also resulted in a deeper understanding of how bodily structures and processes facilitated or limited performance. The technology for adapting devices and environments to the needs of persons with motor impairment improved. The psychodynamic perspective increased understanding of how emotional problems might interfere with competent performance.

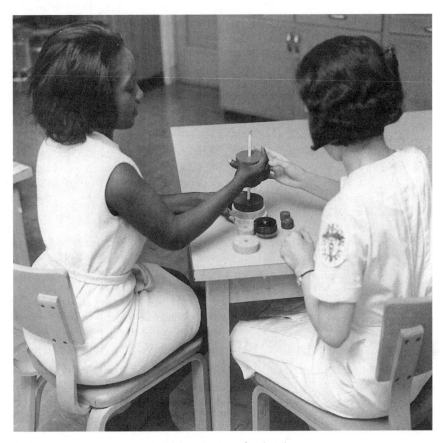

A client engages in grasp and release exercises after hand surgery.

Table 4.1 **Mechanistic Paradigm**

Core Constructs	• The ability to perform depends on the integrity of the neuromotor, musculoskeletal, and intrapsychic systems. • Damage or abnormal development in the inner systems can result in incapacity. • Functional performance can be restored by improving/compensating for limitations in inner systems.
Focal Viewpoint	• Precise knowledge and understanding of the inner (intrapsychic, neurological, and kinesiological) workings.
Values	• Value of the inner workings to function. • Value of media as a means to reduce incapacity.

REFERENCES

Ayres, A.J. (1958). Basic concepts of clinical practice in physical disabilities. *American Journal of Occupational Therapy, 12*, 300–302.

Ayres, A.J. (1963). The development of perceptual motor abilities: A theoretical basis for treatment of dysfunction. *American Journal of Occupational Therapy, 17*, 221.

Ayres, A.J. (1972). *Sensory integration and learning disorders.* Los Angeles: Western Psychological Services.

Ayres, A.J. (1974). *The development of sensory integrative theory and practice.* Dubuque, IA: Kendal & Hunt.

Ayres, A.J. (1979). *Sensory integration and the child.* Los Angeles: Western Psychological Services.

Azima, H., & Azima, F. (1959). Outline of a dynamic theory of occupational therapy. *American Journal of Occupational Therapy, 13*, 215–221.

Bobath, K., & Bobath, B. (1964). The facilitation of normal postural reactions and movements in the treatment of cerebral palsy. *Physiotherapy, 50*, 246–262.

Buhler, C. (1962). *Values in psychotherapy.* New York: Free Press.

Conte, W. (1960). The occupational therapist as a therapist. *American Journal of Occupational Therapy, 14*, 1–3.

Fidler, G. (1958). Some unique contributions of occupational therapy in treatment of the schizophrenic. *American Journal of Occupational Therapy, 12*, 9–12.

Fidler, G. (1969). The task-oriented group as a context for treatment. *American Journal of Occupational Therapy, 23*, 43–48.

Fidler, G., & Fidler, J. (1958). *Introduction to psychiatric occupational therapy.* New York: Macmillan.

Fidler, G., & Fidler, J. (1963). *Occupational therapy: A communication process in psychiatry.* New York: Macmillan.

Kuhn, T. (1970). *The structure of scientific revolutions* (2nd ed.). Chicago: University of Chicago Press.

Llorens, L.A., & Young, G.G. (1960). Fingerpainting for the hostile child. *American Journal of Occupational Therapy, 14*, 306–307.

McNary, H. (1958). A look at occupational therapy. *American Journal of Occupational Therapy, 12*, 203–204.

Meyerson, L. (1957). Some observations on the psychological roles of the occupational therapist. *American Journal of Occupational Therapy, 11*, 131–134.

Miller, R.J., & Walker, K.F. (1993). *Perspectives on theory for the practice of occupational therapy.* Gaithersburg, MD: Aspen.

Rerek, M. (1971). The depression years: 1929 to 1941. *American Journal of Occupational Therapy, 25,* 231–233.

Riley, J.N. (1977). Western medicine's attempt to become more scientific: Examples from the United States and Thailand. *Social Science and Medicine, 11*, 549–560.

Rood, M. (1958). Everyone counts. *American Journal of Occupational Therapy, 12*, 326–329.

Smith, H.B. (1978). Scientific and medical bases. In H.L. Hopkins & N.D. Smith (Eds.), *Willard and Spackman's occupational therapy* (5th ed., pp. 82–99). Philadelphia: J.B. Lippincott.

Spencer, E.A. (1978). Functional restoration. In H.L. Hopkins & N.D. Smith (Eds.), *Willard and Spackman's occupational therapy* (5th ed., pp. 335–398). Philadelphia: J.B. Lippincott.

Stockmeyer, S.A. (1972). A sensorimotor approach to treatment. In P. Pearson & C. Williams (Eds.), *Physical therapy services in the developmental disabilities.* Springfield, IL: Charles C. Thomas.

West, W. (Ed). (1959). *Psychiatric occupational therapy.* New York: American Occupational Therapy Association.

CHAPTER 5

Emergence of the Contemporary Paradigm: A Return to Occupation

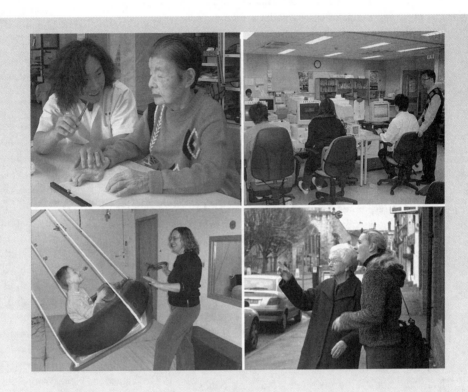

As noted in Chapter 4, the mechanistic paradigm achieved much of its promise to ground occupational therapy in sound medical and scientific concepts. Nonetheless, it also had some unforeseen and undesirable consequences. Occupational therapy's fundamental perspective toward human beings had been altered radically. The early appreciation of the occupation along with the themes of mind-body unity, self-maintenance through occupation, and the dynamic rhythm and balance of occupation were lost. Holistic thinking was replaced with an emphasis on the internal workings of the human psyche and body.

The earlier rationale of therapy, which used such concepts as building morale, regenerating habits, and stimulating interests, was replaced by an emphasis on impairment reduction. This new rationale led to an uncomfortable misfit between the activities used as therapy and the new concepts used to explain them. For example, some therapists maintained the use of such activities as sanding wood, but clients sanded boards solely as a means of exercise and they were never used in woodworking projects. There was increasing use of activities that had a therapeutic purpose (e.g., stacking cones to increase range of motion and strength and working with pegboards to increase fine motor coordination) but lacked meaningful connection to the client's occupational life. Such practices were criticized for ignoring the meaning of the activity to the client (Spackman, 1968).

In other cases, occupational therapists completely dropped participation in meaningful occupation from their therapeutic programs. Within the psychoanalytic approach, activity was seen merely as a method for therapeutic interaction and some concluded that activity was not really necessary at all. Similarly, the use of activity to achieve greater strength was increasingly replaced with pure exercise.

With time, it became apparent that occupational therapy lacked a unifying identity (Gillette, 1967; Gillette & Kielhofner, 1979; Johnson, 1973; King, 1978; Mosey, 1971; Task Force on Target Populations, 1974; West, 1968). The alliance with medicine resulted in a focus on impairment to the neglect of underlying occupational therapy principles (Mosey, 1971; Shannon, 1977). The mechanistic paradigm had diverted the field from its original mission and eclipsed the field's most seminal idea, the importance of occupation as a health-restoring measure (Rerek, 1971; Shannon, 1977).

The Call for a New Paradigm

In the 1960s and 1970s, Mary Reilly and others began to call for a return to the most important elements of the field's first paradigm (Kielhofner & Burke, 1977; Michelman, 1971; Reilly, 1962; Robinson, 1977; Shannon, 1972). Reilly led the development of a renewed focus on occupation. The resulting concepts, referred to as occupational behavior, introduced themes such as the motivation for occupation (Burke, 1977; Florey, 1969), the organization of occupation in time through habits and roles (Heard, 1977; Kielhofner, 1977; Matsutsuyu, 1971; Watanabe, 1968; Woodside, 1976), and the importance of the environment in supporting or impeding adaptation (Dunning, 1972; Gray, 1972; Reilly, 1966; Watanabe, 1968).

The call to resurrect occupational therapy's original focus and ideals began to be echoed by others (Task Force on Target Populations, 1974; West, 1984). For instance, Wiemer (1979) argued:

> Ours is, and must be, the basic knowledge of occupation. It is that knowledge which permits the occupational therapist to look at an activity of daily living in a unique way, and so determine best how to facilitate the patient's or client's goal achievement. Our exclusive domain is occupation. We must refine, research, and systematize it so that it becomes evident, definable, defensible and salable. The "impact of occupation upon human beings" was spelled

> The mechanistic paradigm had diverted the field from its original mission and eclipsed the field's most seminal idea, the importance of occupation as a health-restoring measure.

Mary Reilly

Born in Massachusetts, Mary Reilly graduated from the Boston School of Occupational Therapy. Early in her career she entered military service as Chief Therapist at the Lovell General and Convalescent Hospital at Fort Devens, Massachusetts. Her later work at Fourth Service Command included supervising occupational therapy programs in 11 general, 2 convalescent, and 6 regional and station hospitals. Reilly retired from the army in 1951 with the rank of captain. She earned a doctorate in education in 1959 and later became Chief of the Rehabilitation Department at the Neuropsychiatric Institute at UCLA. She served as a professor at the University of Southern California until retiring in 1977.

As early as 1958, Reilly began to advocate for a change in occupational therapy education and knowledge to incorporate a broader focus on the meaning of productivity and engagement in society and in individual lives. She argued that the human need for engagement in play and work was the foundation and *raison d'être* of the profession. In her 1962 Eleanor Clarke Slagle lecture, Reilly proclaimed occupational therapy to be "one of the greatest ideas of 20th century medicine." She stated that the field's bold hypothesis was that "man, through the use of his hands as they are energized by mind and will, can influence the state of his own health" (Reilly, 1962, p. 2). In this paper, Reilly challenged the field to move beyond its mechanistic focus and recommit to the focus on occupation.

Although Reilly's writings are not extensive, her work was critical in shaping the movement from the paradigm of inner mechanisms to the contemporary paradigm. This was accomplished largely through her work in directing graduate students at the University of Southern California. She led them to develop a body of knowledge that she termed "occupational behavior" to emphasize that the field's knowledge should focus on occupation. She envisioned occupational behavior as the therapeutic framework for practice and education. Reilly contributed to this body of knowledge with her book *Play as Exploratory Learning* (1974). This text was the first serious treatment of the topic of play in the field.

In sum, Reilly was a pivotal figure in shaping the contemporary directions of the field. Her call for a refocus on the theme of occupation came at the time when the field was steeped in the mechanistic paradigm and went unheeded for a period of time. Through her own writings and those of her students, she was able to provide the field with a broad and scholarly understanding of the complex phenomena with which occupational therapists work. Her contribution in shaping the direction of the field places her as one of the most influential scholars in modern occupational therapy history.

out as our sole claim to professionalism by our founders in 1917. It is our latent power if we will but keep it as our focus and direction. (p. 43)

Emergence of a Third Paradigm

As a result of the efforts of many leaders in the field, occupational therapy has presently become "a discipline focused on occupation" (Polatajko, 1994, p. 591). This transformation has required the field to recapture its original orientation and retain important technology accumulated during the mechanistic paradigm. It also has required that the field correct some of the problems that surfaced during the mechanistic paradigm. The focal viewpoint, core constructs, and values of this new paradigm are discussed here.

Focal Viewpoint

The focal viewpoint of the new paradigm reflects not only a return to occupation, but also a particular way of thinking about what factors influence occupational performance. This viewpoint is designed to correct the exclusive emphasis of the mechanistic paradigm on clients' impairments as the primary or sole problems to be addressed in therapy. It also reflects two important influences from outside occupational therapy: disability scholarship and systems theory.

Disability scholars emphasized that disability is not simply a consequence of impairments. They argued that disability is caused by environments that pose physical, attitudinal, economic, and political barriers (Charlton, 1998; Hahn, 1985; Oliver, 1996). Moreover, they pointed out that, if environments are adequately supportive, people with impairments can participate in life in the same ways as their peers who do not have impairments (Crow, 1996; Fine & Asch, 1988; Longmore, 1995; Shapiro, 1993). Albeit from a different vantage point, systems theorists made a similar argument. They noted that human thought, feeling, and action were consequences not only of factors inside the person, but also of characteristics of the person's context including the nature of any task in which the person was engaged (Capra, 1997; Kelso, 1995; Thelen & Ulrich, 1991; Vallacher & Nowak, 1994).

Person, Environment, and Occupation

The focal viewpoint of the current paradigm incorporates elements of both previous paradigms as well as ideas from disability studies and systems theory, as noted earlier. It is focused on the interaction of person, environment, and occupation (Christiansen & Baum, 1997; Dunn, Brown, & McGuigan, 1994). This focal viewpoint emphasizes that all occupational performance is a consequence of the interaction of person, environment, and occupation factors (Fig. 5.1).

Person factors are generally understood to include such things as underlying sensorimotor and cognitive capacities, skills, values, interests, and life experiences, as well as any impairments (American Occupational Therapy Association, 2002). The environment consists of those physical, cultural, social, economic, political, and

<hr>

Box 5.2   Definitions of Occupation

As the field sought to return to a focus on occupation, different definitions have arisen. For instance, Christiansen, Clark, Kielhofner, and Rogers (1995) defined occupation simply as the ordinary and familiar things the people do everyday. Yerxa and her colleagues (1990, p. 1) defined occupation as "specific chunks of activity within the ongoing stream of human behavior which are named in the lexicon of culture." Kielhofner (2008, p. 5) defined occupation as "the doing of work, play, or activities of daily living within a temporal, physical, and sociocultural context that characterizes much of human life." A definition offered by Canadian occupational therapists echoes these themes; it refers to occupation as "the tasks and activities of everyday life, named, organized, and given value and meaning by individuals and a culture" (CAOT, 1997, p. 34). Their definition goes on to note that occupation is everything that people do to occupy themselves, including "looking after themselves (self-care), enjoying life (leisure), and contributing to the social and economic fabric of their communities (productivity) (CAOT, 1997, p. 34).

Most definitions, then, agree that occupation comprises play/leisure, activities of daily living, and productivity. Play/leisure refers to activities undertaken for their own sake; exploring, pretending, celebrating, engaging in games or sports, and pursuing hobbies are all examples (DiBona, 2000; Lobo, 1999; Parham & Fazio, 1997; Passmore, 1998). Activities of daily living are tasks that maintain one's self and lifestyle. They compose much of the routine of everyday life and include self-care, ordering one's life space (e.g., cleaning and paying bills), and getting to resources (e.g., travel and shopping) (Christiansen, 1994). Work includes productive activity (both paid and unpaid) that contributes some service or commodity to others as well as participating in education or training that improves one's abilities to be productive (Kielhofner, 2008).

<hr>

temporal contexts that affect various opportunities for and influences on occupation (Christiansen & Baum, 1997; Dunn, McClain, Brown, & Youngstrom, 2003). The occupation refers to the specific task or activity that the person is doing and/or the goal of that task (Christiansen & Baum, 1997; Nelson, 1988).

Occupational performance is understood to emerge out of the interaction of these person, environment, and occupation factors (Christiansen

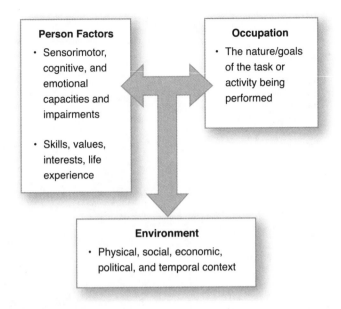

FIGURE 5.1 The focal viewpoint: interaction of person, environment and occupation factors.

& Baum, 1997; Dunn et al., 2003; Trombly, 1993). Thus, person factors alone cannot account for a person's occupational performance since performance also reflects what the person is attempting to do and the context in which it takes place. This viewpoint guides occupational therapists to look beyond impairment to other person factors and also outside the person to the occupation and the context. It also directs therapists to look beyond reduction of impairment to consider how environmental barriers can be removed and/or how occupations can be modified to allow persons to more fully participate in necessary and desired occupations. This perspective represents a return to a more holistic viewpoint.

Core Constructs

As noted earlier, the contemporary paradigm has returned to a focus on occupation. Its core constructs include three broad themes that reflect this focus:

- The importance of occupation to health and well-being
- Recognition of occupational problems/challenges
- Occupation-based practice

The following sections discuss these themes.

The Role of Occupation in Health and Well-Being

There has been a growing recognition that occupation plays a central role in health and well-being. Humans have a strong drive to do things and flourish by engaging in practical, productive, and playful pursuits (Christiansen, 1994; Clark et al., 1991; Parham & Fazio, 1997; Wilcock, 1993). Through occupation (play, activities of daily living, and work), individuals fill their time, create the circumstances of their everyday existence, and make their place in the world (Christiansen, 1996; Wood, 1995). These occupations contribute to development, provide necessary opportunities for physical and mental engagement, and connect people to their social and cultural environment (Clark, 1993; Hasselkus, 2002; Johnsson, Borell, & Kielhofner, 1997). Moreover, participating in occupation creates and affirms meaning in life (Christiansen, 1999; Hasselkus, 2002).

Occupational Problems/Challenges

The contemporary paradigm recognizes problems of participating in occupations as the focus for service (Rogers, 1982). Persons who are denied access to or have restrictions in their occupations

Box 5.3   Contemporary Occupational Therapy Around the World

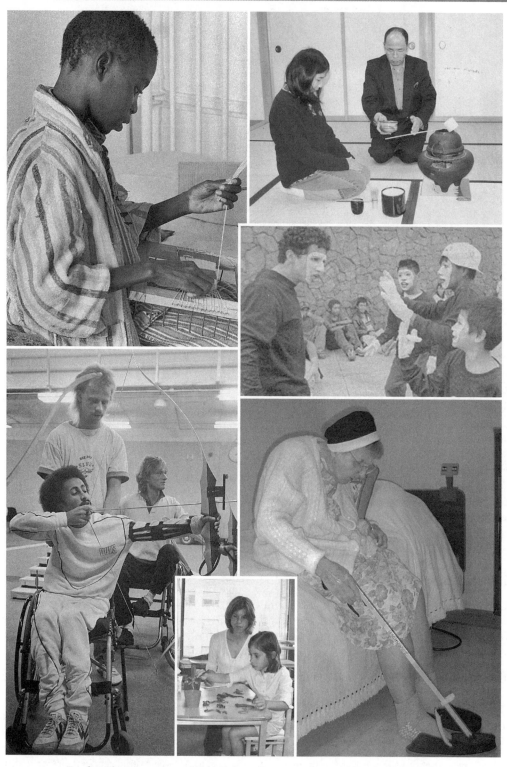

Top five photos courtesy of Bror Karlsson/Banzai Archive and Frank Kronenberg.

Box 5.3   **Contemporary Occupational Therapy Around the World** continued

These images of occupational therapy worldwide demonstrate the field's return to occupation-based practice. In this collage, occupational therapy in Africa, Asia, the Americas, and Europe engages clients in valued occupations. Contemporary therapists view their clients holistically and seek therapeutic gains through the use of activities that are important to their clients.

---

may suffer and/or experience a reduction in quality of life (Christiansen, 1994). A lack or disruption of participation in occupation may also restrict development, resulting in reductions of capacity and leading to maladaptive reactions. Because of the potential negative consequences of such occupational deprivation, it is the central problem to which the field addresses its efforts.

Occupation and the Dynamics of Therapy

The third thematic area of the core constructs addresses the means and the goals of therapy. In the contemporary perspective, the use of occupation to improve health status is once again recognized as the core of occupational therapy (Fisher, 1998; Reilly, 1962; Wood, 1998). As shown in Figure 5.2, therapists employ the therapeutic agency of occupation through four primary pathways:

- Providing opportunities for clients to engage directly in occupations
- Enabling clients to engage in occupations by modifying the task or the environment in which the person performs, including removing architectural and social barriers

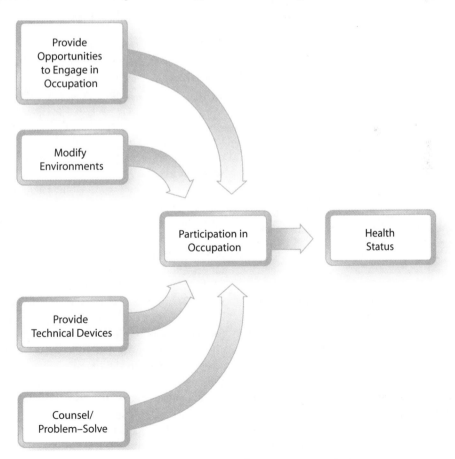

FIGURE 5.2 Pathways to employ occupation as therapy.

(e.g., attitudes, discrimination, unfair policies) (Dunn et al., 1994; Kielhofner, 2002)

• Providing training of clients in the use of various technical devices that extend limited capacity or compensate for lost capacity (Hammel, 1996)

• Providing counseling and problem-solving to facilitate the client's participation in occupations outside of therapy

Underlying these efforts is the recognition that clients' engagement in occupations is the core of therapy. Engagement in occupation involves not only what individuals do but also their subjective experience (Hasselkus, 2002; Yerxa, 1980). Therefore, the client must find meaning in the actions that constitute the therapy. This meaning ordinarily derives from the client's experiential background, the current impact of any impairments on the client's experience, and the significance of the therapeutic activity negotiated between the therapist and the client.

In the end, the meaning that is experienced in the therapeutic process determines the impact of the activity on the individual. Therapy is an event that enters into and becomes part of the client's life story (Helfrich, Kielhofner, & Mattingly, 1994; Kielhofner et al., 2008). The meaning that therapy has for the client is in relation to its relevance and impact upon this story. Moreover, in therapy the therapist helps clients to continue or reinvent that life story (Clark, 1993). Hence, new life meaning can be discovered and enacted in the course of therapy.

Values

With the reorientation of the current paradigm, the centrality of occupation to well-being and quality of life has become a resonant theme in the field (American Occupational Therapy Association, 1993; Fondiller, Rosage, & Neuhas, 1990; Hasselkus, 2002). Related to this, it is recognized that the vision and mission of the field are to promote occupational well-being. Consequently, a core value defining the worth of occupational therapy is its support of clients'

> **In the end, the meaning that is experienced in the therapeutic process determines the impact of the activity on the individual.**

desires to integrate themselves into the mainstream of life through participation in meaningful life occupations (Johnson, 1981; Yerxa, 1983). Contemporary values like this one echo the values of the first paradigm.

A second set of values reflected attempts to correct some of the problems that emerged in the mechanistic paradigm. These problems included the failure to see the client as a whole person and to address what was meaningful to the client, as well as a tendency for therapy to become impersonal and overly technical.

One value emphasized that occupational therapy should always consist of the active and meaning-driven participation of the client, whose actions and investment determined the effectiveness of the therapy (Wood, 1995). This value required a profound respect for and understanding of a client's perspectives, desires, and needs as well as the client's right to make choices and exercise decisions about the therapeutic process (Taylor, 2003; Townsend, 1993). It also meant that occupational therapists had to pay much more attention to their relationship with clients. The mechanistic paradigm also included a psychoanalytic perspective that emphasized the therapeutic relationship, but its emphases were on the therapist as expert and on influencing the client's unconscious processes.

The new paradigm sees the relationship of the occupational therapist with the client in a different light as reflected in the following themes. One important theme, client-centered practice, emphasizes the importance of collaboration with clients (Law, 1998; Law, Baptiste, & Mills, 1995). Client-centered practice emphasizes the importance of recognizing clients' knowledge and experience, strengths, capacity for choice, and overall autonomy. It argues that clients should be treated with respect and considered partners in the therapy process. Client-centered practice also emphasizes the value of client empowerment; that is, providing clients with resources and opportunities to engage in occupations that shape their lives (Law, Polatajko, Baptiste, & Townsend, 1997; Townsend, 2003).

There have also been discussions of the importance of caring in occupational therapy practice (Baum, 1980; Devereaux, 1984; Gilfoyle, 1980; Yerxa, 1980). Caring includes knowing and responding to clients as unique individuals, viewing them holistically, and connecting with them at an emotional level (Stein & Cutler, 1998). Another espoused value is the importance of empathy in the therapeutic encounter (Peloquin, 2002, 2003, 2005). Empathy is characterized by respect for a client's personal dignity, an entry into the client's experience, and a connection with the feelings of the client (Peloquin, 2003). Together, the themes of client-centered practice, caring, and empathy have underscored the importance of the therapeutic relationship in occupational therapy.

> **Together, the themes of client-centered practice, caring, and empathy have underscored the importance of the therapeutic relationship in occupational therapy.**

field's first paradigm was built upon principles of moral treatment and emphasized the importance of occupation to human life and as a therapeutic tool. This paradigm was replaced mid-century with a second paradigm that focused on the inner (neurological, musculoskeletal, and intrapsychic) mechanisms that were thought to determine the ability to perform. The contemporary paradigm has sought to restore the field's original focus on occupation. Its focal viewpoint, core constructs, and values (see Table 5.1 for a summary) shape the professional identities of contemporary occupational therapists.

The contemporary paradigm's influence on professional identities can perhaps best be seen by considering practitioners' reflections on their profession and their own practices. The following reflections on these issues are from four of the occupational therapists introduced in the first two chapters.

Although expressed in different ways, each of these therapists' reflections resonates with the focal viewpoint, core constructs, and values of the contemporary paradigm as they were discussed in this chapter. The therapists' reflections also illustrate that the importance

Discussion: Influence of the Paradigm on Occupational Therapists' Perspectives and Practice

Chapters 3 and 4 along with this chapter provided an overview of how occupational therapy's paradigm has developed for almost a century. The

---

Table 5.1 **The Contemporary Paradigm**

Core Constructs	• The centrality of occupation to health and well-being. • Recognition of occupational problems/challenges as the focus for therapy. • Occupation-based practice (use of occupation to improve health status as the core of occupational therapy).
Focal Viewpoint	• Focuses on the interaction of person, environment, and occupation. • Emphasizes that occupational performance is a consequence of the interaction of person, environment, and occupation factors.
Values	• Importance of occupation to well-being and quality of life. • Importance of supporting clients' desires to integrate themselves into the mainstream of life through participation in occupation. • Importance of active and meaning-driven participation of the client, whose actions and investment determine effectiveness of the therapy. • Importance of the therapeutic relationship, as reflected in the themes of client-centered practice, caring, and empathy.

of this component of the field's conceptual foundations is in how it shapes the way individual therapists understand the nature of their profession and the services they provide to their clients.

Occupational therapists see their clients as occupational beings. They are occupation-focused rather than illness or disability-focused. I view my clients in the context of their environments, personal values, routines, and, most importantly, their occupations. By viewing clients in this wider context, in addition to getting a feel for their performance capacity (strengths and deficits), I have a chance of better understanding why they may be avoiding certain things or taking risks to achieve certain things. I want to find out what truly matters to the person on a daily basis. It is important to carry out a full occupational assessment in order to better understand people's lives rather than jumping on the first impairment or problem that is highlighted. By viewing each client as an occupational "whole," I am able to plan meaningful, motivating intervention.

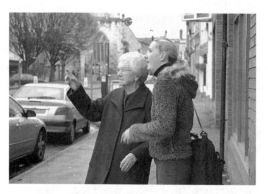

Alice and a client during a therapy session aimed at community re-integration.

What sets occupational therapy intervention apart is the use of practical activities. I might, for instance, support clients to take small risks within an occupation as a stepping stone towards their feeling able to address occupational issues within their own environments. Every case is different, and I do not think there is one set way of addressing problems. With each client, occupational intervention tasks of all ranges are selected (such as shopping, cooking, writing, and gardening at all sorts of different levels according to each client's need). Occupational therapy works because it is not solely tailored to the person's routine, values, and performance skills. Moreover, it is a partnership between the therapist and client, working towards whatever are important or essential for that client.

Occupational therapy recognizes and utilizes clients' strengths. The person who has a memory impairment and difficulty retaining new task information but has knowledge of well-learned tasks can problem-solve, utilize checklists to their advantage, and often continue to carry out important roles. I feel it is important with all therapy to be flexible and problem-solve throughout the therapy process. Getting to know clients as occupational individuals and being interested in more than impairments are important.

When I think of what is important in therapy, I must say that over time, I have increasingly taken the role of "doing" more seriously in my practice, from individual to individual, basing interventions on their values, not mine.

Occupational therapists focus on occupation (day-to-day activities). We use therapeutic activities to assist clients in achieving maximum participation in self-care, work, and play. We have a holistic view of our clients' problems and emphasize how they can use their remaining assets to function and interact with the environment. I consider both the internal and external environments of my clients in deciding how to provide care. To achieve a holistic view, I conduct thorough assessments of my clients in order to understand their expected future life roles, their long-term and short-term goals, and the areas that are of most concern to them for rehabilitation.

We empower our clients to obtain their valued life roles by making the best use of their functional capabilities. We promote quality of life for clients.

Box 5.5   Bacon Fung Leung Ng continued

We also respect clients' choices. Clients should live meaningful lives, but only they can determine what is meaningful for them.

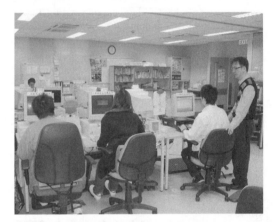

Bacon works with several clients who want to improve their computer skills.

Occupational therapists use diverse approaches to solve identified problems. Different clients require different approaches. Some clients need to acquire skills, some need to develop habits, and some need to be re-motivated. My clients are naturally creative and resourceful and my job is to trust them, provide reflection, and facilitate them to look within themselves and unlock their own strengths and assets. Thus, I emphasize coaching my clients through self-discovery. I always want my clients to gain energy from my assessment and treatment so that they can develop their own goals for the future. Thus, it is important that I can instill hope during treatment.

I make very conscious use of myself in therapy since I believe that the therapeutic relationship is the most critical aspect of my therapy. Because I want my clients to feel a sense of rapport with me, I must be value-free and non-judgmental. I also ask clients for feedback during implementation. My intervention is client-centered; my clients' needs and wants are of highest importance to me.

Box 5.6   Stacey Szklut

Occupational therapists aid their clients in achieving greater confidence and independence in their various occupations. I help children develop skills for the job of life so they can be as successful as possible. Each child, with his or her unique profile, has the potential for success if supported appropriately. My clients' impairments, combined with the effects of lack of success in their interactions with others and the environments they participate in, often hinder their ability to flourish and grow. By minimizing the effects of any impairments and creating support structures in the children's lives, I provide the foundation for more successful social interactions; for emotional, motor, and cognitive development; and for academic learning.

My therapy focuses on tapping a child's inner drive and desire to participate. Occupational therapy is more effective when the child is actively engaged in the process. I use meaningful and fun activities that build on the child's strengths and encourage new development and learning. It is essential to create individual programs for each child and adapt them continuously as the child's skills and needs change. The therapy process is built around what is important to clients and their families. To do this, it is important to appreciate the cultural views that guide my clients' lives and recognize the environments in which they need to be successful. I also consider what is most functionally significant and relevant in the long term for the child to be as successful and independent as possible.

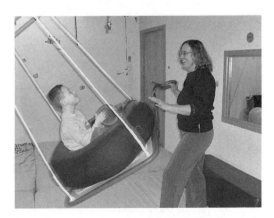

Stacey keeps her client engaged by making therapy fun.

(box continues on page 54)

Box 5.6   Stacey Szklut continued

For me, the therapeutic relationship is key in facilitating meaningful change. I promote the development of self-worth in each client. A child's sense of self is emerging and can be powerfully shaped through having a supportive mentor and positive experiences. The most important thing I can do as a therapist is to appreciate each child's unique gifts and help that child develop confidence as a foundation for all skillful participation. I have been in practice long enough to see many of my clients grow up to be strong, confident, and successful young adults despite their challenges.

Addressing environmental supports is another important part of the therapeutic process. By working collaboratively with the family, I try to assure that the child leaves therapy with a well-developed support network. Together, we create strategies, accommodations, and supports that need to be in place for the child to be a successful part of the family and the community.

Respect and empathy for my clients and their families are critical. Connecting with my clients, having fun with them, finding what is meaningful, and experiencing joy together are what make intervention satisfying and powerful. I am always mindful that success is different for everyone and that each child has unique gifts.

Box 5.7   Hiroyuki Notoh

Occupation includes all those things that are motivated by the client's interests, values, life experiences, skills, context, and so on. Our clients have difficulties doing their occupations. These problems may be due to impairments of body or psychosocial functions or because of environmental circumstances. Occupational therapists try to understand the problems of their clients from the perspective of their doing of meaningful occupations. Occupational therapy is holistic in that it seeks to understand the complexity of each person's problems. Occupational therapists evaluate and intervene at the point where clients have difficulty doing their meaningful occupations. Occupational therapists assist their clients to do their meaningful occupations that, in turn, give clients enjoyment and peace of mind.

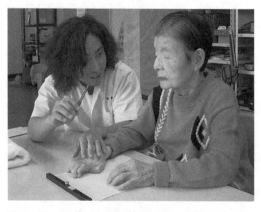

Hiroyuki works on writing with a client whose writing skills diminished after she began using her non-dominant hand for most functions following a stroke.

My clients face threats to functioning independently or being able to return home. It is difficult to accept the fate of going to an institution and giving up the hope that they can live in their home and freely do their meaningful occupations. Even when clients can return home to their families, they do not want to burden their family members. Both groups of clients feel that their impairments threaten their lives and initially want to reduce them as much as possible. So I help them become as functional as possible. I feel that this helps them to find the strength to accept their changed life situations.

I start my therapy by asking clients to tell me about the history of their present impairments and difficulties. Some of them suddenly begin to talk about some topics of hardships in their lives. I listen carefully to what they say. I try to understand my clients' life stories rather than just focusing on their functional problems. After listening to them, I assess their body functions and their cognitive processes and find out what problems they think need to be solved. I always try to know how my clients see their problems. By attending to their perspectives, I can quickly achieve rapport with them and create a feeling of safety in their minds. Once I have a plan for intervention, I ask my clients about it. If they accept it, I start it. If they do not, I talk with my clients to rebuild a plan.

Most of my clients are mourning lost functions. It is important that I try to understand and empathize with their suffering. I always ask myself whether I am empathic, whether I am listening carefully, understanding, and collaborating with my clients. This is the most important aspect of my therapy.

REFERENCES

American Occupational Therapy Association. (2002). Occupational therapy practice framework: Domain and process. *American Journal of Occupational Therapy, 56,* 609–639.

American Occupational Therapy Association. (1993). Core values and attitudes of occupational therapy practice. *American Journal of Occupational Therapy, 47,* 1085–1086.

Baum, C.M. (1980). Occupational therapists put care in the health system. *American Journal of Occupational Therapy, 34,* 505–516.

Burke, J. (1977). A clinical perspective on motivation: Pawn versus origin. *American Journal of Occupational Therapy, 31,* 254–258.

Canadian Association of Occupational Therapists. (1997). *Enabling occupation: An occupational therapy perspective.* Ottawa, Ontario: CAOT Publications ACE.

Capra, F. (1997). *The web of life.* London: HarperCollins.

Charlton, J. (1998). *Nothing about us without us.* Berkeley, CA: University of California Press.

Christiansen, C. (1994). *Ways of living: Self care strategies for special needs.* Rockville, MD: American Occupational Therapy Association.

Christiansen, C. (1996). Three perspectives on balance in occupation. In F. Clark & R. Zemke (Eds.), *Occupational science* (pp. 431–451). Philadelphia: F.A. Davis.

Christiansen, C. (1999). Defining lives: Occupation as identity: An essay on competence, coherence, and the creation of meaning. *American Journal of Occupational Therapy, 53,* 547–558.

Christiansen, C., & Baum, C. (Eds.). (1997). *Occupational therapy: Enabling function and well-being* (2nd ed.). Thorofare, NJ: Slack.

Christiansen, C.H., Clark, F., Kielhofner, G., & Rogers, J. (1995). Position paper: Occupation. *American Journal of Occupational Therapy, 49,* 1015–1018.

Clark, F.A. (1993). Occupation embedded in a real life: Interweaving occupational science and occupational therapy. *American Journal of Occupational Therapy, 47,* 1067–1077.

Clark, F.A., Parham, D., Carlson, M.E., Frank, G., Jackson, J., Pierce, D., et al. (1991). Occupational science: Academic innovation in the service of occupational therapy's future. *American Journal of Occupational Therapy, 45,* 300–310.

Crow, L. (1996). Renewing the social model of disability. In C. Barnes & G. Mercer (Eds.), *Exploring the divide: Illness and disability* (pp. 55–72). Leeds, UK: The Disability Press.

Devereaux, E.B. (1984). Occupational therapy's challenge: The caring relationship. *American Journal of Occupational Therapy, 38,* 791–798.

DiBona, L. (2000). What are the benefits of leisure? An exploration using the leisure satisfaction scale. *British Journal of Occupational Therapy, 63*(2), 50–58.

Dunn, W., Brown, C., & McGuigan, A. (1994). The ecology of human performance: A framework for considering the impact of context. *American Journal of Occupational Therapy, 48,* 595–607

Dunn, W., McClain, L. H., Brown, C., & Youngstrom, M. J. (2003). The ecology of human performance. In E. B. Crepeau, E. S. Cohn, & B. A. B. Schell (Eds.), *Willard & Spackman's occupational therapy* (10th ed., pp. 223–226). Philadelphia: Lippincott Williams & Wilkins.

Dunning, H. (1972). Environmental occupational therapy. *American Journal of Occupational Therapy, 26,* 292–298.

Fine, M., & Asch, M. (1988). Disability beyond stigma: Social interaction, discrimination and activism. *Journal of Social Issues, 44*(1), 3–19.

Fisher, A.G. (1998). Uniting practice and theory in an occupational framework. *American Journal of Occupational Therapy, 54,* 509–521.

Florey, L. (1969). Intrinsic motivation: The dynamics of occupational therapy theory. *American Journal of Occupational Therapy, 23,* 319–322.

Fondiller, E.D., Rosage, L., & Neuhas, B. (1990). Values influencing clinical reasoning in occupational therapy: An exploratory study. *Occupational Therapy Journal of Research, 10,* 41–55.

Gilfoyle, E.M. (1980). Caring: A philosophy for practice. *American Journal of Occupational Therapy, 34,* 517–521.

Gillette, N. (1967). Changing methods in the treatment of psychososical dysfunction. *American Journal of Occupational Therapy, 21,* 230–233.

Gillette, N., & Kielhofner, G. (1979). The impact of specialization on the professionalization and survival of occupational therapy. *American Journal of Occupational Therapy, 33,* 20–28.

Gray, M. (1972). Effects of hospitalization on work-play behavior. *American Journal of Occupational Therapy, 26,* 180–185.

Hahn, H. (1985). Disability policy and the problem of discrimination. *American Behavioral Scientist, 28*(3), 293–318.

Hammel, J. (Ed.). (1996). *Assistive technology and occupational therapy: A link to function* (Section 1). Bethesda, MD: American Occupational Therapy Association.

Hasselkus, B.R. (2002). *The meaning of everyday occupation.* Thorofare, NJ: Slack.

Heard, C. (1977). Occupational role acquisition: A perspective on the chronically disabled. *American Journal of Occupational Therapy, 31,* 243–247.

Helfrich, C., Kielhofner, G., & Mattingly, C. (1994). Volition as narrative: Understanding motivation in chronic illness. *American Journal of Occupational Therapy, 48,* 311–317.

Johnson, J. (1973). Occupational therapy: A model for the future. *American Journal of Occupational Therapy, 27,* 1–7.

Johnson, J. (1981). Old value, new directions: Competence, adaptation, integration. *American Journal of Occupational Therapy, 35,* 589–598.

Johnsson, H., Borell, L., & Kielhofner, G. (1997). Anticipating retirement: The formation of attitudes and expectations concerning an occupational transition. *American Journal of Occupational Therapy, 51,* 49–56.

Kelso, J.A.S. (1995). *Dynamic patterns: The self organization of brain and behavior.* Cambridge, MA: MIT Press.

Kielhofner, G. (1977). Temporal adaptation: A conceptual framework for occupational therapy. *American Journal of Occupational Therapy, 31,* 235–242.

Kielhofner, G. (2002). *A model of human occupation: Theory and application* (3rd ed.). Baltimore: Lippincott Williams & Wilkins.

Kielhofner, G. (2008). *A model of human occupation: Theory and application* (4th ed.). Philadelphia: Lippincott Williams & Wilkins.

Kielhofner, G., Borell, L., Goldstein, K., Jonsson, H., Josephsson, S., Keponin, R., et al. (2008). Crafting occupational life. In G. Kielhofner, *A model of human occupation: Theory and application* (4th ed., pp. 110–125). Philadelphia: Lippincott Williams & Wilkins.

Kielhofner, G., & Burke, J.P. (1977). Occupational therapy after 60 years: An account of changing identity and knowledge. *American Journal of Occupational Therapy, 31,* 675–689.

King, L.J. (1978). Toward a science of adaptive responses. *American Journal of Occupational Therapy, 32,* 429–437.

Law, M. (1998). *Client-centered occupational therapy.* Thorofare, NJ: Slack.

Law, M., Baptiste, S., & Mills, J. (1995). Client-centered practice: What does it mean and does it make a difference? *Canadian Journal of Occupational Therapy, 62,* 250–257.

Law, M., Polatajko, H., Baptiste, S., & Townsend, E. (1997). Core concepts of occupational therapy. In E. Townsend, S. Stanton, M. Law, H. Polatajko, S. Baptiste, T. Thompson-Franson, et al. (Eds.), *Enabling occupation: An occupational therapy perspective* (pp. 29–56). Ottawa, Ontario, Canada: Canadian Association of Occupational Therapists.

Lobo, F. (1999). The leisure and work occupations of young people: A review. *Journal of Occupational Science (Australia), 6*(1), 27–33.

Longmore, P.K. (1995). The second phase: From disability rights to disability culture. *The Disability Rag and ReSource, 16,* 4–11.

Matsutsuyu, J. (1971). Occupational behavior: A perspective on work and play. *American Journal of Occupational Therapy, 12,* 203–204.

Michelman, S. (1971). The importance of creative play. *American Journal of Occupational Therapy, 25,* 285–290.

Mosey, A. (1971). Involvement in the rehabilitation movement: 1942-1960. *American Journal of Occupational Therapy, 25,* 234–236.

Nelson, D. L. (1988). Occupation: Form and performance. *American Journal of Occupational Therapy, 42,* 633–641.

Oliver, M. (1996). *Understanding disability: From theory to practice.* New York: St. Martin's Press.

Parham, L.D., & Fazio, L.S. (Eds.). (1997). *Play in occupational therapy for children.* St. Louis: Mosby.

Passmore, A. (1998). Does leisure support and underpin adolescents' developing worker role? *Journal of Occupational Science (Australia), 5*(3), 161–165.

Peloquin, S.M. (2002). Reclaiming the vision of reaching for heart as well as hands. *American Journal of Occupational Therapy, 56,* 517–526.

Peloquin, S.M. (2003). The therapeutic relationship: Manifestations and challenges in occupational therapy. In E.B. Crepeau, E.S. Cohn, & B.A.B. Schell (Eds.), *Willard & Spackman's occupational therapy* (10th ed., pp. 157–170). Philadelphia: Lippincott Williams & Wilkins.

Peloquin, S.M. (2005). The 2005 Eleanor Clarke Slagle lecture: Embracing our ethos, reclaiming our heart. *American Journal of Occupational Therapy, 59,* 611–625.

Polatajko, H.J. (1994). Dreams, dilemmas, and decisions for occupational therapy practice in a new millennium: A Canadian perspective. *American Journal of Occupational Therapy, 48,* 590–594.

Reilly, M. (1962). Occupational therapy can be one of the great ideas of 20th century medicine. *American Journal of Occupational Therapy, 16,* 1–9.

Reilly, M. 1966. A psychiatric occupational therapy program as a teaching model. *American Journal of Occupational Therapy, 20,* 61–67.

Reilly, M. (Ed.). (1974). *Play as exploratory learning.* Beverly Hills: Sage.

Rerek, M. (1971). The depression years: 1929 to 1941. *American Journal of Occupational Therapy, 25,* 231–233.

Robinson, A. (1977). Western medicine's attempt to become more scientific: Examples from the United States and Thailand. *Social Science and Medicine, 11,* 549-560.

Rogers, J. (1982). Order and disorder in occupational therapy and in medicine. *American Journal of Occupational Therapy, 36,* 29–35.

Shannon, P. (1972). Work-play theory and the occupational therapy process. *American Journal of Occupational Therapy, 31,* 229–234.

Shannon, P. (1977). The derailment of occupational therapy. *American Journal of Occupational Therapy, 31,* 229–234.

Shapiro, J.P. (1993). *No pity: People with disabilities forging a new civil rights movement.* New York: Random House.

Spackman, C. (1968). A history of the practice of occupational therapy for restoration of physical function: 1917-1967. *American Journal of Occupational Therapy, 22,* 67–71.

Stein, F., & Cutler, S.K. (1998). *Psychosocial occupational therapy: A holistic approach.* San Diego: Singular.

Task force on target populations. (1974). *American Journal of Occupational Therapy, 23,* 158–163.

Taylor, R.R. (2003). Extending client-centered practice: The use of participatory methods to empower clients. *Occupational Therapy in Mental Health, 19*(2), 57–75.

Thelen, E., & Ulrich, B.D. (1991). Hidden skills: A dynamic systems analysis of treadmill stepping during the first year. *Monographs of the Society for Research in Child Development, 56* (1, Serial No. 223).

Townsend, E. (1993). Occupational therapy's social vision. *Canadian Journal of Occupational Therapy, 60,* 174–184.

Townsend, E. (2003). Reflections on power and justice in enabling occupation. *Revue Canadienne D'Ergotherapie, 70,* 74–87.

Trombly, C. (1993). The issue is anticipating the future: Assessment of occupational functioning. *American Journal of Occupational Therapy, 47,* 253–257.

Vallacher, R.R., & Nowak, A. (Eds.). (1994). *Dynamical systems in social psychology.* San Diego: Academic Press.

Watanabe, S. (1968). Four concepts basic to the occupational therapy process. *American Journal of Occupational Therapy, 22,* 439–450.

West, W. (1968). Professional responsibility in times of change. *American Journal of Occupational Therapy, 38,* 15–23.

West, W. (1984). A reaffirmed philosophy and practice of occupational therapy. *American Journal of Occupational Therapy, 38,* 15–23.

Wiemer, R. (1979). Traditional and nontraditional practice arenas. In *Occupational therapy: 2001 A.D.* (pp. 42–53) [monograph]. Rockville, MD: American Occupational Therapy Association.

Wilcock, A.A. (1993). A theory of the human need for occupation. *Journal of Occupational Science: Australia, 1*(1), 17–24.

Wood, W. (1995). Weaving the warp and weft of occupational therapy: An art and science for all times. *American Journal of Occupational Therapy, 49,* 44–52.

Wood, W. (1998). It is jump time for occupational therapy. *American Journal of Occupational Therapy, 52,* 403–411.

Woodside, H. (1976). Dimensions of the occupational behavior model *Canadian Journal of Occupational Therapy, 43,* 11–14.

Yerxa, E.J. (1980). Occupational therapy's role in creating a future climate of caring. *American Journal of Occupational Therapy, 34,* 529–534.

Yerxa, E.J. (1983). Audacious values: The energy source of occupational therapy practice. In G. Kielhofner (Ed.), *Health through occupation: Theory and practice in occupational therapy* (pp. 149–162). Philadelphia: F.A. Davis.

Yerxa, E.J., Clark, F., Frank, G., Jackson, J., Parham, D., Pierce, D., et al. (1990). An introduction to occupational science: A foundation for occupational therapy in the 21st century. In J.A. Johnson & E.J. Yerxa (Eds.), *Occupational science: The foundation for new models of practice* (pp. 1–18). New York: Haworth Press.

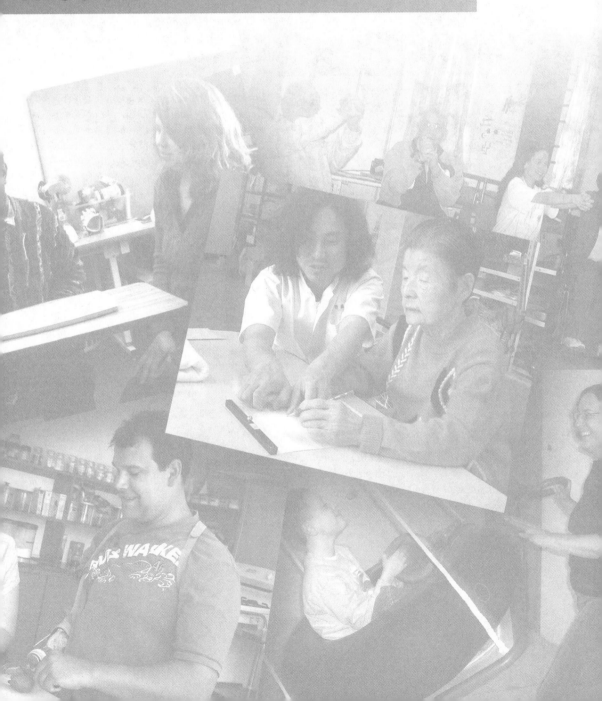

Conceptual Practice Models

CHAPTER 6

The Nature and Role of Conceptual Practice Models

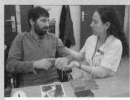 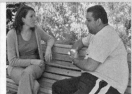

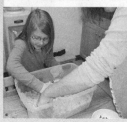 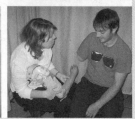

One of my clients was a 29-year-old man from Cyprus who suffered a severe head injury due to a motor vehicle accident and was hospitalized in Jerusalem for seven months. It was very hard to reach him. Nothing interested him.

Maya Tuchner

In working with people who have upper limb amputations, I need to know about how joints work and what muscles do and how to build strength or endurance. I do a lot of work now with technologically sophisticated, externally powered prostheses. This requires that I understand the orientation of muscle fibers within a specific muscle and that I can palpate a muscle belly to feel the contraction that will be used to make a prosthetic hand open or a prosthetic elbow flex. I need to be able to teach clients how to strengthen their muscles and how to improve endurance within a muscle so that they have enough capacity to utilize a prosthesis throughout an entire day for all of the daily activities in which they wish to engage.

Karen Roberts

I work with a young man, Gabriel, who for ten years stayed in his bedroom fantasizing about being a famous Hollywood film producer. Severe and constant mood swings kept him from being able to function. He was unable to sustain any studies or work. He was even unable to pursue artistic projects that he dreamed about. Many years of different therapies had not helped him to get out of his bedroom. He spent his days watching movies, admiring his favorite famous actors, and living vicariously through their lives.

Andrea Girardi

I worked with a girl named Maggie who was in the third grade and had what she called a "bugging problem." Her skin bugged her, especially with certain types of clothing. Maggie could not wear underwear or socks, even on the coldest days. She liked the Velcro straps of her sneakers so tight that she kept ripping the straps off. Maggie wore the same pair of shorts and t-shirt every day and kids were beginning to make fun of her. Maggie had worked with several other specialists and had taken different medications for anxiety. They had not helped the bugging problem.

Stacey Szklut

As each of these therapists' situations and clients illustrate, everyday practice poses challenging puzzles:

- How does one understand the sense of hopelessness in clients who have lost capacities necessary to their accustomed way of life? And, moreover, how does one help these clients retake control of their lives?
- How does one minimize the consequences of clients' sensory, physical, cognitive, or emotional impairments for everyday occupation?
- How does one best interact with mistrustful or withdrawn clients so as to achieve positive outcomes of therapy?

Members of the profession have sought to create explanations for making sense of such puzzles and to develop strategies to solve them. These efforts have resulted in a number of conceptual practice models. These models provide concepts and facts that guide understanding of clients' emotions, thoughts, choices, experiences, capacities, and behaviors. They give insight into the problems faced by clients. Most importantly, they provide

> **Each model provides explanations that make sense of something of practical concern while also providing rationales and practice resources.**

explanations, resources, and evidence that are necessary for good practice.

The Nature and Composition of Conceptual Practice Models

Conceptual practice models all began with a particular problem or circumstance in practice that needed to be understood and addressed. Developers of models sought to create a better understanding of the problem or circumstance and to develop practical means of addressing it. Consequently, each model provides explanations that make sense of something of practical concern while also providing rationales and practice resources. A well-developed model has the following three components:

- Theory that explains something important to practice
- Practice resources (e.g., procedures, materials, and examples) for application
- Research and evidence base that investigate and improve the theory and resources

As shown in Figure 6.1, a model's theory provides the necessary understanding and rationale

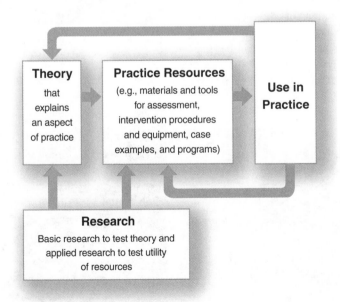

FIGURE 6.1 Components and process of a conceptual practice model.

for practical application. Feedback from practice provides information for further theory development. Basic research examines and leads to improvements in the theory, while applied research examines and leads to improvements in the model's practice resources. This research provides necessary evidence for practice. The following sections examine the characteristics of conceptual practice models in more detail.

Theory

As the examples at the beginning of this chapter illustrated, practitioners often face challenging client problems or circumstances. In order to know what to do about them, it is necessary to have an understanding of them. This is the role of theory. Theories provide an explanation of some problem or circumstance as well as a rationale for what can be done to change it.

Typically, a theory names and defines various factors that are involved and identifies how they are interrelated. For instance, Chapter 11 discusses the concept of volition that helps in understanding a client who is unmotivated. Chapter 13 presents sensory integration theory, which explains why a client may be having extreme difficulty with sensations that interferes with everyday events.

Because the theory in models is developed in response to practical problems, it also addresses the resolution of those problems. Thus, theories also provide an explanation of how the problem or circumstance can be managed or changed. This means that the theory explains an aspect of how the therapy process

works. For instance, Chapter 7 overviews biomechanical theoretical explanations necessary for training a client to use a prosthesis in the place of an amputated arm.

In conceptual practice models, theory is designed as an explanation for application. That is, it provides therapists with an understanding of some problem or circumstance faced in practice and a rationale for what can be done about it. As a result, practitioners can actively use the theory to make sense of their clients and/or therapy circumstances and to made decisions about what to do in therapy. For example, one theory discussed in Chapter 10 will provide explanations of the therapeutic relationship that guides how best to respond to a client's distrust.

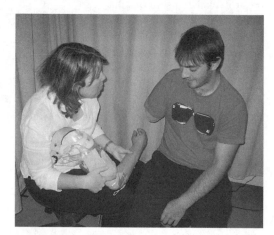

Karen explains how to use a prosthesis to a client with a recent amputation resulting from a car accident.

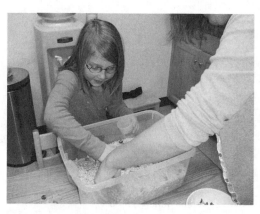

Stacey and a young client play in a tactile bin.

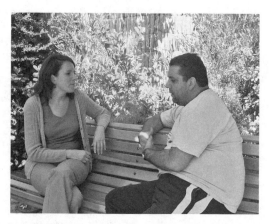

Andrea and a client talk about formulating achievable goals for his future.

Box 6.1   What Is Theory?

Theory is a formal explanation composed of concepts and postulates (Mosey, 1992a). Concepts describe and define some thing (e.g., a type of joint in the body or a kind of thought or feeling), some quality (e.g., the flexibility of a joint or the accuracy of a thought), and/or some process (e.g., moving a body part or problem-solving). Concepts provide a specific way of seeing and thinking about the phenomena to which they refer. Postulates are statements about relationships between concepts. They explain how the characteristics or processes to which concepts refer are organized. For instance, postulates might explain how the components of a joint interact to affect its extent of flexibility or how inaccuracy of thoughts can negatively influence problem-solving.

The key element of theory is explanation. That is, theory must give a useful account for how something works. Thus, theory does more than describe or state what is assumed or important. It provides insight into the nature and workings of specific phenomena that must be dealt with in practice.

Practice Resources

Practitioners who use models require resources to apply them. For instance, therapists must gather and analyze important information about a client or about the therapy process. This process is usually referred to as assessment. Models provide assessments in the form of standardized materials and/or procedures for making sense of critical information. Generally, assessments operationalize one or more of the concepts in the model's theory. As such, they allow the therapists to better comprehend or measure the phenomena explained by the concept. In some cases, a client's score on an assessment can be used to make judgments or predictions that are important for practice.

Application of a model also requires therapists to plan goals for therapy and to plan the intervention process. Most models offer specific procedures or programs with identified goals or outcomes that are expected to result. These are important resources because they make concrete what the theory of a model says should happen in therapy. Intervention procedures and programs are often described in articles or manuals.

Assessment and intervention procedures often involve the use of specific materials or equipment. In the case of assessment, these may include such things as performance tests, instruments for measuring physical abilities, and paper and pencil checklists that are completed by clients. In the case of intervention, a variety of specialized equipment may be used. This ranges from equipment that is used to compensate for limited capacities to equipment that is used as part of the therapy process to provide sensory experiences or exercise certain capacities. The development and availability of these tools for practice are very important parts of conceptual practice models.

The application of conceptual practice models requires judgment on the part of practitioners. Each client represents unique circumstances that require therapists to decide how to apply the theory, how to use available practice resources, and so on. This process of creating individualized interventions is best illustrated through case examples. Through illustrations of particular individuals, they exemplify how the therapy process unfolds and what rationale was used in each step of therapy.

Conceptual practice models are often used as a framework for planning a program of services for a particular client group. Programs are typically designed for a homogeneous group of clients who share a particular diagnosis or occupational problem. Programs are formalized interventions in which the assessment process, the goals, and the interventions are specified and applied uniformly across clients.

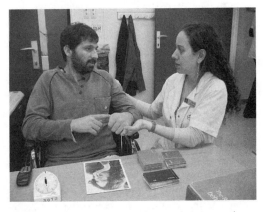

Maya tries to uncover interests in a disinterested client.

In sum, conceptual practice models are most useful to practitioners when they have well-developed resources for application. These practice resources include materials and tools for assessment, intervention procedures and equipment, case examples that illustrate application of the theory in practice, and programs for application of the model to a particular client group.

Research and Evidence Base for Models

Research is used to test a model's theory and its practical utility. Basic research aims to test the explanations offered by a theory, whereas applied research examines the practical results of using a theory to solve problems (Mosey, 1992a, 1992b).

As research evidence mounts, the theory within models can be altered to correct or elaborate existing concepts and propositions. In this way, research improves the usefulness of a model's theory for explaining practical problems and circumstances and what to do about them. Moreover, the existence of a body of research increases the confidence that therapists can place in the theory.

Research that supports the validity of a model's theory and/or provides findings that a model has practical utility is important for guiding evidence-based practice (Holm, 2000). It provides the practitioner with evidence that supports the value of thinking about a problem in a particular way, collecting information using a particular assessment, and/or using certain interventions to achieve therapy goals.

Models in Perspective

Conceptual practice models offer theory that serves as a way of thinking about and doing practice. Moreover, they generate practice resources and guide research that supports evidence-based practice. Since they provide the concepts, practice resources, and evidence that guide and support practice, conceptual practice models greatly influence the quality of occupational therapy

practice. These models are critically important to the profession and to individual practitioners.

In the end, a model should offer insights and tools that enhance practice and produce results desired by clients. This points to the importance of models being developed by collaborating teams of theoreticians, researchers, practitioners, and consumers. A model is only useful if it is thoroughly grounded in practice.

Current Models in Occupational Therapy

In practice, therapists encounter a wide range of impairments, occupational problems, and therapy circumstances. Because of this diversity in the issues that practitioners must address, occupational therapy requires a number of practice models. The following chapters will discuss seven conceptual practice models.

The term model is associated with a variety of frameworks or perspectives in occupational therapy. However, not all of these are conceptual practice models in the sense that they are described in this chapter. The defining characteristics of a conceptual practice model are solid grounding in practice, theory that clearly addresses a unique practice circumstance or challenge, and development of specific practice resources. These are the features that make conceptual practice models indispensable for practitioners.

One of the challenges in writing this book was deciding how to characterize the current conceptual practice models in occupational therapy. In selecting those approaches that can be characterized as conceptual practice models, the following questions were asked:

- Does this model offer theory that addresses a specific and important problem or issue of concern in practice?
- Is this model uniquely grounded in practice? That is, did it emerge out of a practice problem or dilemma and was it developed in close association with practitioners?
- Does this model offer practice resources that are directly useful in practice?

> A model is only useful if it is thoroughly grounded in practice.

- Does this model occupy a unique niche in the field? That is, does it address a unique area or focus of practice and offer an approach distinct from that of others?
- Is there evidence that this model is used in practice?

Based on these criteria, the following seven conceptual practice models were identified as the most prominent and/or promising in the field:

- The biomechanical model
- The cognitive model
- The model of human occupation
- The motor control model
- The sensory integration model
- The intentional relationship model
- The functional group model

Research indicates that the first five of these models are the most frequently used in practice (Brown, Rodger, Brown, & Roever, 2005; Crowe & Kanny, 1990; Haglund, Ekbladh, Thorell, & Hallberg, 2000; Law & McColl, 1989; NBCOT, 2004; Wikeby, Lundgren, & Archenholtz, 2006). The intentional relationship model is a new model that addresses the therapeutic relationship. As noted in Chapter 5, the relationship between therapists and clients has been increasingly recognized as important. Moreover, recent studies indicate that the therapeutic relationship is considered by practitioners to be the most consequential aspect of their therapy (Cole & McLean, 2003; Taylor, Lee, Kielhofner, & Ketkar, in press). Moreover, the American Occupational Therapy Association practice framework recognizes therapeutic use of self as an essential component of therapy (American Occupational Therapy Association, 2002). Because the intentional relationship model addresses an aspect of practice considered critically important but not covered by any existing model, it was selected for inclusion.

The functional group model provides theory and resources related to providing occupational therapy services in groups. Just as the relationship between therapist and client is critical for therapy outcomes, the dynamics and processes of therapeutic groups can also influence the impact of therapy for a client.

Conclusion

This chapter reviewed the nature and composition of conceptual practice models, discussing their importance for occupational therapy practice. It also discussed features that make models most relevant and useful in practice. Seven contemporary models were selected as meeting important criteria for practice relevance and will be presented in the following seven chapters.

REFERENCES

American Occupational Therapy Association. (2002). Occupational therapy practice framework: Domain and process. *American Journal of Occupational Therapy, 56,* 609–639.

Brown, G.T., Rodger, S., Brown, A., & Roever, C. (2005). A comparison of Canadian and Australian pediatric occupational therapists. *Occupational Therapy International, 12*(3), 137–161.

Cole, B., & McLean, V. (2003). Therapeutic relationships re-defined. *Occupational Therapy in Mental Health, 19*(2), 33–56.

Crowe, T.K., & Kanny, E.M. (1990). Occupational therapy practice in school systems: A survey of northwest therapists. *Physical & Occupational Therapy in Pediatrics, 10*(3), 69–83.

Haglund, L., Ekbladh, E., Thorell, L-H., & Hallberg, I.R. (2000). Practice models in Swedish psychiatric occupational therapy. *Scandinavian Journal of Occupational Therapy, 7,* 107–113.

Holm, M. (2000). Our mandate for the new millennium: Evidence-based practice: Eleanor Clarke Slagle lecture. *American Journal of Occupational Therapy, 54,* 575–585.

Law, M., & McColl, M.A. (1989). Knowledge and use of theory among occupational therapists: A Canadian survey. *Canadian Journal of Occupational Therapy, 56*(4), 198–204.

National Board for Certification in Occupational Therapy, Inc. (2004). A practice analysis study of entry-level occupational therapist registered and certified occupational therapy assistant practice. *Occupational Therapy Journal of Research: Occupation, Participation and Health, 24,* S1–S31.

Mosey, A.C. (1992a). *Applied scientific inquiry in the health professions: An epistemological orientation.* Rockville, MD: American Occupational Therapy Association.

Mosey, A.C. (1992b). Partition of occupational science and occupational therapy. *American Journal of Occupational Therapy, 4,* 851.

Taylor, R.R., Lee, S-W., Kielhofner, G., & Ketkar, M. (in press). The therapeutic relationship: A nationwide survey of practitioners' attitudes and experiences. *American Journal of Occupational Therapy.*

Wikeby, M., Lundgren, B., & Archenholtz, B. (2006). Occupational therapists' reflection on practice within psychiatric care: A Delphi study. *Scandinavian Journal of Occupational Therapy, 13*(3), 151–159.

The Biomechanical Model

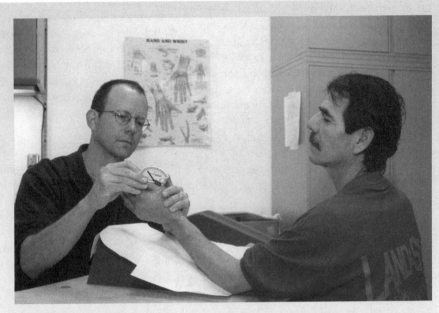

A therapist uses a goniometer (an instrument that measures the degrees of movement in a joint) to measure the finger range of motion of a client whose impairment includes restriction of hand motion. Based on this and other information about the client's movement capacity, the therapist will determine a treatment program aimed at increasing the client's functional use of the hand. This focus on precisely measuring and addressing limitations of functional movement is characteristic of the biomechanical model.

The biomechanical model has been present in some form throughout occupational therapy history. However, this model was most clearly articulated during the period of the mechanistic paradigm that was discussed in Chapter 4. The basic concern of the biomechanical model is with problems related to musculoskeletal capacities that underlie **functional motion** in everyday occupational performance. The model's theory explains how the body is designed for and is used to accomplish motion. At one time this approach was called kinetic occupational therapy, a term that emphasized the goal of restoring abilities for motion (Ogden-Niemeyer & Land Jacobs, 1989).

While much of the underlying theory and research related to the biomechanical model has been developed outside occupational therapy in the fields of anatomy, physiology, and kinesiology, many of the resources for application have been accumulating throughout occupational therapy history. Many of the approaches and devices used today are based on decades of development.

The biomechanical model is applied to persons who experience limitations in moving freely, with adequate strength, and in a sustained fashion. These impairments result from disease or trauma in the musculoskeletal system, peripheral nervous system, integumentary system (i.e., skin), or cardiopulmonary system. Problems of coordinated movement due to central nervous system impairment are more typically addressed through the motor control model or the sensory integrative model. Even in those cases, however, some biomechanical concerns, such as maintaining normal joint movement, are usually addressed.

Theory

The biomechanical approach is based on principles borrowed from the fields of **kinetics** (the study of how forces produce motion in body

> **Whether for manipulation of objects, gesturing in communication, or standing in a line while waiting a turn, all occupations involve persons stabilizing and moving their bodies.**

parts) and **kinematics** (the study of motion of body parts in time). Knowledge of the anatomy and physiology of the musculoskeletal system is also foundational to this model. This knowledge includes understanding of the structure and function of bones, joints, and muscles that underlie motion as well as such processes as tissue healing, muscle strengthening, and the energy cost of activities. Together these processes explain how humans produce and sustain movement. Finally, knowledge of how the cardiopulmonary system supports functioning of the musculoskeletal system is incorporated into this model.

The Basic Concepts of Motion

Motion underlies all occupational performance. Whether for manipulation of objects, gesturing in communication, or standing in a line while waiting a turn, all occupations involve persons stabilizing and moving their bodies. The theory of the biomechanical model concerns the ability to stabilize and move body parts in order to achieve the necessary motion for performing occupations.

The biomechanical model explains how the body produces the stability and movement required to perform occupations using three broad concepts. The first is the potential for motion at the joints, or **joint range of motion.** The second is **strength,** or the ability of muscles to produce tension for maintaining postural control and for moving body parts. The third is **endurance,** which is the ability to sustain motion (i.e., intensity or rate) over the time required to do a particular task.

Joint Range of Motion

Understanding the available motion at each joint comes from knowledge of the structure and function of the joint. Joints are connections between two or more bones. In addition to the two or more surfaces that touch each other, a joint is held in place by ligaments and by muscles that cross the joint. The ways in which joints can move are determined by their structure and surrounding soft tissues (Radomski & Trombly Latham, 2008). For instance, hinge joints such as those of the proximal and distal interphalangeal joints of the fingers (i.e., the two joints nearest the tip of each finger) allow movement in one plane (i.e., extension and flexion). Ball and socket joints, such as the shoulder and hip joints, allow movement in several planes. These joints are not only capable of flexion and extension but also adduction (movement toward the midline of the body), abduction (movement away from the body midline), and rotation (movement about a longitudinal axis). Thus, the structure of each joint determines the movements that are possible at the joint.

The connective tissue (e.g., ligaments), muscle, and skin that surround joints have **elasticity**, which is the ability to stretch and to return to original shape and size after movement. The amount of elasticity of these tissues also affects the extent of possible movement.

Range of Motion

Active range of motion refers to the range of movement that a person can produce using voluntary muscle contraction. **Passive range of motion** refers to the range of movement that is possible when an outside force moves a joint. The potential for motion in the body's joints allows the body to assume positions and engage in actions that are necessary for functional performance. Range of motion makes possible such actions as bending, reaching, pulling, lifting, and grasping.

Strength

Stability and motion are produced when skeletal muscles act on the joints of the body. Muscles cross one or more joints and exert force to control or produce movements allowed by the structure of the joints. Thus, tension produced in the muscles is necessary to stabilize or move joints. Muscles move joints when muscles contract to produce forces that act on one side or aspect of the joint. For example, the muscles that connect to the bones of the fingers on the palm side of the hand flex the fingers, while those muscles

that connect to the finger bones on the back of the hand cause the fingers to extend. For example, as shown in Figure 7.1, the extensor digitorum muscle attaches to the bones of the second, third, fourth, and fifth fingers on the back of the hand and when it contracts it extends the fingers at all three finger joints. Muscles stabilize joints when they produce forces that act with equal tension from all directions in which the joint is capable of moving.

The strength or ability of a muscle to produce tension is heavily influenced by the number and size of fibers in the muscle. The diameter of muscle fibers increases when the muscle is used to produce tension. Thus, the use to which a muscle is put during the course of everyday activities affects its strength.

In daily life, normal movement is not limited to the action of a single muscle across a single

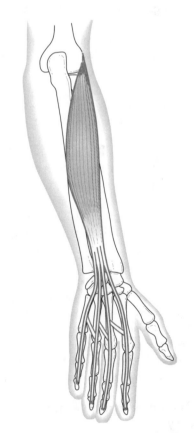

FIGURE 7.1 Extensor digitorum muscle. *From Lippert, L. (2006). Clinical Kinesiology and Anatomy. Philadelphia: F.A. Davis.*

joint. Rather, performance depends on the simultaneous action of muscles across many joints. This produces the combination of stability and movement required for a task. Moreover, groups of muscles work together to produce each movement (Pendleton & Schultz-Krohn, 2006).

The extent of muscle strength determines what kind of functional movement one's body can perform. For example, a certain amount of strength is necessary to lift an arm against gravity. More strength is needed when lifting a heavy object overhead. Along with range of motion, strength determines the extent to which a person is able to execute necessary tasks. To perform optimally, one must have adequate strength to do the tasks that make up one's occupations.

Endurance

The ability to sustain muscle activity (i.e., endurance) is a function of muscle physiology and the underlying cardiopulmonary functions that supply oxygen and energy materials. Thus, endurance is a somewhat more complex phenomenon than strength and motion since it depends on the musculoskeletal system but also entails the functions of other body systems. Two types of endurance are recognized. Muscle endurance refers to the ability of a muscle to contract repeatedly to do work. Cardiorespiratory endurance refers more broadly to the ability to sustain activity over time as when walking or running.

Like range of motion and strength, endurance determines the extent to which persons can do the tasks that make up occupational life. Endurance is most important when an occupation requires repeated motion or sustained effort over time. Walking to school or work, vacuuming or mopping the house, and working on an assembly line are obvious examples of occupations that require one to sustain motion over time. Nonetheless, all activities require a certain amount of endurance since they call for one to stabilize and move oneself for some duration.

The Dynamics of Movement Capacity

Several factors are considered in understanding movement. The potential for movement (joint range of motion) is a function of the anatomy of joints and soft tissues around joints.

Bones constitute a system of rigid levers that are moved by forces produced by the muscles attached to those bones (Hall, 2003). Bones are arranged as levers in which force is applied somewhere along the length of the bone to move it on its pivot point or fulcrum. The production of movement is a function of how muscles act on the levers created by bones. Functional movement requires a complex interaction of forces produced by muscles acting on many levers simultaneously to stabilize and move them according to the task being performed. Endurance while doing a functional activity is a function of muscle physiology and the ability of the body systems to transport needed material into and waste material out of muscle tissue.

Early understanding of how muscles produced movement was based primarily on the anatomical study of their position with respect to the skeletal system (i.e., where the muscles attached to bones and how they crossed joints). Such observations of anatomical organization led to the belief that specific movements and muscles would be used to perform a given task (Radomski & Trombly Latham, 2008).

As more sophisticated methods have become available to study the process of movement, the understanding of how movement is used to accomplish occupations has changed. The actual movements produced during occupational performance can be described in terms of kinematics. For example, movement can be characterized by the actual movement path (e.g., the forward and backward movements such as those used for walking) or displacement of a body part (e.g., the degrees of motion involved in flexing the elbow) and the velocity (i.e., speed) and acceleration (i.e., rate of change in speed).

Kinematics is an important part of the understanding of how the body actually accomplishes functional movements. For example, it is now understood that different persons use different combinations of movements to do the same task and that a person uses different combinations of movements to perform the same task at different times (Trombly, 1995). Despite this complex variability in how functional movements are executed, all movements require the foundation of the potential for range of motion in the structure of the skeletal system and its joints, the necessary strength for accomplishing functional movements provided by muscles, and the endurance to sustain motion over the course of task performance provided by muscle physiology and the supporting cardiopulmonary system.

Maintaining Biomechanical Capacity

One of the most important observations of the biomechanical model is that the capacity for movement (i.e., strength, range of motion, and endurance) not only affects but is affected by occupational performance. That is, muscle strength increases and decreases according to how much muscles are stressed (i.e., used to produce motion) in the course of everyday occupations. Similarly, the structure of bones is positively affected by how much weight-bearing they do, and joint mobility is affected by the nature of ongoing joint movement. Finally, the capacity for endurance waxes and wanes over time with changes in activity level.

While the biomechanical model is used with clients whose musculoskeletal capacities have been compromised due to disease or trauma, the fundamental principle, that biomechanical capacity increases or decreases according to use, is important not only to increasing capacities that have been reduced, but also to ensure that capacities are not decreased through disuse.

Problems and Challenges

The biomechanical model addresses problems and challenges related to producing the stability and movement for the performance of one's occupations. Occupational performance generally requires that we stabilize some part of the body while moving others. For instance, while typing at a keyboard one must keep the back, shoulders, elbow, and wrist relatively stable while the fingers move.

Problems with stability and motion emanate from biomechanical impairments (i.e., restrictions of joint motion, strength, and/or endurance) (Radomski & Trombly Latham, 2008). Thus, the central concern of the model is with problems

that occur when persons cannot generate and/or sustain the stability or movement needed to perform their occupations. A wide range of diseases or traumas may lead to such problems. Additionally, disuse or overuse of the musculoskeletal system can create problems.

Joint range of motion may be limited because of joint damage, edema of tissues around the joint, pain, skin tightness, muscle spasticity (i.e., excess muscle tone producing tightness), or muscle and **tendon** shortening as a consequence of prolonged immobilization. Examples of conditions that affect joint mobility are arthritis, trauma to the joint or to the surrounding connective tissue, and burns that limit the elasticity of skin over the joint.

Muscle weakness (i.e., reduced tension-producing capacity) can occur as a result of disuse or because of disease affecting muscle physiology. Loss of muscle strength may be due to disease (e.g., polio or amyotrophic lateral sclerosis) or trauma (spinal cord or peripheral nerve injury) that affects the nervous system stimulation of muscle contraction. Muscle diseases, such as muscular dystrophy, directly affect muscle tissue and its ability to contract. Finally, extended disuse or immobilization can result in the shrinking of muscle fibers that produces weakness that impairs everyday performance (Pendleton & Schultz-Krohn, 2006; Radomski & Trombly Latham, 2008).

Like strength, endurance can be reduced with any extended confinement or limitation of activity. Other factors, including pathology of the cardiovascular or respiratory systems and muscular diseases, can also reduce endurance.

Sensory Problems

Although problems of sensation are not—strictly speaking—biomechanical, they are often intertwined with movement problems. Tactile sensations or touch are often affected by the same diseases or traumas that affect muscles (i.e., peripheral nerve injuries or spinal cord injuries). Thus, it is very common that sensory loss and loss of motion co-occur. Since tactile sensations are used to direct many movements and to protect the body from harm during performance, they are closely tied to being able to move effectively without injuring oneself (Radomski & Trombly Latham, 2008).

Another important aspect of sensation that is closely tied to movement is pain. While pain ordinarily occurs as a warning against injurious actions, it can be chronically or periodically present in association with disease or trauma that affects the musculoskeletal system. Arthritic pain is a common example. Because pain can affect a person's tolerance for exerting and sustaining movement and because movement can worsen pain, the two must often be considered carefully together.

Rationale for Therapeutic Intervention

Interventions based on the biomechanical model focus on the intersection of motion and occupational performance. These interventions can be divided into three different rationales:

• Preventing deformity and maintaining existing capacity for motion
• Restoring the capacity for motion
• Compensating for limited range of motion, strength, and/or endurance

> **Interventions based on the biomechanical model focus on the intersection of motion and occupational performance.**

These three rationales are often used in combination. The three rationales share the aims of minimizing any gap between persons' existing limited capacity for movement and the movement requirements of their ordinary occupational tasks. The first, preventative, approach seeks to avoid the development of a gap or to prevent the gap from becoming larger. The second, restorative, approach seeks to narrow the gap by increasing the capacity for motion. The third, compensatory, approach seeks to bridge the gap through means external to the musculoskeletal system. Each of these approaches is examined here.

Maintenance and Prevention

As already noted, reasonable use is necessary to maintain function of the musculoskeletal system. The biomechanical model extends this observation to the principle that muscles that are still able to produce contractions and joints that allow motion should be used to maintain their capacity for functional motion. When the person is not able to move joints through muscle contraction, joint range of motion is maintained passively (i.e., by externally manipulating joints through their ranges of motion). Joint positioning, including the use of splints that maintain joints in proper alignment, is also used to prevent joint deformity.

Research has shown, and more people are becoming aware, that many biomechanical problems are caused by how persons perform tasks in their daily occupations. Examples of this are back injury due to use of poor **body mechanics** while lifting and damage to soft tissues due to repetitive motions performed in work (Radomski & Trombly Latham, 2008). This awareness has fueled efforts to prevent occurrence or recurrence of such problems, especially in the workplace and schools. Occupational therapists can teach proper body mechanics or recommend work-task, work-site, or classroom modifications as preventative measures to avoid such biomechanical problems.

Restoration

Restoration aims at increasing available motion, strength, and endurance. Principles of restoration are based on the understanding of normal biomechanical functioning. Because movement maintains normal range of motion, strength, and endurance, movement in therapeutically designed activities or tasks can be used to restore or improve range of motion, strength, or endurance. Strategies for restoring strength, range of motion, and endurance are described later in the chapter (see Intervention).

Goals for increasing motion, strength, and endurance are determined according to the residual potential (i.e., how much improvement a person is likely to be able to achieve based on the nature of the disease or trauma underlying the impairment) and the movement demands of the occupations the person needs and/or wants to perform. For this approach to work, there must be the potential for the person to develop the motion, strength, and endurance necessary for the desired and/or necessary occupations.

For example, a client in occupational therapy who previously had hand surgery may be doing activities designed to restore the active range of motion and strength necessary for typing. Another client recovering from coronary bypass surgery may engage in graded occupations in order to increase endurance to a level required for self-care and leisure activities. Still another client after a work injury may be engaged in simulated work activities designed to increase strength for lifting objects to the level demanded on the job.

Compensation

Many people experience extended, permanent, or progressively greater limitations in the capacity for movement. **Compensatory treatment** (sometimes called the "rehabilitation approach") aims to offset these limitations by bridging the gap between the person's capacity for stability or motion and what is required in everyday occupations (Radomski & Trombly Latham, 2008). Compensation involves one or more of the following strategies:

• Using **prostheses** (devices that replace amputated parts of the body) and **orthoses** (devices attached to the body that substitute for lost stability or movement)
• Modifying or replacing the physical environment and objects (adapted equipment) used to perform routine tasks
• Altering procedures for accomplishing tasks, including the use of other persons as assistants in accomplishing these tasks

Practice Resources

Extensive resources have been developed to support the application of the biomechanical model. Information about these resources exists in a wide variety of published sources, including those that focus on particular kinds of musculoskeletal impairments. While many of the resources for application are generic and can be applied across a wide range of client problems, there are also protocols or approaches that

are tied to a particular impairment (e.g., spinal cord injury or arthritis). Because different impairments mean different underlying causes for movement problems (e.g., de-innervation versus joint deterioration), the implications for what kinds of interventions to use and how to sequence them are different. Moreover, different impairments have different prognoses or expected outcomes that may call for a different balance of preventative, restorative, and compensatory approaches to intervention.

Assessment

Range of motion is one of the most basic measurements done in the biomechanical model. If the client is not capable of moving a joint voluntarily (active range of motion), the therapist passively moves it to evaluate available range (passive range of motion). Flinn, Trombly Latham, and Robinson Podolsky (2008) recommend first doing a functional evaluation of active range of motion that involves asking the client to move various body parts. If observation reveals no obvious limitations that would restrict functional performance, no further evaluation of range of motion is done. However, if problems are noted, then a more detailed range of motion evaluation is completed.

Range of motion is measured in degrees of movement about the axis of a joint. One of the oldest and most common ways of measuring range of motion is with a goniometer, an instrument with a protractor, axis, and two arms that is placed over the joint and aligned with the bones that move about the joint's axis to measure the degrees of range of motion available at that joint.

Strength is normally tested as maximum tension produced under voluntary control (Flinn et al., 2008). The strength assessment used most often is **manual muscle testing,** in which the therapist (alone or using some instrument) tests the ability of the person to produce resistance and/or movement under standardized circumstances. When no instrument is used, the procedure for manual muscle testing is asking the client to move against gravity followed by the break test if the client is capable of moving the body part against gravity. In the break test,

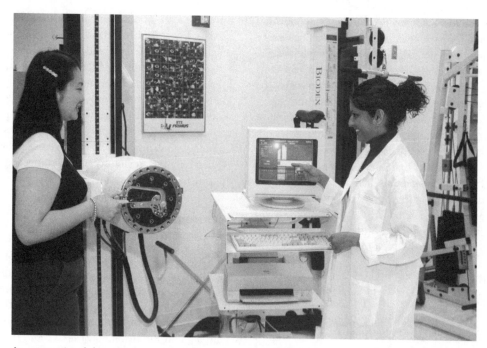

An occupational therapist measures a client's lateral pinch strength using a Baltimore Therapeutic Equipment Work Simulator.

the muscle tested is positioned to give it the most mechanical advantage and the client is asked to hold the position as the therapist increases resistance against it. The extent of effort required for the therapist to break the contraction (i.e., the amount of resistance under which the client can no longer hold the position) is used to grade the client's strength. Strength is graded on an ordinal scale (e.g., normal, good, fair, poor, etc.) or on a numerical scale (0–5).

Another procedure for measuring strength is to use an instrument; this procedure is most commonly used to assess hand strength. A number of instruments exist for this purpose (e.g., a dynamometer that measures hand strength). When using these instruments the therapist asks a client to exert maximal force for a brief period and the instrument measures the extent of force the client produces.

When muscle strength is assessed via manual muscle testing, the results are generally interpreted in terms of what is normal for an individual of the client's age and sex. In addition to examining strength of individual muscles and muscle groups, the evaluator may assess the

pattern of muscle strength and weakness. Another approach to examining strength is to compare a client's ability to do a particular movement against the criteria of how much work is required for a particular kind of task or role. This practice is common in work-oriented evaluations of strength. For instance, a therapist might test a client whose job requires lifting an object that weighs 50 pounds to the height of a normal table by asking the client to perform exactly that action.

Endurance can be measured either dynamically or statically. Static assessment examines how long a client can maintain a contraction. Dynamic assessments of endurance determine the duration or number of repetitions a client can perform before fatigue occurs or by determining the percentage of maximal heart rate that an activity produces.

When measuring endurance, three factors are ordinarily considered: intensity, duration, and frequency. Intensity is a function of both resistance and speed (e.g., how much is being lifted and how fast). Frequency refers to how often the action is repeated and duration to how long it is kept up. As with evaluations of strength, an endurance evaluation can also be done against the criteria of what is required for a particular task or job.

In addition to the more traditional and simple assessments of strength and endurance, several kinds of complex and computer-driven systems are available for muscle strength and endurance testing. These can produce very sophisticated analyses of a person's movement capacities. The methods that a therapist uses will depend on a number of factors including the context and the overall goals of the therapy and resources available.

Intervention

Methods of intervention are clearly delineated in the biomechanical model. When interventions are aimed at maintaining or restoring function, the method must match not only the targeted limitations of motion, strength, and endurance but also their underlying causes, because the latter may determine the most appropriate intervention.

For example, if limited range of motion is due to tightness of soft tissue that is part of the joint, stretching may be used to reduce that tightness and increase range of motion. Stretching is sometimes accomplished actively through movements performed by the client. For example, a person with limited extension in the fingers may be given activities that include picking up objects that require the client to open his hands widely, thus stretching the joints. Stretching can also be done through passive, external means, such as manual stretching that is performed by a therapist or the use of splints that apply pressure that passively stretches the soft tissues of the joint.

However, as stressed earlier, the method of intervention for maintaining or restoring function depends on the underlying cause of the problem. For instance, if limited range of motion is due to edema (swelling of soft tissue surrounding the joint), compression may be used to reduce the edema and, thus, increase range of motion. A similar logic surrounds preventive efforts. For example, active and passive range of motion and appropriate positioning may be used to prevent tightening of soft tissues that would constrict range of motion.

Strength is developed by increasing the stress on a muscle through: (1) the amount of resistance offered to the movement; (2) the duration of resistance required; (3) the rate (speed of movement) of an exercise session; and (4) frequency of sessions. Different types of exercise regimens are available. To increase strength, therapists provide clients opportunities to engage in occupations in which one or more of these demands are gradually increased. These increases in demand result in increases in capacity until a desired level of functioning is reached. Current approaches (such as work hardening) emphasize performing the specific tasks required by the person's occupation (Ogden-Niemeyer & Land Jacobs, 1989).

Endurance is generally addressed by having clients perform activities that require repeated or sustained movement. If the problem is muscular endurance, then activities will stress repeated use of the involved muscles. If the problem is cardiovascular, activities will be designed to place mild stress on the cardiopulmonary system and, thus, increase its capacity.

Occupational therapy intervention that seeks to maintain or restore capacities may also make use of physical agent modalities (e.g., electrical stimulation, paraffin baths, heat or cold packs, and ultrasound). Their use arose primarily in the 1970s and 1980s (Radomski & Trombly Latham, 2008). These are considered adjunctive procedures that are supportive to the main emphasis of using occupations to maintain or restore motion (AOTA, 2003). Occupational therapists also use techniques such as passive manipulation (e.g., massage or joint mobilization) in the same way.

Role of Occupation in Maintenance, Prevention, and Restoration

The traditional view in occupational therapy has been that occupations provide natural and motivating circumstances for maintaining musculoskeletal functioning. This belief is based on the argument that involvement in meaningful occupations employs attention, thereby encouraging greater effort, diminishing fatigue, and diverting attention from pain or fear of movement. Additionally, therapists have argued that occupations provide a form of conditioning that more nearly replicates the normal demands for movement in everyday life. Reflecting this viewpoint, Trombly Latham and Radomski (2002) suggest the following approach to selecting activities used as a therapeutic media:

> The best activity for remediation is one that intrinsically demands the exact response that has been determined to need improvement.... Contrived methods of doing an ordinary activity to make it therapeutic may diminish the value of the activity in the eyes of the patient. (p. 269)

As this quote implies, the therapist requires knowledge of the kind of functional movements that an activity will require from the participant. As noted earlier, it was assumed in the past that a therapist could determine what discrete movements would be required by doing a **biomechanical activity analysis**. Now it is recognized that while it may be possible to determine the overall type of movement required to complete a specific activity, it is not possible to predict the exact pattern of muscle action and joint motion with which a person will accomplish a given task. As Trombly (1995) notes:

> The next time the person does the same thing, his or her muscles may be more warmed up, or there may be a slight difference in placement of task object in relation to the active limb, so a new coordinative structure evolves. That is, different muscles may be recruited, or the same muscles used before may be more or less active in order to accomplish the movement goal in the most efficient way. The motor goal is constant or invariant and requires a constant or invariant response, but this response can be fulfilled by a varying set of muscular contractions. (p. 965)

Thus, contemporary biomechanical activity analysis is less concerned with specific motions and, instead, focuses on functional movements. That is, therapists pay more attention to the functional purpose of a task, because purpose does appear to exert an organizing influence on movement (Trombly, 1995). This also means that when therapists analyze activities, they need to think about requisite movement in functional terms such as holding, grasping, lifting, climbing, pressing, and carrying. These are the kinds of functional movements that tend to remain stable within occupations while the underlying combinations of muscle action and joint motion that accomplish the functional movements may vary considerably.

While the process of analyzing an activity is viewed differently than in the past, it is still an important element of this model since therapists need to modify occupational activities in order to achieve therapeutic goals. Activities may be modified so as to reduce or alter task demands and thereby prevent musculoskeletal problems.

Therapists may also adapt activities to better match permanently reduced musculoskeletal capacity. Finally, activities may be progressively modified to intensify task demands that will increase musculoskeletal capacity. Therapists have several ways to modify an activity including:

1. Positioning the task
2. Adding weights or other devices that provide assistance or resistance to movements performed in the activity
3. Modifying tools to reduce or increase demands
4. Changing materials or size of objects used
5. Changing the method of accomplishing the task

In doing activity adaptation, Trombly Latham and Radomski (2002) caution that the therapist should not contrive the activity so much that it becomes meaningless. In all cases of using adapted activities, it is important that the client be involved in occupational performance that has some meaning and relevance.

Compensatory Intervention

Compensatory interventions are used for clients who will live with a disability either temporarily or permanently. Underlying such intervention is the principle that when persons do not have the biomechanical capacity to perform daily living, leisure, and work tasks in ordinary ways, special equipment and modified procedures can compensate. They are used to close the gap between the person's capacities and the task demands. The desired goal of the treatment is for clients to be able to use their remaining capacities (and by so using, maintain them) while being able to participate in the occupations they wish to do.

Evaluation includes assessment of actual performance in activities of daily living (e.g., toileting, bathing, feeding, grooming, dressing, mobility, and communication), leisure, work, and community living. When assessment is completed and the person's inability to perform necessary tasks is identified, the therapist determines the biomechanical limitations and assets. With this information, the therapist can recommend and train persons in the use of special equipment, modified procedures, or altered environments that make it possible for the person to perform the task. A wide range of adaptive equipment (commercially available or fabricated in therapy) is used to assist persons in performing every aspect of their daily occupations.

Compensatory intervention falls into three broad categories:

- Use of orthoses and prostheses
- Use of adaptive equipment
- Task and/or environmental modification

Orthoses can align a body part in proper position, reduce stress to a joint by providing stability, compensate for weak muscles, or provide a low-grade stretch. The earliest orthoses were fabricated by occupational therapists and while therapists still engage in splint fabrication, a wide variety of prefabricated splints are commercially available. Orthoses support, immobilize, or position a joint or joints and are used to correct for deformities and/or to increase function. An orthosis may be temporary or permanent. Orthotic splints either use existing movements to achieve functional motion or rely on sources of power external to the body. Occupational therapists are also involved in training clients to use prostheses.

Adaptive equipment exists to interface between musculoskeletal capacities and environment and task demands. Some equipment is quite simple, involving modification of ordinary tools and implements to make them easier to grasp and be manipulated. Some involves modification of the environment (i.e., adding ramps and grab bars) to make it easier for persons with limited biomechanical capacity to get around. There also exists more sophisticated equipment such as motorized wheelchairs, special communication

Box 7.1   Improving Functioning Through Use of a Prosthesis

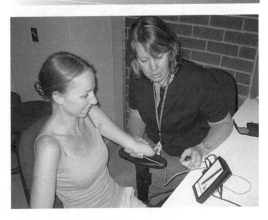

In this photo Karen Roberts is working with a client to prepare her to use a myoelectric prosthesis. Jacqueline had an amputation when she was a teenager and only wore a prosthesis for a very short time. During the past 15 years Jacqueline has developed overuse problems in her back and her right arm that manifest as pain when she completes her daily occupations. She hopes that a prosthesis may enable her to engage in some bimanual activities with improved posture and decreased discomfort. To operate this type of prosthesis, Jacqueline's muscles need sufficient strength to enable the prosthesis to open and close; she also needs to increase her muscle endurance so that she can use a prosthesis throughout an entire day. The myoelectric training program involves using a type of biofeedback machine that measures the strength of a muscle contraction. Karen can measure endurance over time based on how long Jacqueline is able to continue performing adequate contractions. Jacqueline works on her muscle capacity through a home exercise program and in time they will use a training prosthesis to practice daily occupations.

devices, environmental controls, and modified workstations.

The occupational therapist identifies, in collaboration with the client, the most appropriate device and/or modified procedure to use in occupational tasks. The therapist also provides instruction and practice in how to make use of compensatory devices and procedures. This can include instructing persons in how to organize their tasks and time to make the best use of existing capacity to accomplish their occupational tasks.

The occupational therapy setting is often used for persons to try out adapted equipment and procedures. Also, as therapists increasingly provide services in homes, schools, and workplaces, they can work even more specifically in the natural setting in which the task is to be performed. Therapists may assist individuals in planning changes in their homes (if this is financially feasible) and in learning to access specialized transportation and community facilities.

Work Hardening

Work hardening is an individualized biomechanical approach to treatment aimed at returning an individual to work, usually to a specific job. One of the main methods used in work hardening is **physical reconditioning**, the use of simulated and real work activities along with exercise to improve the person's ability to perform specific work tasks.

Work hardening programs employ a range of equipment, including exercise and aerobic conditioning equipment, work capacity evaluation devices (that simulate the required movements of work tasks), work samples and workstations that simulate real jobs, and individualized simulations that reproduce a specific job requirement (Basmajian & Wolf, 1990; Riccio, Nelson, & Bush, 1990).

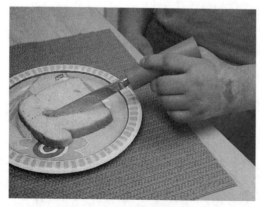

A client with a hand injury uses a knife with a built-up handle to spread peanut butter on a piece of bread.

Research and Evidence Base

Research related to the biomechanical model is substantial and continues to grow. Interdisciplinary investigators study muscle physiology, the effects of exercise, the dynamic role of muscles and muscle groups in movement, and movement or exercise-based interventions for a variety of patient populations (Basmajian & Wolf, 1990; Lippert, 2006). As this body of knowledge develops, it influences the use of the biomechanical model in occupational therapy.

Occupational therapy research related to the biomechanical model is primarily related to the interface of movement and occupation and to this model's practice resources. One area of study is the relationship between musculoskeletal functioning and success in occupations. Such studies have examined, for instance, the ability of measures of physical capacities to predict injured workers' return to work (Kircher, 1984); the potential for persons with muscular dystrophy to participate in specific occupational tasks (Schkade, Feilbelman, & Cook, 1987); the relationship of wrist muscle tone to self-care abilities (Spaulding, Strachota, McPherson, Kuphal, & Ramponi, 1989); and the relationship of grip strength to functional outcomes and work performance following hand trauma (Wahi Michener et al., 2001).

Other studies examine the actual muscle action and kinematics patterns used in different task conditions (Baker, Cham, Cidboy, Cook, & Redfern, 2007; Follows, 1987; Ma & Trombly, 2004; Mathiowetz, 1991; McGrain & Hague, 1987; Trombly & Cole, 1979; Trombly & Quintana, 1983; Wu, Trombly, & Lin, 1994). Such research helps to clarify how movement is produced and used in occupational performance.

Studies are used to validate and develop assessments used with this model (Broniecki, May, & Russel, 2002; King & Finet, 2004). Studies also examine the impact or outcomes of biomechanically based interventions (Driver, 2006; Lieber, Rudy, & Boston, 2000; Schinn, Romaine, Casimano, & Jacobs, 2002).

One final area of inquiry related to the biomechanical model includes studies that examine how the purpose or meaning of activities affects therapy compliance, effort, fatigue, and improvement in movement capacity. One such study demonstrated the advantages of a dance program over normal range of motion exercises (Van Deusen & Marlowe, 1987a; Van Deusen & Marlowe, 1987b). A study of elderly women supported the conclusion that adding imagery to movement is more effective than rote exercise in eliciting frequency and duration of movement (Riccio et al., 1990). A study of women demonstrated that perceived exertion was less in a task with purpose than in a purposeless task in which the same effort was exerted (Kircher, 1984). Based on such research, Nelson and Peterson (1989) argue that activities that add purpose to movement may enhance the quality of exercise both by increasing the goal orientation of the client and by providing environmental support that guides the client's attention and motor planning.

> **What makes the biomechanical model a unique model of practice in occupational therapy is the way biomechanical principles are applied to understanding and enhancing occupational performance and the use of occupations to influence changes in range of motion, strength, and endurance.**

Discussion

The use of biomechanical knowledge is not unique to occupational therapy. For example, physical therapy also applies biomechanics. What makes the biomechanical model a unique model of practice in occupational therapy is the way biomechanical principles are applied to understanding and enhancing occupational performance and the use of occupations to influence changes in range of motion, strength, and endurance. Growing emphasis on the functional outcomes from intervention (e.g., whether the person will return to work or remain living at home) encourages the use of occupations that present clients with real-life demands.

There is evidence that the biomechanical model is the most widely used model in occupational therapy (National Board for Certification in Occupational Therapy,

Box 7.2

Biomechanical Model Case Example: BONNIE

Bonnie, a 56-year-old right-handed math professor, injured her dominant hand when she stumbled and fell while holding a water glass. The glass shattered, lacerating Bonnie's right palm. Several tendons in her hand were cut as were the digital nerves to the thumb and index fingers. Bonnie underwent surgical repair of all injured structures. After her operation, Bonnie's hand surgeon referred her to occupational therapy. Mike Littleton, Bonnie's occupational therapist, works with patients who have limitations in functional movement due to illness or injury. Mike used the biomechanical model to address Bonnie's limited movement in her hand.

Bonnie was first seen for her initial evaluation 10 days after her surgery. During Bonnie's initial visit, Mike's approach was preventative; he fabricated a splint to protect the repaired structures in her hand and to promote healing of those structures. Approximately two weeks later, Bonnie had only minimal ability to close her right hand actively (make a fist) as a result of thickened scar tissue in her palm. She also had difficulty grasping items using this hand. Mike used a sequence of serial static splints to stretch the scar tissue (each new splint stretched the tissue a bit more). Serial splints utilize the concept of low load prolonged stretch (LLPS) to remodel and elongate tight tissues. A splint is fabricated near the maximal stretch point and as the patient gains motion, the splint is re-fabricated at the new end point of motion. He also made use of physical agent modalities including ultrasound and soft tissue massage to soften and elongate scar tissue. Outside of therapy Bonnie used a continuous passive motion (CPM) machine attached to her hand that helped to increase her range of motion.

(box continues on page 78)

Box 7.1 (continued)

Six weeks after surgery, Mike had Bonnie attempt functional activities in therapy. He noted that she had fine motor problems due to muscle weakness and sensory loss to her thumb and index finger. Work activities such as writing equations on a chalkboard were difficult for Bonnie. Problems using her hand stemmed largely from very limited finger range of motion. Thus, Mike developed and implemented a treatment plan that involved stretching the involved tendons and surrounding scar tissue that were limiting range of motion.

Mike also recommended using large diameter chalk or a chalk holder that would allow for firmer grasp. This allowed Bonnie to write on the chalkboard adequately. Eight weeks after her surgery, Mike measured Bonnie's grip strength and lateral pinch strength using a dynamometer. Her grip strength was found to be 9 pounds per square inch (PSI) in her affected right hand and 46 PSI in her unaffected left hand. Her lateral pinch strength was 4 PSI on her right side and 15 PSI on her left side. These measurements of her right hand were well below average for a woman her age and provided objective evidence that the strength in Bonnie's right hand was significantly compromised. Thus, Mike's next step was to give Bonnie activities to do

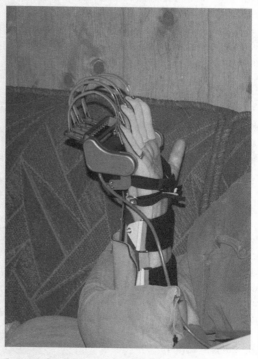

Bonnie's hand in a CPM machine.

that strengthened her hand, focusing on her grip and her ability to pinch with her thumb and forefinger. In addition to goals for increasing strength and range of motion, Mike and Bonnie also set goals to improve her chalkboard writing, computer use, and general fine motor performance.

At 14 weeks post-operation, Bonnie's fingers had enough active range of motion to meet the goal that she and Mike had set. Active range of motion had improved in all of Bonnie's digits. After six months, Bonnie's active range of motion was within normal limits in all of her right finger joints and her grip and pinch strengths were functional. Her grip strength on her right hand had improved to 40 PSI and her lateral pinch on her right side had improved to 10 PSI. Bonnie was performing all work, activities of daily living, and instrumental activities of daily living without difficulty.

As this case illustrates, Mike employed both preventative and restorative intervention strategies. At first, because of the risk of damage following surgery, the focus of therapy was preventative. Later, Mike addressed the range of motion and strength problems that were interfering with Bonnie's occupations. Because they were able to achieve restoration of most of her biomechanical capacities, compensatory strategies were not necessary.

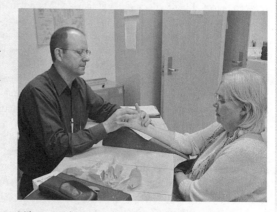

Mike stretching Bonnie's injured hand.

Table 7.1 **Terms of the Model**

Active range of motion	Degree of self-initiated movement possible at a joint.
Biomechanical activity analysis	Examination of the endurance, range of motion, and muscle strength needed for the completion of an activity.
Body mechanics	Position and movements of the body during the performance of occupations.
Compensatory treatment	Therapy involving adaptations to deal with existing limitations.
Elasticity	The capability of tissue to stretch and to return to its original shape and size.
Endurance	The ability to sustain effort over the time required to do a particular task.
Functional motion	Movement required for daily occupations.
Joint range of motion	The potential for motion at the joints.
Kinematics	The study of how the body moves in terms of movement path, velocity, and acceleration.
Manual muscle testing	Examination of an individual's muscle strength by asking the client to produce movement against manual resistance.
Orthosis (pl, orthoses)	Device used to correct joint misalignment or to substitute for lost function.
Passive range of motion	Amount of movement at the joint when the joint is moved by means other than the individual.
Physical reconditioning	The process of returning the body to a state of fitness.
Prosthesis (pl, prostheses)	Device that replaces an amputated body part.
Strength	The ability of muscles to produce tension to maintain postural control and move body parts.
Tendon	Connective tissue that connects a muscle to a bone.
Work hardening	Program applying biomechanical principles by using simulations of the physical requirements of a work situation to recondition persons for work.

2004). Given the centrality of movement problems in occupational therapy clients and the long history of this approach in occupational therapy practice, there is no doubt that the model will continue to be a vital part of occupational therapy science and practice.

SUMMARY: THE BIOMECHANICAL MODEL

Focus

+ Musculoskeletal capacities that underlie functional motion in everyday occupational performance

+ How the body is designed and used to accomplish motion for occupational performance

+ Applied to persons who experience limitations in moving freely, with adequate strength, and/or in a sustained fashion

Theory

+ Kinetic and kinematic principles concerning nature of movement and forces acting on the human body as it moves

+ Anatomy of musculoskeletal system

+ Physiology of bone, connective tissue, and muscle and cardiopulmonary function

+ Capacity for functional motion is based on:
  • Potential for motion at the joints (joint range of motion)
  • Muscle strength (ability of muscles to produce tension to maintain postural control and move body parts)
  • Endurance (ability to sustain effort [i.e., intensity or rate] over time required to do a particular task)

+ Joint range of motion depends on structure and function of joint and integrity of surrounding tissue, muscle, and skin

+ Muscles cross one or more joints and exert force to control or produce movements allowed by the structure of the joints

+ Performance depends on simultaneous action of muscles across many joints producing stability and movement required for a task

+ The ability to sustain muscle activity (i.e., endurance) is a function of muscle physiology in relationship to work being done and supply of oxygen and energy materials from cardiopulmonary system

+ Movements produced during occupational performance are as much a function of dynamic circumstances of performance as they are of structure of the musculoskeletal system

+ Capacity for movement (i.e., strength, range of motion, and endurance) affects and is affected by occupational performance

Problems and Challenges

+ Problems exist when a restriction of joint motion, strength, and/or endurance interferes with everyday occupations

+ Joint range of motion may be limited by joint damage, edema, pain, skin tightness, muscle spasticity (excess muscle tone producing tightness), or muscle and tendon shortening (due to immobilization)

+ Muscle weakness can occur as a result of:
  • Disuse
  • Disease affecting muscle physiology (e.g., muscular dystrophy)
  • Diseases and trauma of lower motor neurons (e.g., polio), spinal cord, or peripheral nerves, which can result in de-innervation of muscles

+ Endurance can be reduced by:
  • Extended confinement or limitation of activity
  • Pathology of cardiovascular or respiratory systems
  • Muscular diseases

+ It is common for sensory loss and loss of motion to co-occur because tactile sensations or touch are often affected by the same diseases or traumas that affect muscles

+ Pain can be chronically or periodically present in association with disease or trauma that affects the musculoskeletal system

Biomechanical Intervention

+ Interventions focus on intersection of motion and occupational performance and can be divided into three approaches:
  • Prevention of contracture and maintenance of existing capacity for motion
  • Restoration by improving diminished capacity for motion

- Compensation for limited motion (sometimes referred to as a rehabilitation approach)

+ Intervention aims to minimize any gap between existing capacity for movement and functional requirements of ordinary occupational tasks

Practice Resources

+ Range of motion is usually measured with a goniometer calibrated to degrees of movement about an axis

+ Strength is normally tested by manual muscle testing in which the therapist (alone or using some instrument) tests the ability of a person to produce resistance and/or movement under standardized circumstances

+ Endurance is usually measured by determining duration or number of repetitions before fatigue occurs

+ Methods of intervention address not only targeted limitations of motion, strength, and endurance, but also their underlying causes because the latter may determine the most appropriate intervention

+ Strength is developed by increasing stress on a muscle through:
  - Amount of resistance offered to the movement
  - Duration of resistance required
  - Rate (speed of movement) of an exercise session
  - Frequency of sessions

+ Occupations
  - Provide natural and motivating circumstances for maintaining musculoskeletal functioning
  - Employ attention, thereby encouraging greater effort, diminishing fatigue, and diverting attention from pain or fear of movement

- Provide conditioning that more nearly replicates normal demands for movement in everyday life

+ Attention to functional purpose of a task is important because purpose does appear to exert an organizing influence on movement

+ Activity may be modified to:
  - Reduce or alter task demands and prevent musculoskeletal problems
  - Match permanently reduced musculoskeletal capacity
  - Intensify task demands that will increase musculoskeletal capacity

+ Ways to modify an activity include:
  - Positioning the task
  - Adding weights or other devices that provide assistance or resistance to movements performed in the activity
  - Modifying tools to reduce or increase demands
  - Changing materials or size of objects used
  - Changing method(s) of accomplishing task

+ When using adapted activities it is important that the client be involved in occupational performance that does have some meaning and relevance

+ When persons do not have biomechanical capacity to perform daily living, leisure, and work tasks in ordinary ways, special equipment and modified procedures can compensate (i.e., close the gap between a person's capacities and task demands)

+ Prescription, design, fabrication, checkout, and training in use of orthoses may be employed to support, immobilize, or position a joint to prevent/correct contractures and/or enhance function

+ Current approaches (such as work hardening) emphasize strengthening by having the client perform tasks required by that person's occupation

REFERENCES

American Occupational Therapy Association. (2003). Physical agent modalities: A position paper. *American Journal of Occupational Therapy, 57,* 650–651.

Baker, N.A., Cham, R., Cidboy, E.H., Cook, J., & Redfern, M.S. (2007). Kinematics of the fingers and hands during computer keyboard use. *Clinical Biomechanics, 22,* 34–43.

Basmajian, J.V., & Wolf, S.L. (1990). *Therapeutic exercise* (5th ed.). Baltimore: Williams & Wilkins.

Broniecki, M., May, E., & Russel, M. (2002). Wrist strength measurement: A review of the reliability of manual muscle testing and hand-held dynamometry. *Critical Reviews in Physical and Rehabilitation Medicine, 14*(1), 41–52.

Driver, D.F. (2006). Occupational and physical therapy for work-related upper extremity disorders: How we can influence outcomes. *Clinical and Occupational and Environmental Medicine, 5*(2), 471–482

Flinn, N.A., Trombly Latham, C.A., & Robinson Podolski, C.R. (2008). Assessing abilities and capacities: Range of motion, strength, and endurance. In M.V. Radomski & C.A. Trombly Latham (Eds.), *Occupational therapy for physical dysfunction* (6th ed., pp. 92–185). Philadelphia: Lippincott Williams & Wilkins.

Follows, A. (1987). Electromyographical analysis of the extrinsic muscles of the long finger during pinch activities. *Occupational Therapy Journal of Research, 7,* 163–180.

Hall, S.J. (2003) *Basic biomechanics* (4th ed.). New York: McGraw Hill.

King, P.M., & Finet, M. (2004). Determining the accuracy of the psychophysical approch to grip force measurement. *Journal of Hand Therapy, 17,* 412–416.

Kircher, M.A. (1984). Motivation as a factor of perceived exertion in purposeful versus nonpurposeful activity. *American Journal of Occupational Therapy, 38,* 165–170.

Lieber, S., Rudy, T., & Boston, J.R. (2000). Effects of body mechanics training on performance of repetitive lifting. *American Journal of Occupational Therapy, 54,* 166–175.

Lippert, L.S. *Clinical kinesiology and anatomy* (4th ed.). Philadelphia: F.A. Davis.

Ma, H., & Trombly, C. (2004). Effects of task complexity on reaction time movement kinematics in elderly people. *American Journal of Occupational Therapy, 58*(2), 697–687.

Mathiowetz, V.G. (1991). *Informational support and functional motor performance.* Unpublished doctoral dissertation, University of Minnesota, Minneapolis.

McGrain, P., & Hague, M.A. (1987). An electromyographic study of the middle deltoid and middle trapezius muscles during warping. *Occupational Therapy Journal of Research, 7,* 225–233.

National Board for Certification in Occupational Therapy, Inc. (2004). A practice analysis study of entry-level occupational therapist registered and certified occupational therapy assistant practice. *Occupational Therapy Journal of Research: Occupation, Participation and Health, 24,* S1–S31.

Nelson, D.L., & Peterson, C.Q. (1989). Enhancing therapeutic exercise through purposeful activity: A theoretical analysis. *Topics in Geriatric Rehabilitation, 4,* 12.

Ogden-Niemeyer, L., & Land Jacobs, K. (1989). *Work hardening: State of the art.* Thorofare, NJ: Slack.

Pendleton, H.M., & Schultz-Krohn, W. (Eds.). (2006). *Pedretti's occupational therapy practice skills for physical dysfunction* (6th ed.). St. Louis: C.V. Mosby.

Radomski, M.V., & Trombly Latham, C.A. (Eds.). (2008). *Occupation therapy for physical dysfunction* (6th ed.). Philadelphia: Lippincott Williams & Wilkins.

Riccio, C.M., Nelson, D.L., & Bush, M.A. (1990). Adding purpose to the repetitive exercise of elderly women. *American Journal of Occupational Therapy, 44,* 714–719.

Schinn, J., Romaine, K., Casimano, T., & Jacobs, K. (2002). The effectiveness of ergonomic intervention in the classroom. *Work, 18,* 67–73.

Schkade, J.K., Feilbelman, A., & Cook, J.D. (1987). Occupational potential in a population with Duchenne muscular dystrophy. *Occupational Therapy Journal of Research, 7,* 289–300.

Spaulding, S.J., Strachota, E., McPherson, J.J., Kuphal, M., & Ramponi, M. (1989). Wrist muscle tone and self-care skill in persons with hemiparesis. *American Journal of Occupational Therapy, 43,* 11–24.

Trombly, C.A. (1995). Occupation: Purposefulness and meaningfulness as therapeutic mechanisms. *American Journal of Occupational Therapy, 49,* 960–972.

Trombly, C.A., & Cole, J.M. (1979). Electromyographic study of four hand muscles during selected activities. *American Journal of Occupational Therapy, 33,* 440–449.

Trombly, C.A., & Quintana, L.E. (1983). Activity analysis: Electromyographic and electrogoniometric verification. *Occupational Therapy Journal of Research, 3,* 104–120.

Trombly, C.A., & Radomski, M.V. (Eds.). (2002). *Occupation therapy for physical dysfunction* (5th ed.). Philadelphia: Lippincott Williams & Wilkins.

Van Deusen, J., & Marlowe, D. (1987a). A comparison of the ROM dance, home exercise/rest program with traditional routines. *Occupational Therapy Journal of Research, 7,* 349–361.

Van Deusen, J., & Marlowe, D. (1987b). The efficacy of the ROM dance program for adults with rheumatoid arthritis. *American Journal of Occupational Therapy, 41,* 90–95.

Wahi Michener, S.K., Olson, A.L., Humphrey, B.A., Reid, J.E., Stepp, D.R., Sutton, A.M., & Moyers, P.A. (2001). Relationship among grip strength, functional outcomes, and work performance following hand trauma. *Work, 16,* 209–217.

Wu, C-Y., Trombly, C.A., & Lin, K-C. (1994). The relationship between occupational form and occupational performance: A kinematic perspective. *American Journal of Occupational Therapy, 48,* 679–687.

CHAPTER 8

The Cognitive Model

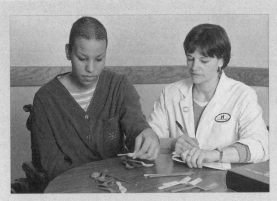

A client recovering from brain damage is seated with an occupational therapist. She is engaged in a task of sorting knives, forks, and spoons. After this she will engage in a task of making a phone call to a store and getting certain information. By observing things such as how the client approaches these tasks, what mistakes she makes, and what aspects of the task are more challenging and why, the therapist will derive a picture of the client's cognitive processes and problems. This understanding of the client's cognitive strengths and limitations in task performance will be used to design an intervention that may include alterations in the tasks being done, teaching the client strategies to overcome or compensate for her limitations, and/or altering the environment to enhance cognitive performance.

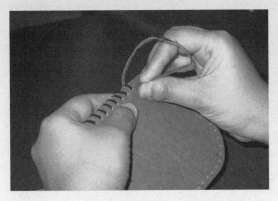

Another client with a psychiatric disability works with a small piece of leather with pre-punched holes. Following instructions given by the therapist, the client attempts to complete a leather lacing stitch. Based on the client's performance in this task, the therapist will draw preliminary conclusions about the extent of the client's cognitive impairment. Based on this and other assessments the therapist will identify the client's level of cognitive functioning and make recommendations for the type of environment in which the client could best function after discharge.

These are two examples among several approaches that have been developed by occupational therapists to address problems related to cognition. Each draws on interdisciplinary concepts to explain cognition and cognitive problems. The common emphasis of all these approaches is the way that cognition and cognitive problems affect task performance and participation. While each approach has unique concepts, terminology, and resources, there is significant overlap among their concerns, concepts, assessments, and intervention strategies.

This chapter emphasizes the key concepts and strategies that are common or generic while also acknowledging some of the unique approaches. Thus, the chapter discusses a cognitive model that is inherent across these approaches, characterizing how cognition and cognitive problems are understood and how the latter are assessed and addressed in occupational therapy. Table 8.1 provides an overview of the major occupational therapy cognitive approaches that are synthesized in this chapter.

Theory

Cognitive concepts and related interventions used in occupational therapy are based on the work of neuroscience, neuropsychology, and psychology (in particular, learning theory that stresses information processing) (Abreu, 1981; Katz 2005; Levy, 2005a). This section characterizes the range of concepts that are used to understand cognition and cognitive problems. Together they constitute six important themes about cognition:

• The Definition of Cognition
• The Composition of Cognition
• The Cognition-Motor System Connection
• Influence on the Social Context on Cognition
• Information-Processing Function of Cognition
• The Dynamic Nature of Cognition

Taken together these definitions identify cognition as a process of identifying, selecting, interpreting, storing, and using information to make sense of and interact with the physical and social world, to conduct one's everyday activities, and to plan and enact the course of one's occupational life.

The Definition of Cognition

Several definitions of cognition are found in the literature. A very broad definition stresses that cognition is the process of experiencing and engaging in the complexities of everyday life (Lazzarini, 2005). A more specific definition indicates that cognition refers to the processes by which sensory input is transformed, reduced, elaborated, stored, recorded, and used (Levy & Burns, 2005). Yet another definition posits that cognition is the capacity to take in, organize, assimilate, and integrate new information with previous experience and to adapt to environmental demands by using previously acquired information to plan and structure behavior for goal attainment (Toglia, 2005). Taken together these definitions identify **cognition** as a process of identifying, selecting, interpreting, storing, and using information to make sense of and interact with the physical and social world, to conduct one's everyday activities, and to plan and enact the course of one's occupational life.

The Composition of Cognition

Cognition is not a singular or linear process. Rather, it is "a complex amalgam of different component systems" (Levy & Burns, 2005, p. 322). While it is broadly recognized that cognition is the composite of many interacting components or processes, no single accepted formulation or taxonomy of those components or processes exists.

(text continues on page 92)

Table 8.1 **Characteristics of Occupational Therapy Cognitive Approaches**

Approach/author(s)[intended population]	Interdisciplinary Concepts	View of Cognition	View of Impairment/Problems	Assessment Strategy	Intervention Approach
Cognitive Disabilities (Allen, Levy, & Burns) [severe psychiatric illness, dementia]	Originally based on Piaget's concepts of cognition. Reformulated emerging theory and concepts from cognitive neuroscience	Based on a conceptualization of information processing, offers a hierarchical description of different levels of functional performance capabilities and limitations	Neurological injury or disease impairs cognition, imposing restrictions on performance and learning potential	Identify/monitor level of cognitive function based on an ordinal classification scheme that identifies six levels of cognitive functioning	Centers on current capabilities, providing the just-right challenge, and adapting the task and environment to the individual
Dynamic Interactional Approach (Toglia)	Dynamical systems theory	Cognition is a product of the dynamic interaction among the person, activity, and environment	Examines abilities and problems in terms of underlying strategies, ability to monitor performance, and potential for learning	Use cues and task alterations to identify a person's potential for change. Alter task and environmental variables to enhance ability to process, monitor, and use information	Remedial: change the person's strategies and self-awareness. Compensatory: modify external factors such as activity demands and environment or simultaneously focus on person, task, and environment systematically
Higher-Level Cognition (Katz & Hartman-Maeir)	Interdisciplinary literature of higher-level cognitive functions	Focus on higher-level cognition: awareness and executive functions	Unawareness of limitations. Difficulties with executive functions (planning, problem-solving, monitoring, and adjusting performance)	*Awareness.* Compare client's estimation of ability, prediction of performance with actual abilities/performance; examine on-line awareness to choose appropriate tasks and detect/correct errors.	*Awareness.* Remedial (for mild-to-moderate unawareness): educate client or allow client to experience impairment in task performance, provide support to face emotionally difficult information.

				Evaluation	Intervention
				Executive functions. Use a battery that combines tabletop, functional, and observational measures	Compensatory: environmental adaptations and behavior approaches. *Executive functions.* Remedial: provide persons with opportunities to choose, select, plan, and self-correct. Compensatory: provide external support or strategies
Quadraphonic Approach (*Abreu*)	Information processing, teaching-learning, neurodevelopment and biomechanics, and narrative concepts	Stresses the mind-body connection (i.e., the relationship of cognition and the motor system) and the life history context in which cognition occurs	Disruption of cognitive and motor systems with impact on client's life story	Micro evaluation: cognitive and motor control strategies, assessment of cognitive processes (e.g., attention, memory, problem-solving, motor planning). Macro evaluation: the client's subjective sense of satisfaction and adaptation. Identifies client's level of functional performance (seven levels)	Focus on the client-learner, therapist-teacher, and training-compensatory environment. Emphasis of intervention is based on client's functional performance level and integrates cognition, movement, and client's personal narrative. Approach depends on client's functional level

(table continues on page 88)

Table 8.1 Characteristics of Occupational Therapy Cognitive Approaches continued

Approach/ author(s)/[intended population]	Inter-disciplinary Concepts	View of Cognition	View of Impairment/ Problems	Assessment Strategy	Intervention Approach
Cognitive Rehabilitation (*Averbach & Katz*) [stroke and TBI]	Incorporates ideas of neuro-plasticity	Through learning and experience one can: (1) improve ability to evaluate and be aware of abilities and avoid entering situations beyond one's capacities, (2) create alternative cognitive strategies		Assess cognitive abilities/disabilities, level of awareness and executive functioning abilities, occupational information, and preferred learning patterns	Broaden capacity to process information, transfer, and generalize to functional areas
Neurofunctional Approach (*Giles*) [clients with several cognitive deficits]	Behavioral and cognitive theories of learning, movement science, and OT, dynamical systems perspective		In clients with severe cognitive impairment, learning potential is very constrained by inability to generalize and use higher-order compensatory skills. Learning must be specific, clearly guided, and practiced until highly habituated to result in functional gains	Determine current level of functioning under conditions similar to expected living situation. Standardized testing can be used to identify specific reasons why performance may break down	Training in highly specific compensatory strategies. Assist performance of a specific functional behavior through specific task training
Cognitive Orientation to daily Occupational Performance (*Polatajko & Mandich*)		Thinking patterns drive behavior and new thinking patterns can result in behavior change. New skills emerge from the interaction	Does not describe cognitive impairments, as cognition is used as a strategy for addressing performance difficulties due	Daily activity log. Activity card sort (things done and not done). COPM. Performance Quality Rating scale: observation scale for	CO-OP is a client-centered, performance-based, problem-solving approach that enables skill acquisition. It uses: (1) a strategic

[children with developmental coordination disorder]	of the child, the task, and the environment	to motor coordination problems	repeatedly measuring performance and change (research tool). Dynamic performance analysis (observation-based process of identify performance problems or performance breakdown)	sequence of identifying a goal, planning, doing, and checking, and (2) a process of guided discovery in which the child is supported to find out how to do the task at hand
Dynamic Cognitive Intervention (Hadas-Lidor & Weiss) [all populations]	Luria's and Feuresten's notion that cognition is influenced by social mediation	Cognition is shaped and mediated by learning experiences (i.e., how stimuli emitted by the environment are transformed by a mediating agent [e.g., parent] who selects, frames, filters, and schedules stimuli)	Low performance is linked to learned cognitive structures that can be more important than cognitive impairment due to etiological factors	Focuses on modifiability of cognition and attempts to understand cognitive functions responsible for deficiencies in cognition (which may be motivational, emotional, as well as cognitive)	Change cognitive structures that determine low performance through mediated learning experience. Seeks to transform client into an autonomous independent thinker capable of initiating and elaborating actions

The most widely accepted perspective is that cognition includes:

• Higher-level processes (also referred to as metacognition or metacognitive processes)
• Specific or basic cognitive functions (Katz & Hartman-Maeir, 2005; Unsworth, 1999)

Higher-Level Cognitive Processes

The higher-level (metacognitive) processes include **awareness** and **executive functions** (Katz & Hartman-Maeir, 2005). Awareness is the ability to perceive oneself in relatively objective terms. It includes both awareness of one's capacities that exist prior to performance and on-line awareness, which includes self-monitoring and self-regulation within tasks (Toglia, 2005). Executive functions are linked to intentionality, purposefulness, and complex decision-making; they include identifying, initiating, and pursuing goals, planning strategies and sequencing steps of action, solving problems, monitoring progress, and adjusting one's behavior to circumstances (Katz & Hartman-Maeir, 2005; Levy & Burns, 2005).

Specific or Basic Cognitive Functions

There is no universally accepted taxonomy of basic cognitive capacities. Traditionally, cognitive capacities were identified as discrete aspects of the cognitive process such as:

• Attention
• Concentration
• Memory
• Perception of spatial relations
• Visual attention and visual scanning of the field of vision
• Thinking (categorization, sequencing) (Katz & Hartman-Maeir, 2005; Quintana, 1995; Zoltan, Seiv, & Freishtat, 1986)

Levy and Burns (2005) offer a different way of denoting specific cognitive abilities that underscores them as functional abilities:

• Maintain attention and focus
• Learn and retain information
• Perform calculations and solve problems
• Accurately recognize objects
• Determine where objects are
• Understand and use language

Assessments of specific cognitive abilities are abundant and are often used to understand what impairments exist in basic capacities. However, there is a growing tendency to place less emphasis on these more specific areas of cognitive ability and focus instead on underlying cognitive processing strategies and environmental conditions that influence performance (Toglia, 1992, 2005; Toglia & Finkelstein, 1991).

The Cognition-Motor System Connection

Cognition arises out of interaction of the brain and body with the environment (Lazzarini, 2005). Thus, cognition is part of a mind-body system in which cognitive functions cannot be understood fully without reference to the motor system (Abreu & Peloquin, 2005). Information coming into the cognitive process is gathered by the body through the senses as well as being generated through bodily actions. Thus, the quality of cognition is affected by various physical impairments that limit sensation or movement. Additionally, the translation of cognition into action requires that intentions, plans, and goals be enacted through the body.

Box 8.1   Perception as a Component of Cognition

Many processes previously referred to as perceptual are increasingly referred to as lower-level cognitive operations. It has long been recognized that perception and cognition are best considered as two ends of a continuum of abilities (Abreu & Toglia, 1987). On one end are processes that involve immediate apprehension and appreciation of sensory data; these were often referred to as perceptual processes. Recognizing the smell of coffee, the taste of ice cream, and the sight of a flower are examples. On the other end of the continuum are more abstract and reflective processes that involve the formulation of intentions and action plans. Making coffee, deciding between chocolate and strawberry ice cream, and arranging flowers in a bouquet all involve more abstract processes. Since no clear line can be drawn between perceptual and cognitive processes, it is more common now to recognize them as all part of a complex cognitive process.

Influence of the Social Context on Cognition

Cognition involves a long developmental process that begins as children first encounter and learn about their environment. Importantly, what one takes in from the environment and how one makes sense of this information are shaped by parents, caretakers, teachers, and others (Hadas-Lidor & Weis, 2005). The influence of others on how cognition develops is referred to as **social mediation.** The way one learns to process information is a product of social mediation. For example, language provides ways of labeling and categorizing objects in the environment. What objects people recognize, what they understand about them, what they know how to do with them, and what significance they assign to them are all influenced by social mediation. The entire process of education is a formalized process of social mediation that is designed to influence both how and what students think.

Information-Processing Function of Cognition

A central aspect of cognition is information processing. Levy (2005a) proposes that cognition involves processing of information through three distinct stages:

• Sensory-perceptual memory
• Short-term working memory
• Long-term memory

As shown in Figure 8.1, information is first processed through sensory-perceptual memory before reaching short-term working memory. It is then processed in short-term working memory before reaching long-term memory. Information stored in long-term memory can be retrieved and used within either sensory-perceptual memory or short-term working memory.

Sensory-perceptual memory is the recall of sensory information (e.g., sight, sound, touch) just long enough for it to be analyzed and filtered. Sensory-perceptual memory monitors the vast amount of incoming information at any moment. Based on experience, only the most relevant information is perceived and organized into meaningful perceptual patterns. That information is selected for storage in working memory. The rest rapidly decays from memory.

Short-term working memory is what one is thinking about at the moment; thus, it is also referred to as conscious attention. It consists of chunks of information that the mind can consciously attend to and process at any one time. It involves a thorough process of holding information in mind and working on or processing that information to locate its underlying meaning and prepare it for storage. During working memory processing, executive control serves an oversight function, selecting and regulating the flow of information. Additionally, language and visual-spatial functions aid in the processing of auditory and visual information. Irrelevant patterns of thought and action are also inhibited. The most relevant information is passed on for retention in long-term memory.

Long-term memory is information that is available for recall over an indefinite period. It includes implicit and explicit memory. Implicit memory includes:

• Procedural information (i.e., the memory of how to do things)
• Perceptual priming (a non-conscious form of memory in which exposure to a stimulus predisposes one to perceive the same or a related stimulus)
• Priming (a process in which exposure to a stimulus makes certain memories related to that stimulus more available)
• Conditioning, which refers to motor and emotional memories formed automatically through classical conditioning (pairing one stimulus with another) or operant conditioning (pairing a certain behavior with a consequence)

Explicit memory includes:

• Episodic memory (remembering personally relevant facts and events)
• Semantic memory (knowledge and beliefs about facts and concepts stored in the form of language, visual spatial images (e.g., perception of objects in space), or visual perceptual images (e.g., face recognition)

This conceptualization of cognition illustrates how it is made up of a collection of interacting systems that influences how one attends to,

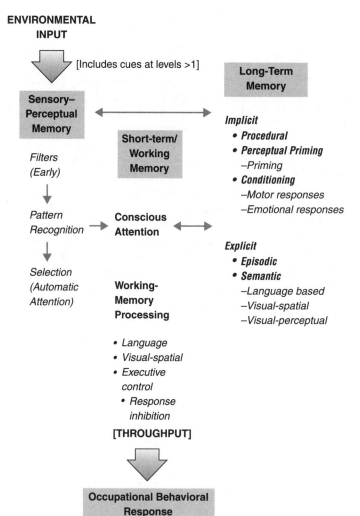

ENVIRONMENTAL INPUT

[Includes cues at levels >1]

Sensory–Perceptual Memory

Short-term/ Working Memory

Long-Term Memory

Filters (Early)

Pattern Recognition → **Conscious Attention**

Selection (Automatic Attention)   **Working-Memory Processing**

Implicit
- *Procedural*
- *Perceptual Priming*
  –*Priming*
- *Conditioning*
  –*Motor responses*
  –*Emotional responses*

Explicit
- *Episodic*
- *Semantic*
  –*Language based*
  –*Visual-spatial*
  –*Visual-perceptual*

- *Language*
- *Visual-spatial*
- *Executive control*
  - *Response inhibition*

[THROUGHPUT]

Occupational Behavioral Response [OUTPUT]

FIGURE 8.1 Information Processing Model of Cognition. *From: Katz, N. (Ed). Cognition and occupation across the life span: Models for intervention in occupational therapy. Bethesda, MD: AOTA Press.*

registers, makes sense of, stores, and recalls a variety of information.

The Dynamic Nature of Cognition

Cognition is dynamic and results from multiple factors both inside and outside of the person interacting together (Hadas-Lidor & Weiss, 2005; Toglia, 2005). According to Toglia (2005), cognition involves the simultaneous and dynamic interaction of the following factors:

- Structural capacity (a person's limits in processing and interpreting information)

- Personal context (an individual's unique characteristics such as personality, coping style, beliefs, values, expectations, lifestyle, motivation, and emotions)
- Self-awareness (recognition of personal strengths and weaknesses; ability to judge task demands; anticipate problems; and monitor, regulate, and evaluate performance)
- Processing strategies (small units of behavior that contribute to the effectiveness and efficiency of performance such as the use of attention, visual processing, memory, organization, and problem-solving)

- Characteristics of the activity being done such as complexity, familiarity, and meaningfulness
- Social, physical, and cultural aspects of the environment

Thus, a person's cognitive performance is a reflection of the dynamic interaction of all these factors (as shown in Fig. 8.2) and a change in any one of these factors can produce changes in cognition.

Problems and Challenges

Most cognitive approaches are concerned with difficulties related to structuring and organizing and using information for task performance. Cognitive impairments are reflected in decreases in the efficiency of processing strategies to select, discriminate, organize, and structure incoming information (Toglia & Finkelstein, 1991). For instance, a person with cognitive problems "may not automatically attend to the relevant feature of a task, group similar items together, formulate a plan, or break the task down into steps" (Abreu & Toglia, 1987, p. 441).

Cognitive problems may include difficulties with:

- Selecting and using efficient processing strategies to organize and structure incoming information

- Anticipating, monitoring, and verifying accuracy of performance
- Accessing previous knowledge when needed
- Flexibly applying knowledge and skills to different situations (Toglia, 2005)

These problems might be in a specific area such as visual processing or they may be more generalized (Toglia, 2005). Often, information-processing abilities, learning abilities, and higher-order cognitive functions (metacognition) are impaired together as part of an overall cognitive disability (Neistadt, 1994; Toglia, 1998).

Cognitive problems are also recognized as dependent on task and environmental context (Neistadt, 1994; Toglia, 1998). For example, persons with cognitive problems may not have difficulty processing information in simple tasks but may show problems in more complex tasks. Similarly, a person may function well in a familiar environment but show difficulty when the environment is novel.

Cognitive impairments routinely lead to problems in occupational performance. Hence, difficulties throughout a person's work, play, and self-care can result from impairment of cognitive capacities. For example, memory loss or poor problem-solving may impair function throughout a whole range of occupational tasks.

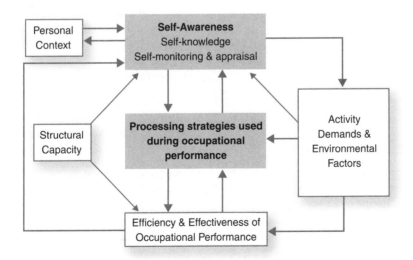

FIGURE 8.2 The dynamic interactional model of cognition. *From: Katz, N. (Ed). Cognition and occupation across the life span: Models for intervention in occupational therapy. Bethesda, MD: AOTA Press.*

Rationale for Therapeutic Intervention

The explanation for cognitive interventions falls into two major categories:

• Remedial (sometimes referred to as restorative)
• Compensatory (sometimes referred to as adaptive)

The kind of learning of which a person is capable determines which of these two broad types of interventions will work best (Katz, 2005; Zoltan, 2007). The ability to learn is affected by the status of higher-level cognitive processes (awareness and executive control) (Toglia, 1998). For example, problems with awareness of limitations, assessing task difficulty, selecting appropriate cognitive strategies, and monitoring performance can limit learning (Toglia, 1991). The extent to which a person can transfer learning from one situation to another also influences the choice of intervention (Neistadt, 1994). Persons with limited ability to transfer learning are generally candidates for only compensatory intervention.

Remedial (restorative) interventions aim to retrain or restore specific cognitive skills (Katz & Hartman-Maeir, 2005; Neistadt, 1990). Such interventions are used with persons with a greater capacity for learning; these people have intact higher-level cognitive processes and the ability to transfer learning from one situation to another.

Compensatory (adaptive) interventions help persons to capitalize on their existing potentials. They are applied to clients who have less capacity for learning. There are three types of compensatory interventions:

• Process-oriented and dynamic strategy learning
• Specific skill training
• Task and environmental modification

Process-oriented and dynamic strategy learning interventions seek to make individuals aware of their cognitive limitations and help them learn to compensate for their problems using their remaining abilities. This intervention approach is used when persons have some remaining capacity for learning and some higher-level cognitive processes. When learning and higher-level cognitive processes are more severely affected, the specific skill-training intervention and the task and environmental modification are used.

Specific skill training involves teaching a very specific compensatory strategy or a specific functional task. This intervention requires learning to perform simple procedures under controlled conditions with sufficient repetition so that behavior becomes highly habituated and automatic (Giles, 2005).

Task and environmental modification does not seek to change functional capacity but instead seeks to identify conditions under which a person can safely and successfully perform (Allen, 1992; Levy, 2005b). It consists of identifying the extent of a client's current cognitive limitation and adapting tasks the client does and the client's environment accordingly.

Practice Resources

The area of cognition is characterized by a wealth of assessments and intervention strategies. While each approach is unique, many share common assessments and interventions. The following sections illustrate the range of assessment and intervention strategies.

Assessment Strategies and Methods

The main strategies of cognitive assessment are:

• Assessment of the occupational/functional consequences of impaired cognition
• Assessment of cognitive components
• Dynamical assessment
• Determination of level of cognitive impairment/function

Each of these strategies follows a particular logic to assessment as is discussed later. Within the strategies, therapists use a variety of assessment methods. Specific assessment methods include:

• Observation during task performance to note processing strategies, functional impairment, and overall cognitive level
• Interview (to gather information on the client's awareness of cognitive impairments, lifestyle, and narrative)
• Standardized tests (verbal, paper and pencil, and tabletop) that range from screening for cognitive problems and determining cognitive

Box 8.2 Improving Cognitive Functioning

Laila, 23 years old, came to Cathleen Jensen for occupational therapy after she was assaulted on a city street and suffered blunt head trauma. General testing of Laila's process skills and mental functions revealed moderate impairments in memory with attention deficits. Cathleen incorporated strategies involving list-writing and visual reminders into Laila's therapy to improve her cognitive skills. One activity involved preparation of a three-part meal while using a to-do list with tasks that Laila could cross off as they were completed during progression of the activity.

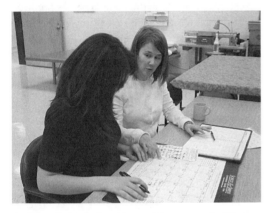

Cathleen helps Laila with cognitive strategies like making lists and using a planner.

On Laila's final day of treatment, she was given the address and an appointment card for her follow-up visit to a neurosurgery clinic. Laila was able to find her way to the clinic successfully within her provided time limit by using strategies of preplanning by reviewing the map, verbal rehearsal, and visual cues including the address card and a small map.

Box 8.3 Cognitive Assessment

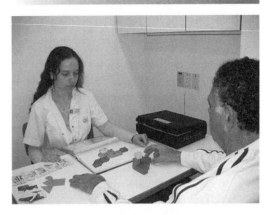

Standardized cognitive assessment is an important component of the cognitive model. Detailed assessment provides a clear picture of the client's cognitive impairment and helps the occupational therapist tailor an individual and efficient treatment plan.

level (extent of impairment) to assessing specific cognitive abilities and examining multiple cognitive factors

Occupational/Functional Assessment

Occupational/functional assessments look at how cognitive impairments affect function, satisfaction, lifestyle, and personal narrative (Abreu & Peloquin, 2005; Katz, 2005; Zoltan, 2007). The point of these assessments is to place the impairment in the occupational context. They determine: (1) the extent to which cognitive limitations restrict independence and affect safety, and (2) the impact of the impairment on the larger occupational life of the person. Strictly speaking, these assessments do not describe or measure cognition but rather its consequences. Consequently, some of the assessments used for occupational functional assessment may not be unique to the cognitive model. Typical assessments are time logs, interviews and observations of task performance, gathering information from caretakers and/or relatives, and cognitive tests that simulate daily tasks or are done while performing daily activities.

For example, the A-One is an assessment that links functional performance in occupations to neurobehavioral deficits (Arnadottir, 1990). It identifies both the level of independence in five activities of daily living (ADLs) and the presence and severity of specific neurobehavioral impairments through analysis of how the impairments affect ADL tasks.

Component Assessment

Component assessments are used to identify the extent and nature of underlying cognitive deficits to understand why performance is breaking down. These assessments can focus on higher-level cognitive functions (executive functions and awareness) as well as lower and specific cognitive functions.

Awareness Assessment

Problems of awareness must be inferred by comparing a client's verbal report or rating of impairment with a more objective measure, by comparing a client's predicted performance with actual task performance, and/or by examining a person's ability to choose tasks within abilities and to detect and correct errors.

Executive Function Assessment

Assessment of executive functions can include a wide range of strategies. Katz and Hartman-Maeir (2005) recommend that evaluators use a battery that combines tabletop, functional, and observational measures. Assessments that involve functional tasks are the preferred and most ecologically valid means of assessing executive functions.

Assessment of Basic/Specific Cognitive Functions

Lower level cognitive functions are generally assessed through standardized tests. An array of such tests are available and they address a variety of specific cognitive functions such as visual and spatial perception, orientation, praxis, memory, attention, and unilateral neglect (Averbuch & Katz, 2005). An example is the Loewenstein Occupational Therapy Cognitive Assessment (LOTCA) (Cermak et al., 1995; Itzkovich, Elazar, Averbuch, & Katz, 1990). It consists of four major areas (orientation, perception, visuo-motor organization, and thinking operations) represented by a total of 20 subtests.

Dynamical Assessment

Dynamical assessment reflects the principle that personal, task, and environmental variables all contribute to cognition (Toglia, 2005; Zoltan, 2007). This approach aims to uncover abilities and problems in terms of the client's awareness and the cognitive strategies the client employs during task performance. Dynamical assessment also emphasizes carefully considering conditions of the activity or task and environment and relevance to the person's real life. Dynamical assessment uses a strategy of determining changes in

performance that occur when the therapist offers cues, mediation, feedback, or task alterations. The therapist does these things and observes their impact on the client's cognition to provide information about cognitive modifiability or learning potential. Thus, dynamical assessment provides a window into what intervention might accomplish; it is a process of problem-discovery (identifying where and how performance breaks down) and problem-solving (identifying and testing strategies for solving problems that occur in performance (Polatajko & Mandich, 2005).

Toglia (2005) indicates that dynamic assessment should unfold as follows. First, the therapist should determine the client's self-perception of performance and abilities prior to task performance. During task performance, the therapist observes and seeks to facilitate changes in performance by using cues, strategy teaching, and changes in the task. After the task, the therapist asks for the client's perception of his/her performance. By asking about performance before and after the task, the therapist gets a picture of the client's self-awareness. This picture is guided by a decision tree that offers a series of questions about the client's performance and the influence of the environment on performance.

Assessment of the Level of Cognitive Impairment/Functioning

Examination of the person's level of cognitive impairment or functioning is a strategy associated with the quadraphonic and cognitive disabilities approaches (Abreu & Peloquin, 2005; Allen, Earhart, & Blue, 1992; Levy & Burns, 2005). In the quadraphonic approach, seven functional levels identify the client's degree of dependence or independence (Abreu & Peloquin, 2005). The functional level is determined from a variety of sources of information and is used as a basis for identifying goals and intervention strategies.

The cognitive disabilities approach proposes a continuum of cognitive impairment and functioning divided into six levels (seven if the coma is included) (Allen, Kehrberg, & Burns, 1992):

- Coma (prolonged state of unconsciousness with a lack of specific response to stimuli)
- Automatic Actions (invariable responses to a stimulus initiated by someone else)

- Postural Actions (self-initiated gross body movements)
- Manual Actions (use of the hands and occasionally other parts of the body to manipulate material objects)
- Goal-Directed Actions (completion of a series of steps to match a concrete sample or a known standard of how the finished product should appear)
- Exploratory Actions (discoveries of how changes in neuromuscular control can produce different effects on material objects)
- Planned Actions (represents normal functional status)

Assessments used to determine at which level the client is functioning include the Allen Cognitive Level test, the Routine Task Inventory, and the Cognitive Performance Test. The Allen Cognitive Level (ACL) test uses performance in a single activity to provide a quick estimate of the client's cognitive level. Leather lacing is the activity; the cognitive level is determined by the complexity of leather lacing stitch that the client can imitate.

The Routine Task Inventory (RTI-E) is administered by interviewing the client or by observing the client's performance. The RTI-E (Katz, 2006) consists of 32 routine activities such as grooming, dressing, bathing, shopping, and doing laundry as well as more general behavior items such as following instructions, cooperating, and supervising. Each task is described according to each of the six cognitive levels of performance. Matching the client's reported or observed performance to the descriptions under each task enables the therapist to determine the client's level of cognitive functioning.

The Cognitive Performance Test (CPT) (Burns, 2006) is composed of seven activities of daily living tasks: dress, shop, toast, telephone, wash, travel, and medication. Each task employs standardized equipment and administration. For example, the dress task consists of asking a client to choose the appropriate attire for a cold, rainy day. The client chooses between a man and woman's heavyweight raincoat, a man and woman's robe, a man's straw hat, a man's rain hat, a woman's plastic rain scarf, a woman's sheer scarf, and an umbrella. The client's choices and behavior in putting on appropriate clothing are used to determine the cognitive level at which the client is functioning.

Choosing Assessment Strategies and Methods

There are no universally accepted strategies of assessment. Each of the approaches shown in Table 8.1 has its own recommended strategies and methods of assessment. The client's characteristics will also determine which assessments are possible and useful. Recently, Hartman-Maeir, Katz, and Baum (2009) have suggested the following sequence for accomplishing a comprehensive cognitive functional evaluation process:

- Interview and background information including an occupational history
- Cognitive screening and baseline status tests in order to acquire a basic knowledge of the cognitive abilities and deficits of the client
- General cognition and executive functions in task performance to determine the impact of cognitive problems on the person's occupations
- If warranted, cognitive tests to identify the nature and extent of problems in specific cognitive domains (e.g., spatial neglect, attention, memory, and executive functions)
- Observation/measure of the impact of specific cognitive deficits on daily functions
- Determination of resources and barriers in the client's environment

In sum, therapists addressing cognitive problems have a wide range of strategies and tools available for assessment. The case at the end of this chapter illustrates how a therapist might use results from several cognitive assessments to get a thorough understanding of a client's cognitive problems.

Intervention

As discussed earlier, remedial (restorative) cognitive interventions seek to improve cognition through task involvement and training while compensatory approaches seek to help persons capitalize on their existing potential by using remaining abilities, learning specific skills, or through task and environmental modification.

This section overviews a number of specific interventions. Some address a specific problem or aim; others are designed for particular populations. While some approaches are clearly remedial or compensatory, some blend both types of intervention.

Treatment of Awareness and Executive Functions

When treating problems of awareness, remedial approaches (suitable for those with mild to moderate unawareness and capacity to learn) include:

• Providing information to the client about his/her impairment
• Helping the client experience the impairment in activities that highlight problems but do not overwhelm the client
• Using the therapeutic relationship to help the client to acknowledge and face emotionally difficult information about his/her impairment (Averbuch & Katz, 2005).

For those with a severe awareness problem, a compensatory approach is used; it stresses environmental adaptations and using behavioral techniques to extinguish maladaptive behaviors stemming from unawareness.

Remedial treatment of executive functions involves providing persons with opportunities to choose, select, plan, and self-correct; it may include unfamiliar unstructured problems with graded task demands. The compensatory approach involves providing external support or strategies to allow adequate performance (Averbuch & Katz, 2005).

Dynamical Strategy Treatment

Dynamical strategy treatment is process-oriented and dynamic (Toglia, 2005; Zoltan, 2007). It is based on the principle that performance can be modified by changing any or all of the following:

• The activity demands
• The environment
• The person's use of strategies and self-awareness

This approach emphasizes the interaction of personal, task, and environmental conditions (Toglia,

1998, 2005). It considers how and under what conditions a client shows a problem, the strategies a client uses to process information, and how such strategies succeed and fail under different tasks and environmental conditions. The therapist identifies task and environmental dimensions that create difficulty for the client as well as client information-processing difficulties that create problems across different kinds of tasks. Treatment is then individualized. Activity analysis to identify opportunities for task modification is also important to this approach. Finally, the approach involves practice in multiple contexts to enhance transfer of learning. The dynamical approach is used with clients at a variety of levels of cognitive functioning but is best suited for those with adequate awareness and learning potential.

Cognitive Retraining

Cognitive retraining is an approach designed for persons with stroke and traumatic brain injury (Averbuch & Katz, 2005). This mostly remedial approach aims to broaden a client's capacity to process information and to be able to transfer and generalize to functional areas. This approach aims to improve the client's ability to evaluate and be aware of abilities, avoid entering situations beyond capacities, and use alternative, more effective cognitive strategies. This approach uses the following methods:

• Enhancing clients' remaining abilities by using supports to maximize success and minimize frustration
• Individual or group training in suitable cognitive strategies
• Using specific structured teaching-learning strategies
• Training in procedural strategies (i.e., how to do specific routine tasks in a structured environment)

Neurofunctional Training

For clients with severe cognitive impairments, neurofunctional training (Giles, 2005) uses two main compensatory strategies:

• Training clients in highly specific (task and/or context) compensatory strategies in which there is little expectation of generalization

- Specific task training to assist clients to perform a given functional behavior

This intervention focuses on achieving automatic performance of behavior. It focuses the client's attention on a specific behavior or area of skills deficit. The desired behavior is learned in repeated short practice sessions in a controlled environment until it becomes habituated. The approach uses activity analysis and behavior techniques of cueing, chaining, and reinforcement. It also emphasizes avoiding errors since the clients targeted by this approach do not learn from mistakes and perpetuate their errors.

Dynamic Cognitive Intervention

The dynamic cognitive intervention approach is potentially relevant to all populations (Hadas-Lidor & Weiss, 2005). It emphasizes how environmental stimuli can be transformed by a mediating agent who selects and organizes information from the environment. Thus, the mediator (therapist) aims to:

- Increase intentionality and raise awareness of the ways one acts
- Help the client go beyond immediate needs or concerns to make generalizations
- Raise the awareness and understanding, making explicit the reasons and motivations for doing things
- Support a sense of competence and ability in task performance

This approach aims to change the basic cognitive structures of low performance and transform clients into autonomous independent thinkers capable of initiating and elaborating actions. The approach combines remedial and compensatory interventions that directly and simultaneously enhance participation while seeking to improve and expand learning ability and self-perception.

Cognitive Orientation to daily Occupational Performance (CO-OP)

CO-OP is a cognitive intervention for improving motor performance in children with developmental coordination disorder (Polatajko & Mandich, 2005). Thus, the approach is unique in that it does not directly target improvements in cognition but rather uses cognition as a means to achieve better performance.

The approach uses a global strategic sequence of identifying a goal, planning, doing, and checking. It emphasizes talking to enhance cognitive mediation of performance. It also uses a process of guided discovery that seeks to scaffold learning; the child is supported to find out how to do the task at hand. The therapist asks guiding questions and coaches the child toward finding strategies to improve performance. Intervention unfolds in the following sequence:

- Preparation, which is focused on ensuring parental commitment to the process, identifying client-chosen goals, and verifying baseline performance
- Acquisition, in which dynamic performance analysis is used to identify performance problems or performance breakdown. The child is supported to identify and use cognitive strategies to enhance performance
- Verification, which involves checking that goals have been met and measuring change

Research and Evidence Base

Research related to this model includes a large body of interdisciplinary research on cognition as well as research by occupational therapists related to specific approaches discussed in this chapter. One active area of research in occupational therapy is the development and testing of assessment tools (Baum & Edwards, 1993; Boys, Fisher, Holzberg, & Reid, 1988; Cermak, 1985; Katz, Hartman-Maeir, Ring, & Soroker, 2000; Van Deusen, Fox, & Harlowe, 1984; Van Deusen & Harlowe, 1987). Other studies have evaluated the incidence of cognitive-perceptual deficits in persons with various kinds of neurological impairment. One such project was a study of the patterns of impairment in motor planning, language, and memory in persons with Alzheimer's disease (Baum, Edwards, Leavitt, Grant, & Deuel, 1988).

Other studies have sought to demonstrate the impact of cognitive deficits on occupational performance. They have shown that cognitive deficits are related to problems of self-care performance (Abreu & Hinajosa, 1992; Kaplan & Hier, 1982;

Titus, Gall, Yerxa, Roberson, & Mack, 1991). Studies supporting the usefulness of cognitive interventions are available in interdisciplinary literature (Katz, 2005). There is less research on the outcomes of specific approaches that make up this model.

Discussion

Although the cognitive model has been developing for some time, it is still a multifaceted and loosely connected collection of concepts and approaches rather than a single well-integrated model. Nonetheless, this model is important to the field, given the pervasiveness of cognitive impairments in occupational therapy clients. Moreover, the variety of concepts and approaches that fall within the cognitive model provide a multidimensional understanding and approach to cognitive impairments.

Nevertheless, using the cognitive model in practice will require one to become familiar with the various approaches discussed in this chapter in order to identify those most relevant to one's client population. Additionally, learning the specific concepts and becoming proficient in the use of practice resources associated with these approaches will be necessary. While these tasks are made challenging by the lack of cohesion among the various approaches, they are helped by the fact that most of them are gathered under one cover in Katz's (2005) text, *Cognition and Occupation Across the Life Span: Models for Intervention in Occupational Therapy* (2nd edition).

Box 8.4

Cognitive Model Case Example: SHALOM

Shalom is a 43-year-old male with severe traumatic brain injury (TBI). He sustained a right acute subarachnoid hemorrhage from a fall at work and subsequently underwent a craniotomy. Shalom lives with his wife and three children in an apartment. Before the injury, he worked as a driver for a high-ranking public officer. His wife managed the household functioning and he assisted in cleaning, dishwashing, and laundry. Both he and his wife describe their family life as satisfying before the injury.

Shalom began rehabilitation three weeks after the injury. At this point he had mild weakness of his left side and mild imbalance during ambulation. He also suffered from hemianopsia (i.e., blindness in one-half of the perceptual field). Shalom's language skills were intact and he communicated effectively with individuals in his environment, including other clients, family members, and therapists. Shalom had severe cognitive impairments. He was independent in eating and grooming but required supervision or assistance in dressing, bathing, toileting, and walking using a walker. He was unable to engage in his previous major occupational roles.

Maya Tuchner, his occupational therapist, used the dynamic interactional approach (Toglia, 2005) along with Goal Management Training (GMT) (Levine et al., 2000), a specific executive strategy developed for treating individuals with executive function impairments, and related knowledge from neuropsychology to address his cognitive problems.

The main problem areas identified by cognitive testing and functional observations were in planning and performing complex tasks. Shalom approached tasks in an impulsive manner, was easily distracted from his goal, lost concentration quickly, and had difficulty monitoring and adapting his performance accordingly.

Maya decided to administer the following comprehensive cognitive battery of tests to get an in-depth picture of his cognitive problems.

- **The COGNISTAT**—Neurobehavioral Status Examination (Kiernan, Mueller, & Langston, 1995), which is a screening test to determine the cognitive status of the client. The test assesses orientation, attention, language, constructional ability, memory, calculations, and reasoning. According to the COGNISTAT, Shalom had mild-to-moderate impairments in attention, memory, and abstract thinking.

Box 8.4 (continued)

- **The Clock Drawing Test** (Rouleau, Salmon, Butters, Kennedy, & McGuire, 1992) is a brief test that measures constructional abilities and cognitive processes and includes quantitative and qualitative analysis of a clock drawing (11:10). The test showed that Shalom had difficulty in planning ability.
- **The Rivermead Behavioral Memory Test (RBMT)** (Wilson, Cockburn, & Baddeley, 1985) is a battery designed to assess memory abilities in everyday tasks. The RBMT revealed that Shalom had mild impairment in memory, mainly in prospective memory (i.e., the ability to remember things in the future. An example is remembering to ask a question at the end of the test).
- **The Self-Awareness of Deficit Interview (SADI)** (Fleming, Strong, & Ashton, 1996) is a structured interview that provides comprehensive information of a person's awareness of his or her deficits and their consequences, as well as the ability to set realistic goals for the future. The SADI showed that Shalom had partial to good awareness of his cognitive deficits and current functional limitations but questionable ability to set realistic goals for the future. For example, he thought he would be able to resume driving in the near future.
- **The Behavioral Assessment of the Dysexecutive Syndrome (BADS)** (Wilson, Alderman, Burgess, Emsile, & Evans, 1996) is an instrument consisting of six subtests that measure executive functions: shifting, planning, strategy use, and temporal judgment. According to the BADS, Shalom showed mild impairments in shifting (between two rules in the test) and moderate to severe impairments in planning and strategy use.
- **The Kettle Test** (Harel, Mizrachi, & Hartman-Maeir, 2007; Hartman-Maeir, Armon, & Katz, 2005, 2007) is a brief cognitive performance-based assessment that includes making two cups of hot drinks. On The Kettle Test Shalom exhibited impulsive behavior with difficulties in planning.

This evaluation battery showed that Shalom demonstrated significant cognitive deficits in attention and executive functioning that impeded his participation in most occupational areas. He was aware of most of his deficits and their implications and was highly motivated to engage in rehabilitation.

The course of the treatment began with supporting Shalom to identify short-term goals. He identified that he wanted to be independent in self-care activities (dressing and bathing), preparing a hot drink, preparing a meal, and money management; he also wanted to learn how to play a new game that he could do for leisure and to spend time with his children.

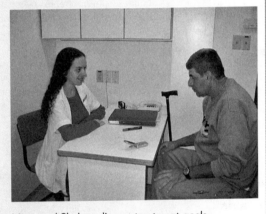

Maya and Shalom discuss treatment goals.

Maya also knew that it was important for Shalom to practice executive strategies across these activities. She introduced a structured intervention for addressing executive problems, the designated global executive strategy (which uses a *stop-define-list-check* strategy to help remediate executive problems). She introduced the intervention in two stages. Because of Shalom's impulsivity she begin with the inhibitory component (stop and define the goal), which was introduced visually via a stop sign that was presented in all therapeutic activities (including basic ADLs at the beginning). Eventually, Maya was able to use only a verbal cue to stop and define the goal and with time Shalom had internalized the strategy and used it regularly. The second stage of the training involved acquiring the "*List*" and "*Check*" strategy that required Shalom to write down in advance the steps and materials for each activity and check off each step during and after performance. This global strategy was practiced across all activities in the rehabilitation setting with Maya's support. Shalom felt the strategy was useful and clearly demonstrated benefits within each session and across sessions; he became empowered by this and was motivated to use the strategy at home as well.

(box continues on page 102)

Box 8.4 (continued)

In addition, Shalom's wife, who occasionally took off from work and joined the sessions or was debriefed by phone, was included in the process as much as possible. She was encouraged to allow her husband to begin participating in these activities at home, with her support. At first she said it was easier for her to do them by herself, but in time she realized the importance of letting Shalom participate in daily activities and previous roles.

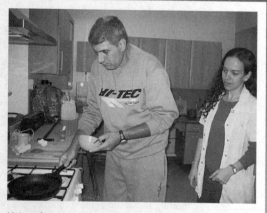

After four months, Shalom was reassessed with the battery of the cognitive assessments that was used for initial evaluation. On these tests, he showed improvements in attention, memory, and planning. He also acted less impulsively. However, he was still having difficulties in planning and monitoring when undertaking complex or new tasks.

Using the strategies he has learned in therapy, Shalom cooks a meal with Maya's supervision.

At this point, Shalom began to raise the issue of return to work. Shalom was in a role of family provider and it was very important for him to be able to return to work in the future. However, because of expected permanent impairments, alternatives to professional driving would be necessary. Before working as a driver, Shalom worked in a governmental archive (mainly sorting and filing papers). He felt that this was a reasonable goal for him. Consequently, as preparation for vocational rehabilitation, his occupational therapy started to include sorting and filing tasks within which he continued to implement his newly learned executive strategies.

At the time this case was written, Shalom had received occupational therapy for almost six months. He gained independence in basic activities of daily living. He had partially returned to his previous roles (i.e., helping his wife in the household activities and playing with his children). He had not returned to work and was still receiving treatment in outpatient rehabilitation. His main goal was to return to work and he was still practicing executive strategies in various activities relating to possible work in the future.

Table 8.2 **Terms of the Model**

Awareness	The ability to perceive oneself in relatively objective terms.
Cognition	A process of identifying, selecting, interpreting, storing, and using information to make sense of and interact with the physical and social world, to conduct one's everyday activities, and to plan and enact the course of one's occupational life.
Executive functions	Higher-level cognitive processes linked to intentionality, purposefulness, and complex decision-making; includes identifying, initiating and pursuing goals, planning strategies and sequencing steps of action, solving problems, monitoring progress, and adjusting one's behavior to circumstances.
Long-term memory	The lasting implicit and explicit recall of information.
Sensory-perceptual memory	Recall of sensory information (e.g., sight, sound, touch, and proprioception) just long enough for it to be analyzed and filtered.

Table 8.2   **Terms of the Model** continued

Short-term working memory	The conscious recall of information (what one is thinking about at the moment) that locates its underlying meaning and prepares it for storage.
Social mediation	The influence of others on how cognition develops.

SUMMARY: THE COGNITIVE MODEL

Theory

+ Defines cognition as a process of identifying, selecting, interpreting, storing, and using information to make sense of and interact with the physical and social world, to conduct one's everyday activities, and to plan and enact occupational life

+ Cognition includes:
  • Higher-level processes (metacognition) of awareness (ability to perceive oneself in relatively objective terms) and executive functions (e.g., identifying, initiating and pursuing goals, planning strategies and sequencing steps of action, solving problems, monitoring progress, and adjusting behavior to circumstances
  • Specific or basic cognitive functions (e.g. attention, concentration, memory)

+ Cognition is part of a mind-body system in which cognitive functions cannot be understood fully without reference to the motor system

+ Cognition involves a long developmental process influenced by social mediation

+ A central aspect of cognition is information processing through three distinct stages:
  • Sensory-perceptual memory (the recall of sensory information [e.g., sight, sound, touch] just long enough for it to be analyzed and filtered)
  • Short-term working memory (what one is thinking about at the moment)
  • Long-term memory (information that is available for recall over an indefinite period)

+ Cognition is dynamic and results from multiple factors both inside and outside of the person interacting together

Problems and Challenges

+ Most cognitive approaches are concerned with difficulties relating to structuring, organizing, and using information for task performance (in a specific area such as visual processing or more generalized)

+ Cognitive problems may include difficulties with:
  • Selecting and using efficient processing strategies to organize and structure incoming information
  • Anticipating, monitoring, and verifying accuracy of performance
  • Accessing previous knowledge when needed
  • Flexibly applying knowledge and skills to different situations (Toglia, 2005)

+ Cognitive problems:
  • Are dependent on task and environmental context
  • Routinely lead to problems in occupational performance

Rationale for Therapeutic Intervention

+ The explanation for cognitive interventions falls into two major categories:
  • Remedial (sometimes referred to as restorative)
    ▪ Aims to retrain or restore specific cognitive skills
    ▪ Used with persons with greater capacity for learning, with more intact higher-level

cognitive processes and the ability to transfer learning
- Compensatory (sometimes referred to as adaptive)
  - Helps persons to capitalize on their existing potentials
  - Applies to clients who have less capacity for learning
  - Three types of compensatory interventions
    - Process-oriented and dynamic strategy learning (learning to compensate for their problems using their remaining abilities)
    - Specific skill training (teaching a very specific compensatory strategy or a specific functional task)
    - Task and environmental modification (identifying the extent of cognitive limitation and adapting tasks and environment accordingly)

Practice Resources

Assessment

+ The main strategies of cognitive assessment are:
  - Assessment of the occupational/functional consequences of impaired cognition
  - Assessment of cognitive components to identify the extent and nature of underlying cognitive deficits to understand why performance is breaking down
  - Dynamical assessment that reflects the principle that person, task, and environmental variables all contribute together to cognition
  - Determination of level of cognitive impairment/function

+ Specific assessment methods include:
  - Observation during task performance (to note processing strategies, functional impairment, and overall cognitive level)
  - Interview (to gather information on the client's awareness of cognitive impairments, lifestyle, and narrative)
  - Standardized tests (verbal, paper and pencil, and tabletop) that range from screening for cognitive problems, determining cognitive level (extent of impairment), and assessing specific cognitive abilities, to examining multiple cognitive factors

Intervention

+ Remedial treatment of awareness problems includes:
  - Providing information to the client on impairment
  - Helping the client experience the impairment in activities that highlight problems but do not overwhelm the client
  - Using the therapeutic relationship to help the client to acknowledge and face emotionally difficult information about impairment

+ Remedial treatment of executive functions involves providing persons with opportunities to choose, select, plan, and self-correct

+ Compensatory approach to awareness stresses environmental adaptations and using behavioral techniques to extinguish maladaptive behaviors stemming from unawareness

+ Compensatory approach involves providing external support or strategies to allow adequate performance

+ Dynamical strategy treatment is based on the principle that performance can be modified by changing:
  - Activity demands
  - Environment
  - Person's use of strategies and self-awareness
  - Task and environmental dimensions that create difficulty for the client as well as information-processing difficulties that create problems across different kinds of tasks

+ Cognitive Retraining
  - Mostly remedial approach designed for persons with stroke and traumatic brain injury
  - Aims to improve:
    - Capacity to process information
    - Ability to transfer and generalize to functional areas
    - Awareness of abilities
  - Uses the following methods:
    - Enhancing remaining abilities through supports to maximize success and minimize frustration
    - Individual or group training
    - Using specific, structured teaching-learning strategies
    - Training in procedural strategies

◆ Neurofunctional Training
  • For clients with severe cognitive impairments
  • Uses two main compensatory strategies:
    ▪ Training in highly specific (task and/or context) compensatory strategies
    ▪ Specific task training to assist clients to perform a given functional behavior

◆ Dynamic Cognitive Intervention
  • Combines remedial and compensatory interventions that directly and simultaneously enhance participation while seeking to improve and expand learning ability and self-perception
  • The mediator (therapist) aims to:
    ▪ Increase intentionality and raise awareness of the ways one acts

    ▪ Help go beyond immediate needs or concerns to make generalizations
    ▪ Raise the awareness and understanding, making explicit the reasons and motivations for doing things
    ▪ Support a sense of competence and ability in task performance

◆ Cognitive Orientation to daily Occupational Performance (CO-OP)
  • A cognitive intervention for improving motor performance in children with developmental coordination disorder
  • Uses a global strategic sequence of identifying a goal, planning, doing, and checking
  • Emphasizes talking and uses a process of guided discovery that seeks to scaffold learning

REFERENCES

Abreu, B.C. (1981). *Physical disabilities manual.* New York: Raven Press.

Abreu, B.C., & Hinajosa, J. (1992). The process approach for cognitive-perceptual and postural control dysfunction for adults with brain injuries. In N. Katz (Ed.), *Cognitive rehabilitation: Models for intervention in occupational therapy* (pp. 167–194). Boston: Andover Medical.

Abreu, B.C., & Peloquin, S.M. (2005). The quadraphonic approach: A holistic rehabilitation model for brain injury. In N. Katz (Ed.), *Cognition and occupation across the life span: Models for intervention in occupational therapy* (2nd ed., pp. 73–112). Bethesda, MD: American Occupational Therapy Association Press.

Abreu, B.C., & Toglia, J.P. (1987). Cognitive rehabilitation: A model for occupational therapy. *American Journal of Occupational Therapy, 41,* 439–448.

Allen, C. (1992). Cognitive disabilities. In N. Katz (Ed.), *Cognitive rehabilitation: Models for intervention in occupational therapy* (pp. 1–21). Boston: Andover Medical.

Allen, C., Earhart, C., & Blue, T. (1992). *Occupational therapy treatment goals for the physically and cognitively disabled.* Rockville, MD: American Occupational Therapy Association.

Allen, C., Kehrberg, K., & Burns, T. (1992). Evaluation instruments. In C.K. Allen, C.A. Earhart, & T. Blue, *Occupational therapy treatment goals for the physically and cognitively disabled.*

Rockville, MD: American Occupational Therapy Association.

Arnadottir, G. (1990). *The brain and behavior: Assessing cortical dysfunction through activities of daily living.* St. Louis: C.V. Mosby.

Averbuch, S., & Katz, N. (2005). Cognitive rehabilitation: A retraining model for clients with neurological disabilities. In N. Katz (Ed.), *Cognition and occupation across the life span: Models for intervention in occupational therapy* (2nd ed., pp. 113–138). Bethesda, MD: American Occupational Therapy Association Press.

Baum, C., & Edwards, D.F. (1993). Cognitive performance in senile dementia of the Alzheimer's type: The Kitchen Task Assessment. *American Journal of Occupational Therapy, 47,* 431–436.

Baum, C.M., Edwards D., Leavitt, K., Grant, E., & Deuel, R. (1988). Performance components in senile dementia of the Alzheimer type: Motor planning, language, and memory. *Occupational Therapy Journal of Research, 8,* 356–368.

Boys, M., Fisher, P., Holzberg, C., & Reid, D.W. (1988). The OSOT perceptual evaluation: A research perspective. *American Journal of Occupational Therapy, 42,* 92–98.

Burns, T. (2006). *Cognitive performance test (CPT).* Pequannock NJ: Maddak.

Cermak, S.A. (1985). Developmental dyspraxia. In E.A. Roy (Ed.), *Advances in psychology: Neuropsychological studies of apraxia and related disorders* (vol. 23, pp. 225–248). North Holland, NY: Elsevier Science.

Cermak, S., Katz, N., McGuire, E., Peralta, C., Maser-Flanagan, V., & Greenbaum, S. (1995). Performance of Americans and Israelis with cerebrovascular accident on the Loewenstein Occupational Therapy Cognitive Assessment (LOTCA). *American Journal of Occupational Therapy, 49,* 500–506.

Fleming, J.M., Strong, J., & Ashton, R. (1996). Self-awareness of deficits in adults with traumatic brain injury: How best to measure? *Brain Injury, 10,* 1–15.

Giles, G.M. (2005). A neurofunctional approach to rehabilitation following severe brain injury. In N. Katz (Ed.), *Cognition and occupation across the life span: Models for intervention in occupational therapy* (2nd ed., pp. 139–165). Bethesda, MD: American Occupational Therapy Association Press.

Hadas-Lidor, N., & Weiss, P. (2005). Dynamic cognitive intervention: Application in occupational therapy. In N. Katz (Ed.), *Cognition and occupation across the life span: Models for intervention in occupational therapy* (2nd ed., pp. 391–412). Bethesda, MD: American Occupational Therapy Association Press.

Harel, H., Mizrachi, E., & Hartman-Maeir, A. (2007). *Validity and reliability of The Kettle Test – A test for identifying cognitive problems in daily functions in post-stroke geriatric patients.* Paper presented at Israeli Society for Physical and Rehabilitation Medicine, Tel-Aviv, Israel, November.

Hartman-Maeir, A., Armon, N., & Katz, N. (2005). *The kettle test: A cognitive functional screening test.* Paper presented at Israeli Society of Occupational Therapy Conference, Haifa, Israel.

Hartman-Maeir, A., Armon, N., & Katz, N. (2007). *The kettle test: A brief cognitive-functional measure.* Test protocol is available from the first author, School of Occupational Therapy, Hebrew University Jerusalem, Israel.

Hartman-Maeir, A., Katz, N., & Baum, B. (2009). Cognitive functional evaluation (CFE) process for individuals with suspected cognitive disabilities. *Occupational Therapy in Health Care, 23*(1), 1–23.

Itzkovich, M., Elazar, B., Averbuch, S., & Katz, N. (1990). *LOTCA: Loewenstein occupational therapy cognitive assessment manual.* Pequannock, NJ: Maddak.

Kaplan, J., & Hier, D.E. (1982). Visuo-spatial deficits after right hemisphere stroke. *American Journal of Occupational Therapy, 36,* 314–321.

Katz, N. (Ed.). (2005). *Cognition and occupation across the life span: Models for intervention in occupational therapy* (2nd ed.). Bethesda, MD: American Occupational Therapy Association Press.

Katz, N. (2006). *Routine task inventory—RTI manual.* Unpublished.

Katz, N., & Hartman-Maeir, A. (2005). Higher-level cognitive functions: Awareness and executive functions enabling engagement in occupation. In N. Katz (Ed.), *Cognition and occupation across the life span: Models for intervention in occupational therapy* (2nd ed., pp. 3–25). Bethesda, MD: American Occupational Therapy Association Press.

Katz, N., Hartman-Maeir, A., Ring, H., & Soroker, N. (2000). Relationship of cognitive performance and daily function of clients following right hemisphere stroke: Predictive and ecological validity of the LOTCA battery. *Occupational Therapy Journal of Research, 20,* 3–17.

Kiernan, R.J., Mueller, J., & Langston, J. (1995). *Cognistat: The neurobehavioral cognitive status examination manual.* Fairfax, CA: The Northern California Neurobehavioral Group.

Lazzarini, I. (2005). A nonlinear approach to cognition: A web of ability and disability. In N. Katz (Ed.), *Cognition and occupation across the life span: Models for intervention in occupational therapy* (2nd ed., pp. 211–233). Bethesda, MD: American Occupational Therapy Association Press.

Levine, B., Robertson, I.H., Clare, L., Carter, G., Hong, J., Wilson, B.A., et al. (2000). Rehabilitation of executive functioning: An experimental-clinical validation of goal management training. *Journal of the International Neuropsychological Society, 6*(3), 299–312.

Levy, L.L. (2005a). Cognitive aging in perspective: Information processing, cognition, and memory. In N. Katz (Ed.), *Cognition and occupation across the life span: Models for intervention in occupational therapy* (2nd ed., pp. 305–325). Bethesda, MD: American Occupational Therapy Association Press.

Levy, L.L. (2005b). Cognitive aging in perspective: Implications for occupational therapy practitioners. In N. Katz (Ed.), *Cognition and occupation across the life span: Models for intervention in occupational therapy* (2nd ed., pp. 327–346). Bethesda, MD: American Occupational Therapy Association Press.

Levy, L.L., & Burns, T. (2005). Cognitive disabilities reconsidered: Implications for occupational therapy practitioners. In N. Katz (Ed.), *Cognition and occupation across the life span: Models for intervention in occupational therapy* (2nd ed., pp. 347–388). Bethesda, MD: American Occupational Therapy Association Press.

Neistadt, M.E. (1990). A critical analysis of occupational therapy approaches for perceptual deficits in adults with brain injury. *American Journal of Occupational Therapy, 44,* 299–304.

Neistadt, M.E. (1994). The neurobiology of learning: Implications for treatment of adults with brain injury. *American Journal of Occupational Therapy, 48,* 421–430.

Polatajko, H.J., & Mandich, A. (2005). Cognitive Orientation to daily Occupational Performance with children with developmental coordination disorder. In N. Katz (Ed.), *Cognition and occupation across the life span: Models for intervention in occupational therapy* (2nd ed., pp. 237–259). Bethesda, MD: American Occupational Therapy Association Press.

Quintana, L.A. (1995). Evaluation of perception and cognition. In C. Trombly (Ed.), *Occupational therapy for physical dysfunction* (4th ed., pp. 201–223). Baltimore: Williams & Wilkins.

Rouleau, I., Salmon, D.P., Butters, N., Kennedy, C., & McGuire, K. (1992). Quantitative and qualitative analyses of clock drawings in Alzheimer's and Huntington's disease. *Brain and Cognition, 18*(1), 70–87.

Titus, M.N., Gall, N.G., Yerxa, E.J., Roberson, T.A., & Mack, W. (1991). Correlation of perceptual performance and activities of daily living in stroke patients. *American Journal of Occupational Therapy, 45,* 410–417.

Toglia, J.P. (1991). Generalization of treatment: A multicontext approach to cognitive perceptual impairment in adults with brain injury. *American Journal of Occupational Therapy, 45,* 505–516.

Toglia, J.P. (1992). A dynamic interactional approach to cognitive rehabilitation. In N. Katz (Ed.), *Cognitive rehabilitation: Models for intervention in occupational therapy* (pp. 104–143). Boston: Andover Medical.

Toglia, J.P. (1998). A dynamic interactional model to cognitive rehabilitation. In N. Katz (Ed.), *Cognition and occupation in rehabilitation: Cognitive models for intervention in occupational therapy* (pp. 4–50). Bethesda, MD: American Occupational Therapy Association.

Toglia, J.P. (2005). A dynamic interactional approach to cognitive rehabilitation. In N. Katz (Ed.), *Cognition and occupation across the life span: Models for intervention in occupational therapy* (2nd ed., pp. 29–72). Bethesda, MD: American Occupational Therapy Association Press.

Toglia, J.P., & Finkelstein, N. (1991). *Test protocol: The dynamic visual processing assessment.* New York: New York Hospital–Cornell Medical Center.

Unsworth, C. (Ed.). (1999). *Cognitive and perceptual dysfunction: A clinical reasoning approach to evaluating and intervention.* Philadelphia: F.A. Davis.

Van Deusen, J., Fox, J., & Harlowe, D. (1984). Construct validation of occupational therapy measures used in CVA evaluation: A beginning. *American Journal of Occupational Therapy, 38,* 101–106.

Van Deusen, J., & Harlowe, D. (1987). Continued construct validation of the St. Mary's CVA Evaluation: Bilateral awareness scale. *American Journal of Occupational Therapy, 41,* 242–245.

Wilson, B.A., Alderman, N., Burgess, P.W., Emsile, H., & Evans, J.J. (1996). *Behavioral assessment of dysexecutive syndrome.* St. Edmunds, UK: Thames Valley Test.

Wilson, B., Cockburn, J., & Baddeley, A. (1985). *The Rivermead behavioral memory test: Manual.* London: Thames Valley Test.

Zoltan, B. (2007). *Vision, perception, and cognition* (4th ed.). Thorofare, NJ: Slack.

Zoltan, B., Seiv, E., & Freishtat, B. (1986). *Perceptual and cognitive dysfunction in the adult stroke patient.* Thorofare, NJ: Slack.

CHAPTER 9

The Functional Group Model

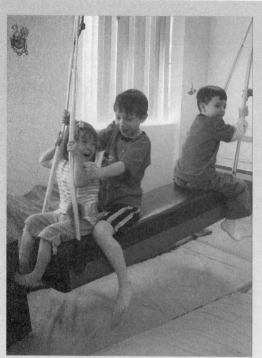

In a center that provides services to clients with sensory processing disorders, children often play together in small groups, with guidance from the therapist as needed. At times the groups are planned and other times they form informally as children ask to join an activity that looks fun to them. They might enter an imaginative play scenario, such as going on a safari, cooperatively plan an obstacle course, play a board game, or participate in a competitive game of bumper tires. Within these groups children work on turn-taking, sharing, working together, and being a good friend. They build valuable skills that will help them become successful outside of the therapy session.

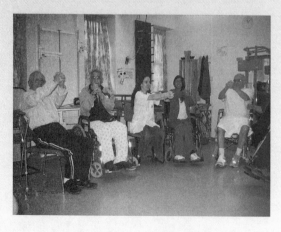

Maya Tuchner runs a hemiplegia group designed for clients following cerebrovascular accident (CVA) who are in daycare or inpatient rehabilitation. The group is led every day by an occupational therapist for about half an hour. The group focuses on motor and cognitive functioning. The group starts with basic orientation in time and place and mention of special events like holidays. Then, there are several exercises that include bilateral and symmetric movements along with balance exercises. Participation in the group requires the ability to imitate movements but does not require comprehension, so that clients with aphasia can also participate. The group also provides basic social stimulation.

As demonstrated in these examples, occupational therapists frequently use groups of clients interacting together as a means of providing therapy. The use of groups has always been part of occupational therapy, as Chapters 3 and 4 illustrated. There are distinct advantages to addressing some client problems or needs and to providing some kinds of services in groups. For instance, groups are a natural context for addressing clients' interpersonal problems and groups can be a source of social support and feedback needed by clients. Moreover, certain kinds of services, such as those that are designed to impart information, improve understanding, or teach skills, can be enhanced by being delivered in groups where clients can share relevant knowledge and experience. Finally, services offered in groups are less expensive than those offered on a one-to-one basis. For these and other reasons, groups are increasingly used in occupational therapy (Duncombe & Howe, 1985; Howe & Schwartzberg, 1986), creating the need for knowledge on how to conduct therapeutic groups.

Groups are often used to achieve goals related to other conceptual practice models discussed in this text. For instance, as seen in Chapter 8, some cognitive interventions are provided in groups. A variety of groups based on the model of human occupation have been developed (Baron, 1987; Braveman, 2001; Gusich & Silverman, 1991; Kaplan, 1986; Knis-Matthews, Richard, Marquez, & Mevawala, 2005). Exercise and range of motion groups also are used to achieve biomechanical goals of increasing range of motion or endurance. In these instances the content of the group is guided by these models. However, the effectiveness of such groups can be either hindered or enhanced depending on how group dynamics and processes are managed to influence the individual members. It is to these aspects of groups that the functional group model is addressed.

The functional group model was first introduced in 1986 (Howe & Schwartzberg) as an approach to guide occupational therapy group intervention. Functional groups, in which members participate in occupation, are distinguished from group psychotherapy and related activity groups, which focus on using discussion and group dynamics to resolve intrapersonal and interpersonal difficulties by achieving insight and working through issues. A functional group seeks to enhance occupation (Schwartzberg, Howe, & Barnes, 2008). Functional groups are considered appropriate for clients who need to:

- Evaluate their own ability to carry out life roles
- Acquire skills and role behaviors
- Develop communication and interaction skills to enhance occupational performance
- Prevent loss or deterioration of skills and behaviors
- Improve health, wellness, or quality of life (Schwartzberg et al., 2008)

Theory

Concepts Related to Groups

Schwartzberg et al. (2008) first discuss features that are common to all groups. These concepts address the definition, characteristics, and features of groups and serve as a context for thinking about the more specific, functional group.

Definition of Groups

Schwartzberg et al. (2008) note that the term group refers to a collection of people interacting together in order to achieve a common aim or purpose. They note, however, that true groups include:

- Interaction among their members
- A common goal
- A relationship between size and function (the size of the group is related to what the group is supposed to accomplish)
- Members' desire or consent to participate in a group
- A democratic capacity for self-determination

When these features are present, a true group exists. Thus, five people waiting in line at the grocery store do not constitute a group. On the other hand, five high-school students working together to decorate the gym for a dance do constitute a group.

Characteristics of Groups

All groups are characterized by structure, cohesion, and stages of development. **Group structure** refers to "the combination of mutually connected and dependent parts of the group that form its existence" (Schwartzberg et al., 2008, p. 7). Group structure includes the organization and procedures of the group. It is influenced by its context, climate, composition of members, purpose, and goals. Group structure is also influenced by how the leader and members interact and the size and norms of the group.

Group cohesion refers to the intensity of feeling for and identification with the group among its members; it is reflected in a sense of group solidarity in how much the members value and care about the group. Cohesion is affected by how members mutually understand, accept, and support each other and by the extent of trust between members.

Stages of group development refer to the phases a group passes through during its existence. These stages are dynamic and unpredictable and may be characterized by fluctuations. While formulations of group stages have been identified, they all share a common trajectory in which the group must first be formed, followed by building of relationships, deciding aims and procedures, accomplishing tasks, and then terminating.

Features of Groups

Two features are common to all groups: content and process. **Content** refers to tasks done during the group and what is said or discussed. For example, if an occupational therapy group cooks a common meal, the activities involved in cooking and the necessary conversation about getting the cooking done is the content. **Process** refers to how things are said and done and how the group goes about accomplishing its goals. For instance, how members of the group decide together what to cook and whether everyone has a say in the decision-making are parts of the process.

Two types of group behavior contribute to the group process:

• Group task functions that enable the group to accomplish its aims related to content (Bales, 1950)

Box 9.1 Levels of Group Development

Mosey (1970) identified five levels of group development in which each level represents an increasingly cohesive, balanced, and self-determining group.

• Parallel groups in which members pursue individual tasks with minimal interaction
• Project groups in which members engage in short-term activities that are related and that require some interaction
• Egocentric cooperative groups in which members cooperate together on a long-term activity and are able to respond to each other emotionally but still need a leader to keep the group together
• Cooperative groups in which members address each other's social and emotional needs along with the activity goals of the group and are largely self-determining
• Mature groups in which members balance achieving the group's goals with meeting social and emotional needs and leadership comes from co-equal members

• Group-building and maintenance functions that help create and sustain relationships and connections between members (Bales, 1950)

Members can take on different roles in groups that contribute to these functions. For example, the initiator-contributor comes up with and suggests new ideas or procedures while the energizer prods the group to action. These roles both contribute to group task functions. Group-building and maintenance functions are supported by such roles as the encourager (who gives praise and agrees with others), the harmonizer (who helps resolve difference between members), and the gatekeeper (who facilitates communication between members). Group members may also take on individual roles such as dominator, playboy (clown), or aggressor (Benne & Sheats, 1978) that may become detrimental to the group process if not addressed.

Concepts Specific to the Functional Group Model

The functional group model is based on concepts of interaction analysis, group membership and leadership functions, group dynamics, the phases of group development, and the impact of group process on individual growth. Based on these concepts, the functional group model reflects the principles that groups:

- Encompass a common goal and dynamic interaction of their members
- Have capacity for self-direction
- Can become increasingly independent of designated leadership
- Can address individual needs
- Provide multiple types of feedback and support
- Can support members' growth and change (Schwartzberg et al., 2008)

The functional group model also recognizes that members bring to groups an innate drive for competence (White, 1959, 1971) and a hierarchy of needs (i.e., physiologic, safety, belonging and love, esteem and self-actualization) (Maslow, 1970). Central to the functional group model is the idea that purposeful activity or doing can provide opportunities for persons to adapt (King, 1978), exhibit goal-oriented behavior (Fidler & Fidler, 1978; Reed, 1984), and experience feelings of personal satisfaction (Barris, Kielhofner, & Hawkins, 1983).

> **Central to the functional group model is the idea that purposeful activity or doing can provide opportunities for persons to adapt, exhibit goal-oriented behavior, and experience feelings of personal satisfaction.**

Drawing on these ideas, the functional group model asserts the following about the interrelatedness of groups, therapy, and occupation:

- Functional groups provide members with a here-and-now reality orientation that encourages growth and change—that is, when people engage in meaningful occupations in groups they can learn to function independently. Groups can also provide opportunities for persons to learn to adapt to the environment as well as a modified environment that supports individuals' performance capabilities
- Functional groups are designed to give the amount and type of feedback and support that address members' needs
- Group activities and discussions can be structured to encourage group-centered

leadership, giving members an opportunity to learn about their own capabilities and about how the environment or context influences them
- Through participation in activities and discussion, functional groups encourage and promote growth and change; they give opportunities for learning, practicing skills, and achieving mastery and competency
- Functional groups can be structured or organized to accommodate many levels of human development and functioning. They enable members to lead the process of doing and, thus, empower the group's capacity for self-direction

The basic concepts of the functional group model are **adaptation** (adjustment of the environment) and **occupation** (i.e., action or behavior of a member in the group). According to this model, adaptation is brought about through the member's action within the group. Thus, the functional group model is action-oriented and promotes adaptation through action (Schwartzberg et al., 2008). According to this model, four types of action that promote adaptation can occur in a functional group:

- Purposeful action
- Self-initiated action
- Spontaneous (here-and-now action)
- Group-centered action (Schwartzberg et al., 2008)

Purposeful action occurs when a member perceives the group activity as being congruent with the member's characteristics (e.g., needs and goals). Factors that influence the experience of purposeful action are:

- Social and cultural relevance to the member
- Match to the member's skill level
- Meanings evoked by the objects used, interaction with other participants, and the general context

When there is congruency between a member's characteristics and characteristics of an activity, there is a greater likelihood that the member of a group will experience pleasure and satisfaction, and that learning or positive change will occur. In a functional group, the leader seeks to facilitate purposeful action through careful selection of meaningful occupations in which group members can engage and through group discussions about action (i.e., planning, processing, and reflecting on group action) (Schwartzberg et al., 2008).

Self-initiated action refers to a member's volitional efforts to be a part of the group and to benefit from participation. Members differ in the extent to which they are capable of self-initiated action. Self-initiated action occurs when members view the goals of the group as congruent with their own goals. Facilitating self-initiated action is an important element of the functional group model (Schwartzberg et al., 2008).

Spontaneous (here-and-now) action refers to behaviors that emerge instinctively from the group process and contribute to members' experiential learning. For example, members might discover through the group process which behaviors evoke desired outcomes and which evoke unwanted outcomes. Spontaneous action also allows a member to exercise and improve perception, judgment, and decision-making. Functional groups should be designed to provide a safe and supportive context for members to function spontaneously (i.e., to explore, practice skills, and/or carry out relevant tasks and roles) (Schwartzberg et al., 2008).

Group-centered action is action that takes into consideration the emotional and social needs of all members and that contributes toward a common task and goal. In a functional group, the group leader aims to create an environment that encourages interdependent action requiring group members to function as members of the group and not just as individual agents. Group-centered action can influence a member's sense of individual and group identity and help the member learn to manage personal behavior to accommodate the needs and goals of other members and of the group as a whole.

These four types of action underlie members' involvement in the functional group. Moreover, it is the role of the leader to facilitate each of these four types of action in the functional group. The functional group model has a number of assumptions (see Box 9.2) that can serve as guides to the leader for how to facilitate action that will lead to positive adaptation.

Rationale for Therapeutic Intervention

Groups generate their own dynamic that influences the behavior of the group as a whole (Schwartzberg et al., 2008). The members of the group are also influenced by this group dynamic. The functional group seeks to enhance occupational behavior and thus adaptation by mobilizing these dynamic group forces that have the potential to positively shape people's understanding of themselves or their abilities. For example, groups provide persons with choices for activity and encourage people to assume responsibility for meeting their needs.

> The functional group seeks to enhance occupational behavior and thus adaptation by mobilizing dynamic group forces that have the potential to positively shape people's understanding of themselves or their abilities.

Groups can also provide a sense of identity and self-worth to their members. Further, they offer social positions (roles) that can meet a variety of individual needs and, at the same time, require persons to respond to environmental expectations. Moreover, groups provide a structure that guides individual participation along with socializing influences that are necessary for learning adaptive occupational behavior. In these and other ways, functional groups offer interactions that, through the nature of the action (purposeful, self-initiated, spontaneous, or group-centered), elicit adaptive responses from members and influence the individual to participate positively and, thereby, change.

Box 9.2   Assumptions of the Functional Group Model

The functional group model reflects a number of underlying assumptions (Schwartzberg et al., 2008) that are summarized below.

People Assumptions
- People:
  - Are bio-psycho-social systems
  - Are social beings that exist in groups
  - Are action or "doing" oriented and motivated toward competency
  - Have needs that can be met through a group
  - Communicate both verbally and nonverbally
  - Grow and change
  - Are unique, complete individuals with congruence between emotion and action

- Groups
  - Model the social behavior patterns in the larger society
  - Mobilize forces that affect people's sense of identity, safety, and self-esteem and may be experienced as valuable or burdensome

Functional Group Assumptions
In general, groups:

- Have a common goal and dynamic interaction of members
- Can provide multiple sources of feedback and support
- Can promote independence from the leader
- Can support growth and change of members
- Can be self-directive
- Can satisfy individual needs and social demands

Specifically, functional groups:

- Provide a here-and-now, reality orientation to encourage growth and change
- Give feedback and support according to members' needs
- Can be structured to encourage group-centered leadership
- Can lead to individual growth and change
- Can accommodate different levels of development and functioning
- Can address individual needs and provide necessary learning

The Occupational Nature of a Functional Group
- Groups can enhance the use of occupations to help people function independently to accommodate to or adapt to the environment

- Doing and social participation involve feedback and support
- By structuring activities, objects, and the environment, members are enabled to learn about their context and their own capabilities
- Activities should provide opportunities to practice and learn skills and to achieve mastery and competence
- Giving possibilities for doing empowers the group's capacity for self-direction
- Group activity demands and contextual features influence participation and can maintain, improve, or enhance individuals' occupational performance

Health
- Health involves mind and body in interaction with the social and physical environment
- Purposeful activity supports the health of mind and body
- Health involves independence and capacity for self-direction
- Health involves interdependence and capacity for relatedness

Occupation
- Meaningful occupations in a group encourage the persons to assume responsibility for their own needs
- Purposeful activities involve individual and group choice or volition
- Purposeful activities used in a group can improve performance, adaptive behavior, and the potential for meeting individual responsibilities
- Active doing in a group encourages social participation and enhances self-care, productive, and leisure skills
- Active doing in a group can promote self-appraisal and sense of self-worth
- Lack of meaningful occupation leads to disorientation and breakdown in useful habits and threatens the health of mind and body
- Engaging in meaningful occupations positively influences one's sense of well-being
- An adaptive response requires:
  - Active participation
  - Meeting environmental and task demands and expression of needs or goals
  - Integrating and organizing a response that leads to self-reinforcement
- By meeting biological, psychological, and social needs, meaningful occupations can influence change in the person's state of health

(box continues on page 114)

Box 9.2   **Assumptions of the Functional Group Model** continued

Social Systems Assumptions

* Functional groups:
  * Include both therapy groups and naturally occurring groups (e.g., families or work groups)
  * Provide structure and goals to guide participation and address the social and emotional needs
  * Provide beneficial socialization that shapes the learning of behavior
  * Build on strengths of members
  * Parallel individual needs and societal demands
  * Are structured so that members have the opportunity to help each other and experience feelings of self-worth

Change Assumptions

* Functional groups:
  * Are structured to motivate purposeful and meaningful action
  * Provide experiential learning in a supportive environment structured to practice daily living skills
  * Aim to move members toward independence/interdependence and adaptation

Functional Assumptions

* Functional groups:
  * Provide a place to function in the reality of the present, learn and practice skills, and address other areas of needed growth
  * Are concerned with elements of performance in work, play, social participation, and self-care
  * Seek to build group cohesiveness necessary to achieve group goals

Action Assumptions

* Functional groups:
  * Emphasize the learning process that occurs through active participation
  * Nurture interpersonal and intrapersonal development
  * Use relations to human and nonhuman environment
  * Require leaders to guide the activity of the group according to individual needs for self-motivation and mastery

Box 9.3   **A Pain Management Group**

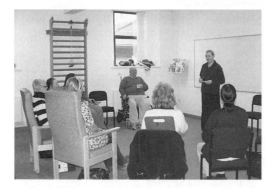

Alice works with a group of clients who share the experience of chronic pain.

The pain management program that Alice Moody runs is a 12-session group. The aim of this group is to reduce the disability and distress associated with chronic pain and increase quality of life. The group follows an educational format and the occupational element involves members carrying over what they learn into everyday life activities. Occupational therapy topics include, for instance, activity pacing, seating and posture, beds, bending and lifting, physical relationships, and ADLs in general. Overall, the content of the group is guided by the biomechanical model and by concepts and resources of cognitive behavioral treatment.

The process of the group follows principles and procedures of the functional group model. For instance, this group has ground rules for members that are designed to encourage group cohesiveness. The group is structured so that members feel supported and inspired to make changes within their lifestyle in a purposeful, meaningful manner. This is achieved through the following elements:

* Facilitated group discussions regarding subject matter are presented. Open and interactive sessions are encouraged along with sharing of ideas and experience
* Informal discussions and sharing of experiences with team members and peers during coffee breaks

Box 9.3   **A Pain Management Group** continued

• Goal setting as a group exercise. Meaningful and personal individual goals are set by group members with support to encourage active experimentation and learning of new strategies/material. It is then up to group members to complete goals outside of the group. Goals are reviewed within the group, and associated learning by actual experience is discussed openly within the group. Feedback, support, and further ideas are often offered to further promote experimentation and adaptive

change. As noted in the functional group model, the group is founded on the principle that member involvement in goal setting reinforces a sense of control and mastery

• Members are encouraged to practice new life skills such as pacing their sitting/standing within the sessions where they are likely to feel safe, with the aim of feeling more able to do so at work and within other social situations

Practice Resources

Assessment

The assessment instruments used in the functional group include observation, needs assessment, and content and process analysis. The authors of this model offer two basic types of assessments. The first category is assessments developed by psychologists and sociologists for observing group dynamics and group content and process. Examples of group dynamics assessments are a sociogram (a visual representation of member interaction) and a form that indicates types of roles (e.g., task, maintenance, or individual) assumed by different members of the group. These types of group assessment are generally completed by the group leader.

Assessments of group content and process include such things as a meeting evaluation form and a group member feedback form (both are brief forms filled out by members to indicate their feelings about and experience of the group). In addition to these types of forms, observation guides provide a semi-structured approach for leaders' ongoing assessment of group structure and function.

In addition to these generic group assessments, Schwartzberg et al. (2008) have developed a number of forms specifically for the functional group. These include:

• Assessment of Members and Context
• Functional Group Protocol (a form for planning a group)
• Session Plan (a form for planning each session of a group)

• Session Evaluation form (for recording observations about a specific session)

Additionally, they provide formats to structure leader reflection and self-assessment including:

• Leader Self-Assessment forms (for therapists to assess their own leadership)
• Assessment of Activity and Leadership (ideally for peers or supervisors to complete from observation of the leader in a session)

In a functional group, group members are taught and encouraged to be observers and evaluators of group process and progress toward goals. Even if members are only able to understand the evaluation process at a very basic level, this accountability and feedback loop helps leaders verify the accuracy of their assessment of individual and group potential. Finally, the group itself can be used as an arena for evaluation of individual occupational behaviors of members.

Intervention

Most of the practice resources for intervention in the functional group model focus on the role of the group leader that is typically assumed by the occupational therapist. **Leadership** refers to the ability to promote those behaviors that lead to the satisfaction of group needs (Howe & Schwartzberg, 1986). A functional group involves four overall stages in which the group is designed, formed, developed, and concluded (Schwartzberg et al., 2008). During each of these stages the group leader conducts assessment (information gathering) and takes appropriate leadership action in order to ensure that the group is functioning well and positively influencing its members.

Designing a Functional Group

During the design phase, the therapist defines tentative group goals, develops general plans for the group as a whole and for specific sessions, selects the members, and initially outlines a proposed group structure, including tasks to be undertaken in the group. The design balances structure and openness so that the group can be as self-structuring as possible (i.e., not overly dependent on the therapist as the leader).

The design phase of a functional group involves:

- Assessing client needs and available supports (resources) for the group
- Determining group goals and methods, which may involve:
  - A pre-group interview designed to elicit the goals of prospective group members
  - Gathering information on the history of an existing group from records or staff
  - Assessment to determine characteristics of the group's members (e.g., roles, performance capacity and limitations, underlying impairments) and the group's context (e.g., agency location, mission, funding)
  - Developing a session plan to establish the goals and framework for each session
- Establishing group membership criteria and composition (who is suited for and will make up the group) and size
- Planning the group and the tasks that will be performed in the group

Forming the Group

When a group first comes together, a number of factors are involved in how well the group functions. Successful formation of the group requires the group leader to address the following issues:

- Members need to feel a sense of acceptance and belonging
- Relationship of the members to the leader
- Balancing individual with group goals
- Establishing trust

Initial sessions of the group focus on getting everyone acquainted, sharing how the group will function, and developing accepted norms of behavior in the group. Schwartzberg et al. (2008) provide guidelines for how purposeful, self-initiated, spontaneous, and group-centered action can be used to address the issues noted earlier. Moreover, they discuss how the leader can address these issues through setting the group climate to be constructive and supportive, by clarifying norms (e.g., what behavior is expected and encouraged or what is considered important), and setting goals.

Supporting Development of the Group

As noted earlier, groups have unique and unpredictable courses of development. The group leader must strive to create an environment that supports purposeful, self-initiated, spontaneous, and group-centered action throughout. The group leader also evaluates the progress of the group (along with that of members), identifies and manages problems that arise (e.g., addressing issues or affect such as anxiety or anger that may underlie silence, conflict, apathy, or inability to make group decisions). To manage these problems, leaders use a variety of strategies such as self-disclosure, confrontation, modeling desired behavior, providing support or praise, and limit-setting. Problem-solving may also require conflict resolution, involving members in reviewing goals, adapting tasks that the group does, and encouraging a balance in group member roles. Leader self-reflection is crucial to ensure leader effectiveness. The Session Evaluation form is a method to chronicle group and members' progress toward goals and identify changes to integrate into future session plans.

Concluding the Group

Two major tasks for concluding a group involve:

- Reviewing and summarizing the members' experience in the group
- Addressing members' concerns and feelings about the termination (e.g., feelings of sadness, loss, or separation)

A number of additional issues can arise that the leader must address. They may include such things as dealing with unfinished business and helping members transition to new situations.

The leader's role is to ensure that members can go on from the group realizing and retaining their learning and positive changes and with a concrete sense of their accomplishments or how to apply their learning outside the group.

Research and Evidence Base

Schwartzberg et al. (2008) note that "most research deals with *how* to do groups, *how* to achieve the best results, and *how* to manipulate the variables in group practice" (p. 38). There is less research on the outcomes of group intervention. There is growing evidence in occupational therapy and related literature to support many of the tenets of the functional group model (Agazarian & Gantt, 2003; Clark, Carlson, Jackson, & Mandel, 2003; Henry, Nelson, & Duncombe, 1984; Schwartzberg, Howe, & McDermott, 1982; Ward, 2003). Additionally, the functional group model has been used as a framework in research regarding the effectiveness of group intervention (Clark et al., 1997; Jackson, Carlson, Mandel, Zemke, & Clark, 1998; Mandel, Jackson, Zemke, Nelson, & Clark, 1999)

Supporting the outcomes of the functional group, two studies found that activity-based groups were more effective than a verbal group in improving clients' independent functioning and perceptions of their social skills, respectively (DeCarlo & Mann, 1985; Klyczek & Mann, 1986). Another study found that group treatment of patients who had received hip replacements was more cost-effective than individually oriented treatment (Trahey, 1991). Another study found that group-based occupational therapy had a positive impact on functional status of persons with Parkinson's disease while being less labor-intensive than services offered individually (Gauthier, Dalziel, & Gauthier, 1987).

Discussion

The functional group model is a conceptual model of practice that focuses specifically on the process of therapy as it occurs in groups. Thus, the contribution of this model is to an understanding of how group dynamics influence and can be consciously and reflectively used by the occupational therapist to enhance the process and outcomes of therapy. This model recognizes that the central dynamic of occupational therapy is the client's participation in occupations but emphasizes that when this action occurs in a group context, important dynamics influence that action and the impact it has on clients.

This aspect of the use of groups must be differentiated from the use of other practice models to determine the content and goals of groups. As noted at the beginning of this chapter, groups are often used to address cognitive, biomechanical, sensorimotor, and motivational problems. In these instances, other conceptual practice models or related knowledge discussed in this text are used to guide decisions about the specific occupations that will take place in order to address those problems. While it is important in these instances to use other conceptual practice models or related knowledge as a guide to the content and specific aims of the group, the functional group model is used to plan, implement, monitor, and evaluate the group process components. For example, a group that teaches joint protection and energy conservation will have specific content and aims that are guided by the biomechanical model. Nonetheless, because this biomechanical intervention takes place in a group context, the quality of the intervention will be affected by the group process. Thus, a therapist would use the functional group model in combination with the biomechanical model to plan and implement the group intervention. In this way, the functional group model offers additional concepts to help any therapist who is delivering services in a group format.

Box 9.4

Functional Group Model Case Example: A Community-Based Group

Mike, an occupational therapist, and Amanda, an occupational therapy student completing field-work, decided to develop a new group in a community-based day program for adults with intellectual impairments, some of whom also have mental health conditions such as schizophrenia. They decided to use the functional group model as a framework for planning and implementing the group.

Mike and Amanda planned for group membership to be voluntary and composed of clients identified as needing to address pre-vocational issues (work readiness) and to improve social participation. They decided that the group would:

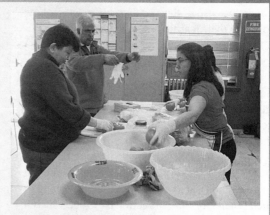

Group members work together to prepare a salad.

• Meet weekly for one hour over a ten-week period
• Be a closed group of six members (two women and four men) aged 22 to 40 years

They decided on a closed group to limit the leader-to-member ratio. Having two leaders with six members would allow for the one-on-one assistance that they anticipated most clients would need at times. They also wanted to have homogeneous membership to promote a sense of commonality among members. They planned that the group activities would be adapted to allow for members' intellectual and motor impairments. This aspect of the group was guided by the biomechanical, cognitive, and motor control models (see Chapters 7, 8, and 12).

All members had difficulties in motor coordination and strength but were able to maintain sufficient balance to perform tabletop activities when seated. Two had difficulty with ambulation and one used a wheelchair. Members also varied in their cognitive abilities. One member could write her full name and read at the elementary school (third to fifth grade) level. Two members were illiterate but able to print their first names. The other three members could read and comprehend material at approximately the middle school (seventh grade) level. One of these clients relied on a laptop with an adapted keyboarding program for communication. Two other members were bilingual and primarily spoke Spanish.

Members' self-care ability ranged from independent to needing verbal cues to partially dependent on assistance. Home health aides, relatives, and/or agency residential staff assisted members who needed help with bathing, dressing, and other personal care needs. Meals were either prepared with supervision or provided for members by agency staff or family members. All members experienced social isolation and exhibited limited role performance and social participation. All were seeking paid work via agency "internships" or supported employment.
To participate in the group, members were asked to agree to a group contract that stated they would:

• Attend every week
• Participate in the group's activities
• Work hard to do their best
• Listen and be kind to others in the group

As part of an orientation to the group's expectations and norms, members were reminded of the center policy that physically or verbally abusive behaviors (hitting, shouting, and swearing) would result in being sent to a calming room with a center staff support person.

Box 9.4 (continued)

General Group Goals

After reviewing the group membership, Mike and Amanda set goals for the group. Accordingly, they decided that members would:

- Interact with others in a socially appropriate manner (i.e., greet each other by name; make eye contact; and demonstrate teamwork by sharing materials, time, and attention)
- Actively participate in the group activities (i.e., sign in attendance, complete tasks, participate in role-play/games, share feedback, and provide positive praise to peers)
- Help set up or clean up group activities
- Talk about what they learned and/or accomplished during the group

While work themes were planned to be inherent in the group tasks, the group process was designed to facilitate interpersonal skill development. Topics for sessions included:

- How to dress for work
- Job interviews
- Job safety
- How to communicate with supervisors
- How to work with others
- How to cope with the stress of job task or social environment

Mike and Amanda planned that themes would be reviewed and repeated weekly to foster and reinforce learning.

Outcome Criteria

Mike and Amanda developed observable outcome criteria for the group. According to these criteria each member would:

- Contribute verbally to the group at least once each session by introducing him or herself, expressing his or her thoughts and feelings in a positive manner to another group member, or commenting to the leader about the group activity
- Engage in group tasks and demonstrate pre-vocational skill development such as signing in for group, attending to a task, asking for help, identifying correct work attire and hygiene, completing agency internship applications with assistance, and role-playing what to do in various work situations
- Show increased personal comfort in the group by staying in the room, making eye contact as appropriate to individuals, smiling, or evidencing signs of decreased anxiety (such as decreased self-stimulation behaviors and decreased perseverative verbalizations)

Group Methods and Procedures

Mike and Amanda also specified that the following group methods and procedures would be used:

- Structured group tasks within the range of member abilities that would promote peer interaction
- Modification of group process and adaptation of tasks as needed
- Crafts, games, sample work tasks, role-play
- Guidance for discussion of action in the present

Leadership Roles and Functions

Mike and Amanda discussed the kind of leadership that they expected would be needed for this group. They decided that the following would be important leadership roles and functions:

- Encouraging and modeling desired group behavior, including: listening, verbally participating, asking for help, being supportive, and giving feedback

(box continues on page 120)

Box 9.4 (continued)

- Providing structured activities as well as limit-setting and redirection to create a safe climate that would encourage member interaction
- Adapting activities to ensure successful participation; attending to and assuming group task and maintenance (socio-emotional) roles (Benne & Sheats, 1978) to support the group process
- Modifying group structure or activities to the changing needs of individual members while simultaneously attending to the needs of the group as a whole; responding to dynamics that emerged during the group sessions
- Establishing a supportive, genuine, and consistent emotional climate via active listening, interactive reasoning, and reinforcement of group and agency rules and norms

The Group Process

Here are three descriptions of group sessions (1, 4, and 10). Each is followed by reflections of the group leaders.

Session One

Amanda welcomed each member as they arrived, asking their names and giving each person a nametag. Once everyone was present, Amanda demonstrated to the members how to put on their nametags. Amanda then placed an enlarged and laminated weekly attendance sheet on the wall. She helped each member put a check mark by his or her name and under the date of the session. Most members were able to follow the verbal instructions but two needed coaching. Additionally, Amanda had to accompany Maria to the board and offered hand over hand assistance. When everyone had signed in, Amanda reviewed the number of sessions remaining (nine) and shared with the group that they would count down each week the number of sessions remaining to help prepare for the day when the group would have its final meeting.

Amanda then introduced Mike who asked her, "How are you today?" Amanda responded, "Fine, thank you. I am excited to be starting our group today." They planned this interaction to model for members the type of personal sharing and social interaction desired in the group. Mike then asked members to introduce themselves. Mike greeted each person by name stating 'Nice to meet you...How are you?" Amanda then read aloud from a prepared poster board on which the group's ground rules and purpose were written:

> In this group we **work hard**, learning about how to **get along** on the job. We **respect** each other's feelings and ideas by listening to each other carefully. We face who is speaking, try not to interrupt, and ask questions to find out more about what the other person is saying. We value **teamwork** and **caring** for others. We show this by greeting each other by name, sharing materials, and giving praise to one another when we have worked hard and done well.

Mike explained that in the first session members were going to make individual collages about their favorite things as a way to get to know one another better and find out everyone's interests. Amanda and Mike showed their own collages depicting their interests as examples. They further explained that each member's individual collage would be used to build a group poster. Mike then pasted his and Amanda's collages to the group poster board to reinforce this goal.

Mike stated that he would like group members to:

- Share supplies and ideas
- Ask for help when needed
- Take turns showing their collages that would be put on the group poster

Mike distributed paper of several colors, asking group members to choose their favorite color. Amanda placed glue sticks, markers, and precut pictures from magazines and store flyers (of things such as animals, plants, clothing, food, movies, sports, and art) in the center of the table. She reminded members they would need to share the supplies, cueing members to pass one another needed items (pictures, glue, and markers). When members spoke about an interest, leaders would ask if others knew about or shared their peer's interest. Responses were used to

Box 9.4 (continued)

facilitate group-centered sharing and discussion (e.g., about surprises, similarities, or differences). Each member showed his or her collage and then added it onto the group poster with assistance as needed.

Reflections on Members' Participation Following Session One

Maria, who typically needs one-on-one attention and assistance, was able to respond to cueing and leader redirection and independently chose pre-cut pictures of animals, sharing with the group that she had a cat. **Jorge**, who is easily frustrated, was able to remain involved in the activity when given minimal assistance from peers to locate desired pictures and frequent reassurance from leaders. **Felicita** was able to ask for assistance from leaders via her augmentative communication device on her laptop. **Elena**, though somewhat echolalic in her vocalizations, willingly shared materials. **Antonia** remained withdrawn and quiet but sorted through materials, collecting items and images and occasionally smiling and nodding when others were speaking about subjects such as animals, sports teams, and food. **Roberto** was friendly and gregarious, but he demonstrated a preoccupation with food, frequently asking for a snack and needing frequent redirection to task as well as prompts to interact with peers instead of leaders.

Maria, Roberto, and Elena expressed their opinions regarding the activity when given options (i.e., what they liked/disliked, found easy/hard, and felt was fun/boring). Maria and Antonia participated in giving one another positive praise either verbally (e.g., "Your picture looks nice") in response to leader modeling. All members willingly participated in a "round of applause" for a job well done, suggested by the leaders when the group composite poster was completed.

Group Leader Self-Reflection

Amanda also discussed with Mike her automatic response of helping Maria to mark the attendance sheet, commenting that she had responded as she would typically to her sibling with Down syndrome. Their observations of Maria's performance suggested that she was capable of the task but would need careful cueing and encouragement to decrease her dependent stance.

Session Four

Mike greeted members as they arrived and cued them to record their attendance on the laminated attendance poster. As in past sessions, Maria asked Amanda to "come with her" to mark the attendance sheet. Amanda gently redirected her, reminding her of last week's group discussion about how she now needed to complete this on her own. She also encouraged Maria by stating that she was sure Maria could do it. Maria asked Antonia to come with her; Antonia looked to the leaders for direction. Mike restated Amanda's limit and suggested that Antonia let Maria know with a nod that she had done a good job when she had finished signing in on the attendance sheet.

The session then began with the opening ritual of reading the group's purpose and goal statement and counting down the seven sessions remaining. Elena repeated each line as read by the leaders. Mike introduced the activity as a game called "Should I wear this to work?" The group was divided into two teams of three members; Maria, Antonia, and Felicita versus Elena, Jorge, and Roberto. For each round, the group was given three enlarged photos of various outfits. Two photos contained attire that was not suitable for work (e.g., formal gowns or torn and stained clothing) and one displaying clothing suitable for many jobs (e.g., neat and clean clothes, functional footwear). The members were asked to:

• Choose which photo they felt was the best choice for work
• Tell the group why it was the best choice
• Point out why the others might not be good choices

(box continues on page 122)

Box 9.4 (continued)

Reflections on Members' Participation Following Session Four

Felicita immediately chose the correct photo for her group and typed out her reason why. Antonia needed encouragement to engage with her team members but was able to identify that one outfit was not suitable for work, stating the clothes were "too dirty." Maria became focused on whether the gown was for someone's wedding and began talking to Amanda about a recent family wedding she had attended. Elena repeated the directions but was unable to focus on the photos. Jorge and Roberto became distracted by the photos and needed frequent reminders from Mike to choose the photo that showed the best clothing choice for what to wear to work. When it came time for each team to share, Maria surprised the leaders by reading out what Felicita had typed. Once Antonia reported her photo as being of an outfit that was "too dirty," Elena chose an outfit with similar characteristics to share, repeating "too dirty." Jorge and Roberto looked to Mike, asking what they should choose. Amanda pointed this out and asked the group to help them out. Maria again surprised the leaders by pointing to the outfit more suitable for work, stating, "You should wear this!" Mike wrapped up the group by laying out the photos of suitable work outfits and declaring that both teams won the game. He thanked Maria for being a good "coach" for Elena, Jorge, and Roberto's team.

Group Leader Self-Reflection

Mike reflected that this activity format was likely too advanced. Amanda suggested they try it again in a parallel format, with members each being given similar smaller photos and asked to sort them into two categories, possibly using a worksheet format onto which they could paste the photos once the group had identified the "dos" and don'ts" of what to wear to work.

Session 10

Amanda greeted members as they arrived and as they independently went to record their attendance on the laminated attendance poster. Maria announced to the group that there were zero sessions remaining. Felicita typed out "I will miss group" and gestured to Maria to read what she had written. Antonia asked Amanda if she could leave the group stating that she felt "bad." Mike encouraged Antonia to take a short break in the hall with him to discuss how she was feeling. Elena began repeated the words, "too bad, too bad" and shaking her head. Amanda asked Roberto to remind the group of its purpose and ground rules, which Roberto recited from memory. She then announced that for the final session of the group they would be having soft drinks and assembling a salad together as it was a special occasion. Members were instructed to don food service gloves. The containers of vegetables were introduced one at a time. Members helped cut up the vegetables and assemble the salad. Members were told they could serve themselves the salad as it was passed around. Roberto repeatedly asked how many salads he could have to eat, needing redirection to attend to the steps of the task. Amanda realized that preparing a second bowl for Mike might be a source of confusion for Roberto, so she told the group she was making a salad for Mike. Maria asked if she could make one for Antonia.

Shortly after this process began, Mike and Antonia rejoined the group. Amanda bridged Mike and Antonia back into the group by informing them that the group had wanted to be sure they each had a bowl of salad. Jorge quietly had offered Felicita assistance by showing her each salad bowl and serving when Felicita nodded. While the group was coming to a close, Maria

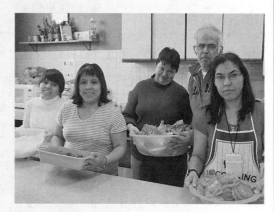

The group shows off its finished salad.

Box 9.4 (continued)

asked if she could read aloud to the group from her new flyer on human rights distributed by the agency. The group agreed. Due to the limited amount of time remaining, Mike suggested that she read aloud her favorite part or page. Maria read about the right to be treated fairly and with respect, stating "this is how we treat each other in group." The group applauded her sponta- neously. Roberto cheered and called out "Maria for president!" Maria told the group she would be starting an internship for eight hours a week for 10 weeks organizing shoes in the shoe department of the retail store next door to the agency.

In bringing the group to a close, Mike told the group that he felt sad it was the last session but glad to have had the chance to work together. He shared memories from each meeting and invited members' reminiscence or feedback. He emphasized examples of teamwork and told the group he felt proud of all they had accomplished. Amanda then officially closed the group by thanking each member for their participation and handing out individualized certificates of achievement.

Leader Reflections Regarding Individual/Group Performance

The cohesion achieved in the final session was evident in the group's ability to manage the anxi- ety of the transition as well as the change from the usual structure to a more open one (making a salad and Maria's reading). With the exception of Antonia's one-on-one time to check in with Mike, the group was able to stay together for the entire session. Members were supportive of each other in their actions and verbalizations. Some were able to identify affect (Felicita: "I'll miss group;" Antonia: feeling "bad"). All were able to tolerate expression of affect and remain task-focused with occasional prompts. All members accepted their certificates, some identifying that they would show them to staff and keep them to remember group. Mike reflected that the leader-member roles had felt more balanced and their co-leadership felt like an equal partner- ship, which is why he felt that it was safe to take time out of the group with Antonia. Amanda felt the closing was symbolic in that it was she who opened the first group session, so it seemed fitting that, as the upcoming graduate, she would close the group and grant each member their certificate.

Conclusion

The functional group model provided a theoretical framework to guide the leaders' reasoning about group member preparation, group composition and member criteria, activity selection and adaptation, and intervention. The four action components of the group were present: purposeful action, self-initiated action, spontaneous (here-and-now) action, and group-centered action. Overall, the group achieved its aims and individual member outcomes were met as measured by specific observable objectives listed under general group goals and outcome criteria.

Mary Alicia Barnes and Sharan Schwartzberg of Tufts University provided the example of this group.

Table 9.1 **Terms of the Model**	
Adaptation	A person's adjustment to the environment.
Functional group	A gathering of people engaged in actions focused on enhancing participants' occupational behavior to support health and well-being.
Group dynamics	Properties of a group that emerge from the interactions among group members.

(table continues on page 124)

Table 9.1 **Terms of the Model** continued

Group history	The story of the group's past structure and functioning.
Group process	How the group functions and communicates.
Group roles	The ways in which members contribute to the overall functioning of the group in terms of group tasks or social-emotional elements.
Group structure	The methods used to facilitate group forming and performing; the combination of mutually connected and interdependent parts of a group.
Leadership	Principles and practices that enhance one's ability to promote behaviors that effectively lead to the satisfaction of group needs and realization of group goals.
Maintenance functions	Processes that strengthen group effectiveness and cohesion.
Psychological field	A property of groups that acts like an energy field, influencing the behavior of the group as a whole and the behavior of individual members of the group.

SUMMARY: THE FUNCTIONAL GROUP MODEL

Theory

+ True groups include:
  • Interaction among their members
  • A common goal
  • A relationship between size and function
  • Members' desire or consent to participate in a group
  • A democratic capacity for self-determination

+ Groups are characterized by structure, cohesion, and stages of development

+ Group structure refers to the combination of parts that form the group

+ Group cohesion refers to the intensity of feeling for and identification with the group among its members

+ Stages of group development refer to the phases a group passes through during its existence

+ Features of groups
  • Content refers to tasks done during the group and what is said or discussed

• Process refers to how things are said and done and how the group goes about accomplishing its goals

+ Two types of group behavior contribute to the group process:
  • Group task functions that enable the group to accomplish its aims related to content
  • Group-building and maintenance functions that help create and sustain relationships and connections between members

+ Concepts specific to functional groups
  • Encompass a common goal and dynamic interaction of their members
  • Have capacity for self-direction
  • Can become increasingly independent of designated leadership
  • Can address individual needs
  • Provide multiple types of feedback and support
  • Can support members' growth and change

+ The basic concepts of the functional group model are adaptation (adjustment of the environment) and occupation (i.e., action or behavior of a member in the group)

✦ Four types of action that promote adaptation can occur in a functional group:
  • Purposeful action
  • Self-initiated action
  • Spontaneous (here-and-now) action
  • Group-centered action

Rationale for Therapeutic Intervention

✦ The functional group seeks to enhance occupational behavior and thus adaptation by mobilizing dynamic group forces that have the potential to positively shape people's understanding of themselves or their abilities

✦ Groups can also provide a sense of identity and self-worth to their members

✦ Further, they offer social positions (roles) that can meet a variety of individual needs and, at the same time, require persons to respond to environmental expectations

✦ Groups provide a structure that guides individual participation along with socializing influences that are necessary for learning adaptive occupational behavior. In these and other ways, functional groups offer interactions that, through the nature of the action (purposeful, self-initiated, spontaneous, or group-centered), elicit adaptive responses from members and influence the individual to participate positively and, thereby, change

Practice Resources

Assessment

✦ Two basic types of assessments
  • Assessments developed by psychologists and sociologists for observing group dynamics and group content and process
  • Assessments of group content and process

✦ Forms specifically for the functional group
  • Assessment of Members and Context
  • Functional Group Protocol
  • Session Plan
  • Session Evaluation form
  • Leader Self-Assessment forms
  • Assessment of Activity and Leadership

Intervention

✦ Leadership refers to the ability to promote those behaviors that lead to the satisfaction of group needs

✦ A functional group involves four overall stages in which the group is designed, formed, developed, and concluded

✦ During each of these stages the group leader conducts assessment (information gathering) and takes appropriate leadership action in order to ensure that the group is functioning well and positively influencing its members

✦ During the design phase, the therapist defines tentative group goals, develops general plans for the group as a whole and for specific sessions, selects the members, and initially outlines a proposed group structure, including tasks to be undertaken in the group

✦ Forming the group involves getting everyone acquainted, sharing how the group will function, and developing accepted norms of behavior in the group

✦ Supporting development of the group involves the group leader creating an environment that supports purposeful, self-initiated, spontaneous, and group-centered action

✦ Concluding a group involves reviewing and summarizing the members' experience in the group and addressing concerns and feelings about the termination

REFERENCES

Agazarian, Y., & Gantt, S. (2003). Phases of group development: Systems-centered hypotheses and their implications for research and practice. *Group Dynamics: Theory, Research, and Practice, 7*(3), 238–252.

Bales, R. (1950). *Interaction process analysis.* Reading, MA: Addison-Wesley.

Baron, K. (1987). The model of human occupation: A newspaper treatment group for adolescents with a diagnosis of conduct disorder.

Occupational Therapy in Mental Health, 7(2), 89–104.

Barris, R., Kielhofner, G., & Hawkins, J.H. (1983). *Psychosocial occupational therapy practice in a pluralistic arena.* Laurel, MD: Ramsco.

Benne, K.D., & Sheats, P. (1978). Functional roles of group members. In L.P. Bradbord (Ed.), *Group development* (2nd ed., pp. 52–61). La Jolla, CA: University Associates.

Braveman, B. (2001). Development of a community-based return to work program for people with AIDS. *Occupational Therapy in Health Care, 13*(3/4), 113–131.

Clark, F., Azen, S.P., Zemke, R., Jackson, J., Carlson, M., Mandel, D., et al. (1997). Occupational therapy for independent-living older adults: A randomized controlled trial. *Journal of the American Medical Association, 278,* 1321–1326.

Clark, F.A., Carlson, M., Jackson, J., & Mandel, D. (2003). Lifestyle redesign improves health *and* is cost-effective. *OT Practice, 8*(2), 9–13.

DeCarlo, J.J., & Mann, W.C. (1985). The effectiveness of verbal versus activity groups in improving self-perceptions of interpersonal communication skills. *American Journal of Occupational Therapy, 39,* 20–27.

Duncombe, L.W., & Howe, M.C. (1985). Group work in occupational therapy: A survey of practice. *American Journal of Occupational Therapy, 39,* 163–170.

Fidler, G.S., & Fidler, J.W. (1978). Doing and becoming: Purposeful action and self-actualization. *American Journal of Occupational Therapy, 32,* 305–310.

Gauthier, L., Dalziel, S., & Gauthier, S. (1987). The benefits of group occupational therapy for patients with Parkinson's disease. *American Journal of Occupational Therapy, 41,* 360–365.

Gusich, R.L., & Silverman, A.L. (1991). Basava day clinic: The model of human occupation as applied to psychiatric day hospitalization. *Occupational Therapy in Mental Health, 11*(2/3), 113–134.

Henry, A.D., Nelson, D.L., & Duncombe, L.W. (1984). Choice making in group and individual activity. *American Journal of Occupational Therapy, 38,* 245–251.

Howe, M.C., & Schwartzberg, S.L. (1986). *A functional approach to group work in occupational therapy.* Philadelphia: J.B. Lippincott.

Jackson, J., Carlson, M., Mandel, D., Zemke, R. & Clark, F. (1998). Occupation in lifestyle redesign: The well elderly study occupational therapy program. *American Journal of Occupational Therapy, 52,* 326–336.

Kaplan, K. (1986). The directive group: Short term treatment for psychiatric patients with a minimal level of functioning. *American Journal of Occupational Therapy, 40,* 474–481.

Klyczek, J.P., & Mann, W.C. (1986). Therapeutic modality comparisons in day treatment. *American Journal of Occupational Therapy, 40,* 606–611.

Knis-Matthews, L., Richard, L., Marquez, L., & Mevawala, N. (2005). Implementation of occupational therapy services for an adolescent residence program. *Occupational Therapy in Mental Health, 21*(1), 57–72.

Mandel, D.R., Jackson, J.M., Zemke, R., Nelson, L., & Clark, F.A. (1999). *Lifestyle redesign: Implementing the well elderly program.* Bethesda, MD: American Occupational Therapy Association Press.

Maslow, A.H. (1970). *Motivation and personality* (2nd ed.). New York: Harper & Row.

Mosey, A.C. (1970). The concept and use of developmental groups. *American Journal of Occupational Therapy, 24,* 272–275.

Reed, K.L. (1984). *Models of practice in occupational therapy.* Baltimore: Williams & Wilkins.

Schwartzberg, S.L., Howe, M.C., & Barnes, M.A. (2008). *Groups: Applying the functional group model.* Philadelphia: F.A. Davis

Schwartzberg, S.L., Howe, M.C., & McDermott, A. (1982). A comparison of three treatment group formats for facilitating social interaction. *Occupational Therapy in Mental Health, 2,* 1–16.

Trahey, P.J. (1991). A comparison of the cost-effectiveness of two types of occupational therapy services. *American Journal of Occupational Therapy, 45,* 397–400.

Ward, J.D. (2003). The nature of clinical reasoning with groups: A phenomenological study of an occupational therapist in community mental health. *American Journal of Occupational Therapy, 27,* 625–634.

White, R.W. (1959). Motivation reconsidered: The concept of competence. *The Psychological Review, 66,* 297–333.

White, R.W. (1971). The urge towards competence. *American Journal of Occupational Therapy, 25,* 271–274.

CHAPTER 10

The Intentional Relationship Model

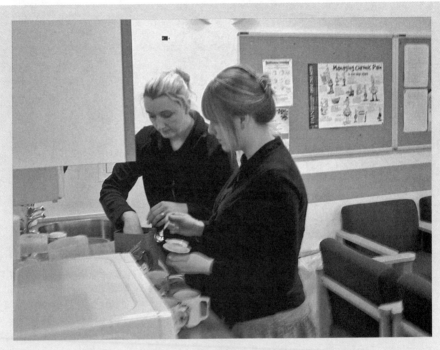

Sarah, a client with chronic pain, arrived late the third time in a row to Alice Moody's pain management group. So far, Sarah had behaved in an aggressive manner toward suggested intervention strategies. Within the group she had refused to engage in the weekly goal-setting that was expected of all members. She had also avoided talking with other group members. Alice felt mildly annoyed at Sarah's late entry and, at the same time, realized that she was occupying the very seat that Sarah had sat in during the last few sessions. Alice was tempted to "stay put," forcing her to sit elsewhere. However, Alice immediately stood up, offered the seat, and produced a welcoming smile. Sarah shrugged, took the offered seat, and explained that she had been having a difficult few days facing some major worries. She then apologized for being late. Alice was initially a bit suspicious about her demeanor, but decided to give Sarah her sincere attention when she engaged Alice in conversation spontaneously during the break for coffee. She began to share with Alice some gripping challenges she and her family were facing. Following this conversation, during which Alice listened and congratulated her for managing to attend the group at all under such difficult circumstances, Sarah offered to come and help Alice make the tea and coffee for the other members of the group.

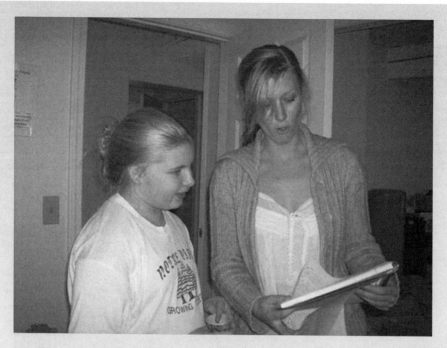

Kortney, an occupational therapy client, has faced many developmental challenges. At first, she was not at all sure about occupational therapy and what it would do for her. Plus, she was tired of having "one thing after another she had to do" and occupational therapy seemed just like "another thing she was going to have to do." Recognizing this and Kortney's needs, Libby Asselin makes use of the collaborating mode in developing goals with Kortney for her weekly occupational therapy sessions. Together, Libby and Kortney developed a weekly plan based on Kortney's goals to increase her speed and endurance so she would be more successful in gym class and while playing with her friends on the playground at school. Libby and Kortney also collaborated on the intervention process by working together on setting up an obstacle course to include activities that are fun for Kortney. The collaborating mode works well to keep this 12-year-old highly motivated in occupational therapy.

As each of these examples illustrates, occupational therapy involves a myriad of interpersonal events (behaviors, feelings, interactions) that require a therapeutic response. It is widely recognized in the field that therapeutic use of self is a highly personal, individualized, and subjective process that can determine whether or not occupational therapy is successful. In the previous examples the occupational therapists made thoughtful and disciplined responses to situations that, if not handled well, may have had detrimental effects on the therapy process. In each of these instances, therapists were using concepts and principles of the intentional relationship model (IRM).

IRM offers a detailed conceptualization of the interpersonal processes of occupational therapy. This model also explains how therapeutic use of self can be utilized in occupational therapy to promote occupational engagement and achieve positive therapy outcomes. It is designed to guide occupational therapists in addressing interpersonal dilemmas and challenges that arise in everyday practice.

Many concepts of IRM have their origins in theory underlying psychotherapy. However, the model distinguishes between traditional psychotherapy, in which interpersonal relating between client and therapist is central, and occupational therapy, which centers on occupational engagement (i.e., undertaking an activity that has a therapeutic aim). Thus, IRM recognizes that the content of occupational engagement in therapy (e.g., doing an activity to increase strength or remediate a cognitive problem) will be guided by other occupational therapy practice models. Importantly, this model underscores the fact that the client's occupational engagement is closely tied to the process of relating that occurs between client and therapist. Thus, the intentional relationship model explains how the relationship between client and therapist affects the overall process of occupational therapy and how that relationship can be used to enhance occupational therapy outcomes.

> The intentional relationship model explains how the relationship between client and therapist affects the overall process of occupational therapy and how that relationship can be used to enhance occupational therapy outcomes.

Theory

As shown in Figure 10.1, the intentional relationship model views the therapeutic relationship as being composed of:

- The client
- The interpersonal events that occur during therapy
- The therapist
- The occupation

The Client

The client is the focal point of this model; IRM emphasizes that it is the therapist's responsibility to develop a positive relationship with the client (Taylor, 2008). In order to develop this relationship and respond appropriately to the client, a therapist must work to understand the client's situational and enduring interpersonal characteristics.

Situational characteristics reflect a client's acute emotional reaction to a specific situation (typically one that is painful, frustrating, or stressful). These characteristics bear no reflection on the client's character or personality. Situational characteristics may be observed, for example, when a newly disabled client exhibits sadness or anger or when a client perceives the therapist to have done or said something that is insensitive. **Enduring characteristics** are stable aspects of the client's interpersonal behavior. They include, for example, a client's preferred style of communication, capacity for trust, need for control, and typical way of responding to change, challenge, or frustration. Enduring characteristics do reflect the client's personality. Knowing which of a client's characteristics are enduring versus situational helps a therapist tailor and modulate responses to the client.

An **interpersonal event** is a "naturally occurring communication, reaction, process, task, or general circumstance that occurs during therapy and that has the potential to detract from or strengthen the therapeutic relationship" (Taylor, 2008, p. 49). The scenarios that opened this chapter are examples of interpersonal events

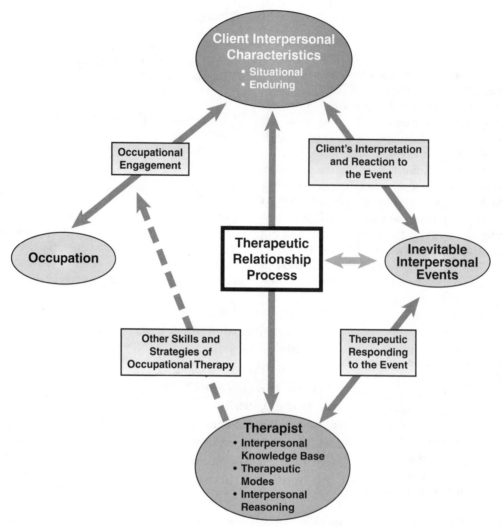

FIGURE 10.1 Model of the intentional relationship in occupational therapy. *From Taylor, R. (2008). The intentional relationship: Occupational therapy and use of self. Philadelphia: F.A. Davis with permission.*

(i.e., coming late to therapy, resistance to participating in therapy); the following are additional examples of interpersonal events:

- A client feels threatened by a therapeutic activity and hesitates to do it
- The therapist asks a question that a client perceives as too emotionally difficult to answer
- A client becomes upset in therapy because of something that is embarrassing
- The client and therapist disagree over some aspect or goal of therapy
- A client questions the value of something the therapist recommends

Of course, these are only a few of an endless number of inevitable interpersonal events that may

occur in the course of occupational therapy. Clients interpret such events based on their unique interpersonal characteristics. Thus, the impact of an event depends on the client involved. When interpersonal events occur, the therapist must be aware of them and respond appropriately.

Interpersonal events are distinguished from other events of therapy by their emotional potential. Consequently, if ignored or responded to sub-optimally, they can threaten both the therapeutic relationship and the client's occupational engagement. When optimally responded to, they are opportunities for positive client learning or change and for solidifying the therapeutic relationship. Because they are unavoidable, a primary task of a therapist using IRM is to respond to these inevitable events in ways that strengthen the therapeutic relationship.

The Therapist

According to IRM, the therapist is responsible for making every reasonable effort to make the relationship work. The therapist brings three main interpersonal capacities into the relationship:

- An interpersonal skill base
- Therapeutic modes (or interpersonal styles)
- Capacity for interpersonal reasoning

The therapist's **interpersonal skill base** includes a continuum of skills that must be judiciously applied by the therapist to build a functional working relationship with the client. Table 10.1 shows the areas of skill addressed by this model. Depending on the therapist's experiences, knowledge, and capacities, some of these skills will come more naturally while others require significant effort and practice to develop.

The second interpersonal capacity therapists bring to the client-therapist relationship is the use of therapeutic modes. A **therapeutic mode** refers to a specific way of relating to a client. IRM identifies six therapeutic modes: advocating, collaborating, empathizing, encouraging, instructing, and problem-solving. Table 10.2 summarizes and gives examples of these modes.

Therapists naturally use therapeutic modes that are consistent with their fundamental personality characteristics. Therapists also vary in their range and flexibility in using modes in relating to clients. Some therapists relate to clients in one or two primary ways, while others draw upon multiple therapeutic modes to suit client characteristics and the therapeutic situation. IRM suggests that therapists should work to increase their comfort in using all six modes. A therapist's **interpersonal style** refers to the therapeutic mode or set of modes typically used when interacting with a client. Multi-modal therapists are able to utilize all six of the modes flexibly and comfortably.

According to IRM, a therapist should choose and apply a particular therapeutic mode or set of modes to match the enduring interpersonal

Table 10.1 Areas of the Interpersonal Skill Base

Area of Skill Base	Content
Therapeutic communication	Communicating verbally and nonverbally, therapeutic listening, asserting, providing clients with direction and feedback, and seeking and responding to clients' feedback
Interviewing skills	Being watchful and intentional in asking a client questions and using strategic questioning (i.e., asking questions in a way that guides clients to think more broadly or differently)
Establishing relationships	Rapport building, matching one's therapeutic style to a client, managing clients' strong emotions, using touch, and cultural competence
Families, social systems, and groups	Understanding and gaining the collaboration of partners, parents, other family, and friends to serve the goals of therapy; understanding the structure, process, and interpersonal dynamics of group therapy
Working effectively with supervisors, employers, and other professionals	Communicating with other professionals about clients; understanding power dynamics and value systems that underlie supervisor/student and employer/employee relationships

(table continues on page 132)

Table 10.1   **Areas of the Interpersonal Skill Base** continued

Area of Skill Base	Content
Understanding and managing difficult interpersonal behavior	Knowing how to respond effectively to behaviors that involve manipulation, excessive dependency, symptom focusing, resistance, emotional disengagement, denial, difficulty with rapport and trust, and hostility
Empathic breaks and conflicts	Knowing how to resolve conflicts and rifts in understanding between client and therapist
Professional behavior, values, and ethics	Knowing how one's values are consistent or inconsistent with the occupational therapy core values, ethical behavior and decision-making, behavioral self-awareness, reliability and dependability, upholding confidentiality, and setting and managing professional boundaries
Therapist self-care and professional development	Knowing, managing, and being accountable for one's emotional reactions to clients, self-reflection, managing personal life and seeking necessary support, and maintaining perspective regarding client outcomes

Table 10.2   **The Six Therapeutic Modes in Occupational Therapy Practice**

Mode	Definition	Example
Advocating	Ensuring that the client's rights are enforced and resources are secured. May require the therapist to serve as a mediator, facilitator, negotiator, enforcer, or other type of advocate with external persons and agencies.	Lobbying with an insurance provider to secure support for a more functional wheel-chair for a client.
Collaborating	Expecting the client to be an active and equal participant in therapy. Ensuring choice, freedom, and autonomy to the greatest extent possible.	Deciding on treatment goals with a client and periodically reviewing and revising these goals with the client.
Empathizing	Ongoing striving to understand the client's thoughts, feelings, and behaviors while suspending any judgment. Ensuring that the client verifies and experiences the therapist's understanding as truthful and validating.	Stopping to listen and taking care to fully appreciate the sense of loss and anxiety about the future of a young client who recently experienced a spinal cord injury.
Encouraging	Seizing the opportunity to instill hope in a client. Celebrating a client's thinking or behavior through positive reinforcement. Conveying an attitude of joyfulness, playfulness, and confidence.	Shouting encouragement to a child who is attempting a new maneuver on a piece of suspended equipment.

Mode	Definition	Example
Instructing	Carefully structuring therapy activities and being explicit with clients about the plan, sequence, and events of therapy. Providing clear instruction and feedback about performance. Setting limits on a client's requests or behavior.	Telling a client exactly how to perform a transfer and giving cues and feedback during his first attempt.
Problem-solving	Facilitating pragmatic thinking and solving dilemmas by outlining choices, posing strategic questions, and providing opportunities for comparative or analytical thinking.	Engaging in trial and error with a client to identify the best work situation to attempt after an on-the-job injury.

characteristics of the client. In addition, certain events or interpersonal events in therapy may call for a **mode shift** (i.e., a conscious change in one's way of relating to a client). As Taylor (2008, p. 52) notes, "if a client perceives a therapist's attempts at problem-solving to be insensitive or off the mark, a therapist would be wise to switch from the problem-solving mode to an empathizing mode so that she can get a better understanding of the client's reaction and the root of the dilemma."

The third skill area is the capacity to engage in an **interpersonal reasoning** (a step-wise process by which a therapist decides what to say, do, or express in reaction to the occurrence of an interpersonal dilemma in therapy). This skill requires vigilance toward the interpersonal aspects of therapy to anticipate dilemmas that might occur, along with reviewing and evaluating options for responding.

The Desired Occupation

The **desired occupation** refers to the task or activity that the therapist and the client have selected for therapy. As noted earlier, selection of the desired occupation and support for occupational engagement are informed by other models discussed in this book. IRM guides the therapist in managing the interpersonal dynamic between the client and the therapist. The therapeutic relationship functions as:

• A support to occupational engagement

• A place where the emotional and coping processes associated with the client's impairment and its implications for occupational performance are addressed

The Therapeutic Relationship

According to Taylor (2008), the **therapeutic relationship** is:

> a socially defined and personally interpreted interactive process between the therapist and a client. It is socially defined in that the therapist and the client are engaged in an interaction within publicly understood roles. The therapist is recognized as bringing a certain kind of expertise, ethical guidelines, and values into a relationship. The client is recognized as a person receiving service to address a particular need. The relationship is understood to exist for the sole purpose of achieving improvement in the client's situation. These parameters are given and provide an important definition of the relationship. (p. 54)

This relationship can be viewed at two different levels or scales:

• Macro-level (i.e., the ongoing enduring rapport and patterns of interaction between client and therapist)
• Micro-level (i.e., the moment-by-moment therapeutic relationship as influenced by interpersonal events of therapy that have the

potential to challenge or enrich the relationship)

The micro and macro scales of therapeutic interaction both play a critical role in the overall process of occupational therapy and they are interrelated. The therapist must appropriately define and keep the boundaries of the therapeutic relationship and maintain a positive climate of interpersonal relating (e.g., trust, mutual respect, and honesty). This both influences and depends on how the therapist responds to the interpersonal events of therapy. The therapeutic relationship is also influenced by characteristics and behaviors that the client and therapist bring to the relationship and by circumstances surrounding the relationship (e.g., the nature of the client's impairment and the context of therapy).

Taylor (2008) notes:

> The stability and success of a therapeutic relationship cannot be assumed. Rather, it begins early in treatment with attempts by the therapist to build rapport, followed by other efforts to develop a relationship that meets the client's immediate interpersonal needs and is appropriate in terms of the circumstances of therapy and the demands of the treatment setting. (p. 55)

Many factors contribute to a successful therapeutic relationship and the therapist must be vigilant to explore, identify, and sustain those factors. Clients also typically bring important characteristics and behaviors into the therapeutic relationship. However, IRM underscores that the occupational therapist must assume the ultimate responsibility for the relationship, thereby creating a space wherein "a client can be vulnerable, distressed, frustrated, or angry without fearing that the relationship will be ruptured" (Taylor, 2008, p. 56).

The following are just a few examples of the myriad of circumstances that can lead to difficulty in the therapeutic relationship:

- The client may bring pre-existing emotional and/or behavioral difficulties into the relationship

- The circumstances of therapy may feel threatening to the client (i.e., performing an evaluation that may influence return to work, discharge placement, or eligibility for disability insurance)
- There may not be a match between the client's and the therapist's interpersonal styles, ages, genders, or ethnic backgrounds
- The client or the therapist may disappoint or fail to meet the other's expectations
- The impact of the impairment or other life changes surrounding it may place the client under extreme stress
- The client or therapist inadvertently says or does something that is perceived as injurious and the situation is not processed and resolved

Inevitable interpersonal events have the potential to intensify difficulties. Simple events such as the therapist's unanticipated need to miss an appointment, a misunderstanding about some aspect of therapy, or a personal crisis or medical exacerbation that causes the client to regress can threaten an already tenuous relationship. How the therapist responds to such events has a powerful influence on the final outcome. Even when the therapeutic relationship is strong, therapists' responses to interpersonal events are critical. Failure to respond adequately to interpersonal events may negatively affect occupational engagement and weaken the therapeutic relationship.

> **The therapist must appropriately define and keep the boundaries of the therapeutic relationship and maintain a positive climate of interpersonal relating.**

Underlying Principles of IRM

Ten fundamental principles underlie this model (Taylor, 2008). They are summarized here.

Critical Self-Awareness Is Key to the Intentional Use of Self

Critical self-awareness involves a general knowledge of one's interpersonal tendencies while interacting with clients of different personalities and under different conditions and circumstances. Interpersonal tendencies include one's emotional reactions and behavior (verbal and nonverbal) and how they are influenced by awkward, tense, or stressful situations. Effective use of self also requires **ongoing critical awareness,** which includes a constant mindfulness about what one is communicating verbally (e.g., choice of words), nonverbally (e.g., positioning of one's body and gestures), and emotionally (e.g., tone, tenor, and volume of voice, and facial expression).

Interpersonal Self-Discipline Is Fundamental to Effective Use of Self

Therapists are responsible for managing and fortifying the therapeutic relationship by attending and responding to ongoing interpersonal feedback from clients. Doing so requires **interpersonal self-discipline** (i.e., anticipating, measuring, and responding to the effects of ongoing communication with a client). Interpersonal self-discipline allows a therapist to develop a stable and predictable relationship in which a client can trust the therapist, who remains focused on what the client wants from the relationship and puts personal reactions and expectations aside. This is particularly important when working with clients that are interpersonally sensitive, difficult, or otherwise vulnerable.

It Is Necessary to Keep Head Before Heart

One cannot assume that as long as one's heart is in the right place, one will naturally react and behave appropriately in therapy. Rather, all therapists have certain tendencies (despite or because of good intentions) that will not always play out positively for clients. Thus, responding from the heart must be guided by critical self-awareness and interpersonal self-discipline.

Mindful Empathy Is Required to Know Your Client

Mindful empathy is "an objective mode of observation in which the therapist comes to feel and understand a client's underlying emotions, needs, and motives, while at the same time maintaining an objective viewpoint" (Taylor, 2008 p. 60). It is a prerequisite to a good therapeutic relationship. Mindful empathy assumes that clients are experts on the meanings they ascribe to their experiences in therapy.

Grow Your Interpersonal Knowledge Base

Interpersonal communication is complex and requires a range of knowledge and skills such as listening effectively, communicating clearly, overcoming basic conflicts and events, and being reliable and predictable. The model provides detailed discussions of a continuum of skills that therapists are encouraged to develop.

Provided That They Are Purely and Flexibly Applied, a Wide Range of Therapeutic Modes Can Work and Be Utilized Interchangeably in Occupational Therapy

Every therapist has unique interpersonal characteristics derived from innate personality and life experiences. These characteristics dispose therapists toward a certain therapeutic mode or modes. No particular mode is superior to another. Moreover, two therapists with very different personalities, who use different combinations of modes, can be equally effective. Nonetheless, certain modes and interpersonal styles tend to work better with different populations and circumstances. Thus, therapeutic use of self requires flexible and appropriate use of modes to address the needs of the client and the situation. Therapists are encouraged and helped by this model to expand their capacity to use different modes.

The Client Defines a Successful Relationship

Clients differ in what they want within the therapeutic relationship. Some prefer a more formal relationship in which the therapist mainly instructs and gives guidance. Other clients desire a more personalized connection and emotional support. Still others wish for an egalitarian and collaborative relationship. Clients may change over time in their desires for the therapeutic relationship. For example, a client who at first wants emotional support and clear directions may later want a more collaborative relationship. Or a client who previously has been very collaborative, when faced with increased disability, may wish to have less responsibility and more support. In the end, success in the relationship is defined by the client, not the occupational therapist.

Activity Focusing Must Be Balanced With Interpersonal Focusing

Activity focusing refers to strategies of responding to interpersonal events that emphasize doing over feeling or relating. **Interpersonal focusing** refers to strategies that emphasize feeling or relating over doing. Balance means that the therapist does not rely too much on using activities to avoid direct discussion of interpersonal issues or, by contrast, does not overemphasize discussion of interpersonal issues to the point that it is uncomfortable or distracts the client from necessary occupational engagement. The balance between activity and interpersonal focusing varies from client to client and over time.

Application of the Model Must Be Informed by Core Values and Ethics

Taylor (2008) emphasizes that occupational therapy core values (AOTA, 1993) and ethics (AOTA, 2005) must inform application of the intentional relationship model in practice.

Cultural Competency Is Central to Practice

Differences in gender, age, race, ethnicity, socioeconomic status, religious views, sexual orientation, disability status, and a wide range of other social and cultural dimensions can affect the therapeutic relationship. Cultural competency (the ability to understand, be aware of, and manage such differences) is central to every therapist's interpersonal knowledge base.

Practice Resources

The resources of the model are focused on helping therapists better understand both their clients' and their own interpersonal characteristics and on helping therapists become more able to monitor and respond to the inevitable interpersonal events of therapy. These resources include the following:

- Materials and procedures for better understanding and monitoring clients' interpersonal characteristics

- Materials and procedures for therapists to better understand their own modes, interpersonal styles, reactions, skills, and knowledge
- Resources for identifying inevitable interpersonal events in therapy
- A format for applying interpersonal reasoning
- Guidelines and materials for developing one's interpersonal skill base (conflict resolution)

Each is discussed here.

Understanding, Monitoring, and Responding to Clients' Interpersonal Characteristics

Actively seeking to know and understand each client's interpersonal characteristics (client emotions, behaviors, and reactions that occur in interactions between the client and therapist) is essential to an intentional and tailored relationship in which the client feels comfortable. As noted earlier, when clients' interpersonal behaviors are inconsistent with how they typically interact with others and largely linked to some other external stressful circumstance, they are referred to as situational. Emotions, behaviors, and reactions that mostly emanate from underlying traits of the client are referred to as enduring interpersonal characteristics. Both types of client characteristics require a therapeutic response, but the nature and extent of the response will vary depending upon whether a client's interpersonal behavior is situational or more enduring. For example, the response to a client who is anxious about a new job would be different from the response to a client who is chronically anxious about any new task or activity.

IRM identifies 12 categories of interpersonal characteristics:

- Communication style
- Capacity for trust
- Need for control
- Capacity to assert needs
- Response to change and challenge
- Affect
- Predisposition to giving feedback
- Capacity to receive feedback
- Response to human diversity
- Orientation toward relating
- Preference for touch
- Capacity for reciprocity

By becoming aware of these categories, a therapist can become more attuned to each client's unique interpersonal characteristics. An Interpersonal Characteristics Rating Scale (Taylor, 2008) can be used to evaluate how clients vary on each these dimensions. In additional to being aware of a client's tendency to display certain interpersonal characteristics, therapists must also be vigilant during therapy to:

- Recognize a client's emotion, reaction, or behavior
- Understand its source
- Consciously and reflectively consider options for how to act
- Monitor the client's response

IRM provides guidance as to the modes that are most likely to be successful in responding to different interpersonal characteristics.

Understanding One's Own Modes, Interpersonal Styles, Reactions, Skills, and Knowledge

IRM emphasizes that self-knowledge and self-discipline are key to becoming an intentional and interpersonally effective therapist. A central component of this self-knowledge is developing an awareness of one's own natural tendency to use certain therapeutic modes. One therapist may learn, for instance, that he is more inclined toward problem-solving and instructing modes while another may be more comfortable and make use of the empathizing and advocating modes. IRM stresses that no mode or therapeutic style (i.e., tendency to use certain comfortable modes) is inherently superior.

However, Taylor (2008) does recommend that therapists:

- Be aware of their dominant modes and their likely impact on clients
- Strive to develop a wider repertoire of mode use
- Achieve greater facility in selecting, utilizing, and changing modes according to client needs and the therapy situation

The ideal is a multi-modal therapist whose use of modes reflects a vigilant understanding of the client's unfolding needs rather than one's personal comfort zone.

A first step in this process is becoming aware of one's current use of modes. Questionnaires and exercises are provided to help therapists learn their comfortable and uncomfortable modes. Taylor (2008) also gives a wide range of examples, exercises, and guidelines for therapists to practice and learn new modes. Finally, she provides examples and guidelines on how to select the appropriate mode or sequence of modes for dealing with different clients and situations.

Identifying and Responding to the Inevitable Interpersonal Events of Therapy

Interpersonal events are distinguished from other therapy events in that they are emotionally charged and ripe with both threat and opportunity. Because these events are inherently emotional, therapists and clients alike can be tempted to ignore them or minimize their significance. However, if ignored, they can lead to difficulties in the therapeutic relationship and negatively affect occupational engagement. On the other hand, if addressed appropriately, these events may lead to positive outcomes that involve feelings such as gratification, fulfillment, satisfaction, or intimacy.

IRM identifies categories of interpersonal events that are shown in Table 10.3 (Taylor, 2008).

How the inevitable interpersonal events of therapy are interpreted by the client is influenced by the circumstances of therapy and the client's unique set of interpersonal characteristics. IRM provides detailed guidance on positive ways that therapists can learn to recognize and deal with the interpersonal events of therapy and clients' reactions to them.

Interpersonal Reasoning

Central to the application of the intentional relationship model is a process of interpersonal

> IRM emphasizes that self-knowledge and self-discipline are key to becoming an intentional and interpersonally effective therapist.

Box 10.1

Dealing With an Interpersonal Event: A Case Example by Hiroyuki Notoh

Yuka is a deaf person in her late seventies. She lives with her husband, who is also deaf. An active woman, her hobbies include athletics, travel, and teaching sign language. She was in a traffic accident and fractured her clavicle, both wrists, several fingers, and her hip. After two weeks of acute care, Yuka moved to a long-term care unit, and I took charge of her occupational therapy.

In the early days of her stay, Yuka's hands were still in casts. Nonetheless, she made great effort to regain her self-care abilities. She also challenged herself to exercise regularly by walking vigorously. Before long, Yuka acquired self-care skills and was walking independently with a cane.

In occupational therapy, Yuka identified the recovery of her hand movements as her primary

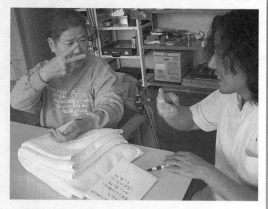

Yuka teaches Hiroyuki how to sign.

goal, since she communicated by sign language. Knowing what Yuka wanted from therapy enabled me to better tailor the treatment to meet her needs. Because she was so able to assert her needs, I found that the collaborating mode generally worked very effectively with Yuka. Once the casts were removed, we decided that our goal was reacquiring hand movements for sign language.

However, Yuka's hands were still swollen and she had contractures. I became aware of how frustrating this was for Yuka when an inevitable interpersonal event occurred. One day, she wanted me to explain why these symptoms had occurred. Since she could not lip-read, I attempted to explain it by using textbooks from anatomy and orthopedics. By the expression on her face I could tell that she did not fully understand. At that point I realized that by not communicating in her language (sign language), I had made an empathic break. In reflecting further about how I had disappointed her, I realized that this was not the only time in which I had burdened Yuka to communicate with me using the written word. I had neglected to realize that there was a fundamental difference in our communication styles that I had not given much weight to because Yuka had never seemed to mind.

I knew I had to do something to resolve this empathic break, so I decided to ask Yuka if she would be willing to teach me some sign language. One day, when Yuka came to the occupational therapy room, she greeted me with sign language and I imitated it. Yuka was delighted, and she grasped my hands to teach me the correct hand movements. I knew I was on my way to mending the empathic break that I had made. After that event, when we had everyday conversation and discussions about therapy, we used more and more sign language. Yuka showed me various signs slowly and repeatedly, and I memorized them. Then another inevitable interpersonal event occurred. After I had learned a sufficient amount of sign language, Yuka made an intimate self-disclosure and told me that although she was able to use a pen to communicate with me she was glad that I had learned sign language because using a pen caused her fingers to hurt more. I told her I was sorry that I had not realized that I needed to learn sign language earlier.

reasoning. **Interpersonal reasoning** is "the process by which a therapist monitors the interpersonal events of therapy, the client's unique interpersonal characteristics, and her or his own behavior in a reflective way to maximize the likelihood that the therapeutic relationship will be successful and supportive of the client's engagement in occupation" (Taylor, 2008, p. 138). It is a process by which therapists decide what to say, do, or express in reaction to

Table 10.3 **Interpersonal Events of Therapy**

Interpersonal Event	Definition
Expressions of strong emotion	External displays of internal feelings that are shown with a level of intensity beyond cultural norms
Intimate self-disclosures	Statements or stories that reveal something unobservable, private, or sensitive
Power dilemmas	Tensions that arise in the therapeutic relationship because of clients' feelings, the situation of therapy, the therapist's behavior, and/or other circumstances that underscore clients' lack or loss of power
Nonverbal cues	Communications that do not involve the use of formal language
Crisis points	Unanticipated, stressful events that distract clients and/or temporarily interfere with clients' occupational engagement
Resistance	Passive or active refusal to participate in some or all aspects of therapy for reasons linked to the therapeutic relationship
Reluctance	Disinclination toward some aspect of therapy for reasons outside the therapeutic relationship
Boundary testing	Behavior that violates or that asks the therapist to act in ways that are outside the defined therapeutic relationship
Empathic breaks	When a therapist fails to notice or understand a communication from a client or initiates a communication or behavior that is perceived by the client as hurtful or insensitive
Emotionally charged therapy tasks and situations	Activities or circumstances that can lead clients to become overwhelmed or experience uncomfortable emotional reactions such as embarrassment, humiliation, or shame
Limitations of therapy	Restrictions on the available or possible services, time, resources, or therapist actions
Contextual inconsistencies	Any aspect of a client's interpersonal or physical environments that changes during the course of therapy

their clients. Interpersonal reasoning involves six steps:

- Anticipate interpersonal events or client behaviors that may test, challenge, or threaten the therapeutic relationship
- Accurately identify interpersonal events and cope (i.e., gain perspective, prepare to do what the client needs, and avoid any impulse toward a response that will not be therapeutic)
- Determine if a mode shift (an intentional change in the way a therapist relates to a client) is required
- Choose a response mode (advocating, collaborating, empathizing, encouraging, instructing, or problem-solving) or a sequence of modes
- Draw upon any relevant interpersonal skills associated with the mode(s) in responding
- Gather feedback (i.e., check in with the client and ask how he or she is feeling about the event and about the way in which the therapist chose to respond to it) and strive toward mutual understanding if the client does not feel the event has been adequately resolved

Interpersonal events typically intensify any underlying vulnerabilities or challenging aspects of a client's interpersonal style, thus increasing the necessity to select the best response. Therapeutic responding and the underlying process of interpersonal reasoning rely heavily upon therapists' use of modes and the extent of development of their interpersonal knowledge base. IRM provides a reasoning tree process that helps guide the therapist through the steps of therapeutic reasoning.

Developing One's Interpersonal Skill Base

Intentional therapists, according to IRM, draw upon nine areas of interpersonal skills. (i.e., therapeutic communication; establishing relationships; interviewing and strategic questioning; understanding families, social systems, and group dynamics; understanding and managing difficult interpersonal behavior; resolving empathic breaks and conflicts; maintaining professional behavior, values, and ethics; working effectively with supervisors, employers, and other professionals; and professional development to become better

therapists). Taylor (2008) provides detailed explanations of each of these skill areas and with them a variety of resources for self-assessment and self-development.

Developing one's interpersonal skills helps one to promote healthy, functional relationships with clients and other members of the treatment team. A therapist's ability to draw upon these skills effectively during therapist-client interactions can enhance the therapeutic alliance and help ensure more positive therapy outcomes. Each therapist has innate areas of strength and weakness for therapeutic interaction. IRM encourages and provides resources (self-assessments, reflection exercises, and examples from other therapists) for therapists to develop awareness of their interpersonal strengths and weaknesses and to strive to develop the capacity for better therapeutic responding over time.

Research and Evidence Base

Because IRM is a new model, research on its concepts and application has yet to be developed. As a prelude to developing IRM, Taylor and colleagues undertook a national study of therapeutic use of self in occupational therapy (Taylor, Lee, Kielhofner, & Ketkar, in press). In this study, over 90% of therapists reported that their relationships with clients affected occupational engagement and over 80% felt that therapeutic use of self was the most important skill in their practice and the key determinant of occupational therapy outcomes. These findings are consistent with claims in the occupational therapy literature about the importance of the therapeutic relationship. The study also found that occupational therapists are frequently challenged to deal with difficult emotions and behaviors in the therapeutic relationship.

Despite the acknowledged importance of the therapeutic relationship, the vast majority of the practitioners in this study did not feel that sufficient knowledge about the therapeutic relationship and therapeutic use of self exists within the field of occupational therapy. Their views strongly supported the need for IRM to be developed.

Another important empirical foundation of IRM is Taylor's (2008) detailed examination of occupational therapists identified as having exceptional skill in the therapeutic use of self. Not only did information about the everyday practice of these therapists inform development of IRM, but these therapists are used extensively in the IRM text to illustrate its concepts.

There is also evidence from other research that supports the importance and content of IRM. Based on their study of occupational therapists in general rehabilitation, Allison and Strong (1994) concluded that good clinical communicators were able to accommodate their interactions to meet their clients' needs as recommended in IRM. Cole and McLean (2003) found that therapists perceived the therapeutic relationship as critical to therapy outcomes and emphasized rapport, open communication, and empathy (all components stressed by IRM) as important. Palmadottir (2006) concluded from her research that occupational therapists needed to have more awareness of how their own attitudes are communicated and acted out in therapy as is emphasized in IRM. Eklund and Hallberg (2001) concluded from their research that verbal interaction was a significant component of the therapeutic relationship, underscoring the IRM assertion that doing and talking need to be balanced in occupational therapy. Further research will be needed to test both the theoretical assertions of this new model and to determine its impact in therapy.

Discussion

Occupational therapy has always emphasized the importance of therapists' interactions with clients. The last three decades have witnessed a growing literature on the therapist-client interaction and, as discussed in Chapter 5, the importance of the therapeutic relationship is central to the field's contemporary paradigm. Despite this, there has not previously been a single coherent approach to conceptualizing the therapeutic relationship in occupational therapy. The intentional relationship model, thus, represents the first systematic explanation of the interpersonal relationship in occupational therapy and the first model to specifically address how to enact the therapeutic relationship.

Box 10.2

Intentional Relationship Model Case Example: JOE

The following case was developed by Emily Ashpole, a newly trained occupational therapist who studied the intentional relationship model from its developer, Dr. Renee Taylor. Emily not only relates how she used the model but also reflects on her therapeutic use of self, which is part of the process of developing one's ability to use the model.

Joe is a 50-year-old Hungarian immigrant who was diagnosed with malignant brain tumors several years ago. He was receiving intensive outpatient occupational therapy services due to impaired function in his right upper extremity. The most noteworthy of Joe's enduring interpersonal characteristics were his affect, communication style, capacity to assert needs, and response to change or challenge. That is, Joe generally presented as cheerful and friendly, smiling at other patients and his therapists. He was thoughtful about communicating his ideas and feelings and would often engage in conversation during therapy. He was not shy about telling people what he needed between sessions. Nor was he reluctant to tell me when an activity was too easy or difficult or when he needed something positioned, for example, to continue with the activity more independently. Joe generally tackled challenging therapeutic activities with effort and determination. He conveyed a strong work ethic and the desire to improve his ability to participate in daily activities.

Joe's treatment day typically began with a short, supervised session in which he engaged in a therapeutic activity that required only set-up. On one particular day, Joe was participating in an activity focused on grasp and release, using his impaired upper extremity. He had performed this activity on many occasions, which had resulted in his own awareness of his progress. This day, however, an interpersonal event of therapy occurred during the activity.

This "typical" grasp and release activity for him became an emotionally charged therapy task. Joe took a lot of pride in the fact that he had built up an ability to complete this task well

(box continues on page 142)

Box 10.2 (continued)

and within a certain time frame. In his own mind, he associated his newfound ability with hope that his cancer was not progressing. I was soon to learn that any setback in his performance of this task threatened this budding sense of hope, and this is why this particular task was emotionally charged for Joe.

Though I did not know it at the time, the difference for Joe on this day was that he was experiencing a severe escalation in fatigue and pain. At this time, the task was not only painful for him, but more importantly Joe was acutely aware that he was not performing the task as well or as quickly as he normally would. Since Joe did not tell me what he was thinking or how he was feeling at the time, I had to rely on my own observations of his affect and other nonverbal cues.

As I observed his performance, I, too, noticed his decreased proficiency with the task. He paused more than usual, cast his eyes downwards, and at one point slumped in his chair. At another point he let out a gasp of exasperation. His frustration and disappointment, and likely his worry, were all evident in his face and behaviors.

In addition to noticing these nonverbal cues, which I considered as interpersonal events in themselves, I realized that Joe was displaying situational interpersonal characteristics that differed from his usual presentation. He appeared discontent and disappointed. In contrast to his usually buoyant and occasionally cheerful attitude, Joe displayed a sullen affect and avoided making eye

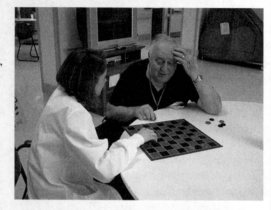

Emily realizes that her client is becoming frustrated with the activity.

contact with me. Different from his typically open and direct communication style, he elected not to tell me about his thoughts or feelings. Moreover, he was unable to communicate what, if anything, he needed in order to continue with the activity. Most importantly, he ultimately gave up during the task, a response that was vastly different than his usual behavior during moments of change or challenge. This collection of behaviors, in addition to the direct observation of his performance, indicated that he was struggling at that point in time.

After observing his nonverbal cues and reasoning that he was overwhelmed, I relied on the empathizing mode, as is recommended in IRM. I showed activity-focused communication by leaning toward him and placing my hand on his arm. I also attempted to show interpersonal-focused communication by verbalizing to him what I thought he was communicating through his expressions and behaviors. I tried to label what I observed by saying to Joe, "You seem overwhelmed by the difficulty you are having with this activity today." After he confirmed the accuracy of my statement by giving a head nod, I stated my concern about his abandonment of the activity since it was atypical behavior for him. These statements served as an opening for Joe to elaborate on how he was feeling and what he was thinking about his current difficulties. We engaged in a discussion that helped me to understand his perceptions of his poor performance and his concerns that his performance difficulties were a potential sign of the spread of his cancer.

As Joe told me about what he had been experiencing and worrying about, I did my best to use the skill of empathic listening, one of the elements of therapeutic listening. When it appeared that we came to an understanding of the event and his nonverbal cues indicated that he was no longer overwhelmed, I knew that a mode shift was needed in order to proceed with the session. That is, I needed to shift to the problem-solving mode in order to discuss with Joe how he should proceed with exploring the possibility that his illness was progressing. After a brief discussion, we decided that Joe would make an appointment to meet with his oncologist to discuss his concerns.

Box 10.2 (continued)

Emily's Reflection

Applying the IRM in practice can be complex. To be able to respond therapeutically in the moment requires many skills and a great deal of awareness. I realized in retrospect that I should have intervened earlier by shifting modes. That is, I might have intervened sooner so that this client did not struggle to the point of feeling overwhelmed and subsequently giving up. Although I recognized that his reaction in therapy was atypical for Joe, I also was aware that he typically communicated his needs, and thus I had learned not to intervene too early. In hindsight, I could have been more attentive to the extent of his increased fatigue and mood and shifted out of the instructing mode earlier.

Table 10.4 **Terms of the Model**

Activity focusing	Strategies of responding to interpersonal events that emphasize doing over feeling or relating.
Critical self-awareness	A general knowledge of one's interpersonal tendencies while interacting with clients of different personalities and under different conditions and circumstances.
Desired occupation	The task or activity that the therapist and the client have selected for therapy.
Emotionally charged therapy task	An activity or situation that can cause clients to become overwhelmed or results in unpleasant emotional reactions like shame, embarrassment, or humiliation.
Enduring characteristics	Stable aspects of the client's interpersonal behavior.
Interpersonal event	A naturally occurring communication, reaction, process, task, or general circumstance that occurs during therapy and that has the potential to detract from or strengthen the therapeutic relationship.
Interpersonal focusing	Strategies that emphasize feeling or relating over doing.
Interpersonal reasoning	A step-wise process by which a therapist decides what to say, do, or express in reaction to the occurrence of an interpersonal dilemma in therapy.
Interpersonal self-discipline	Anticipating, measuring, and responding to the effects of ongoing communication with a client.
Interpersonal skill base	A continuum of skills that must be judiciously applied by the therapist to build a functional working relationship with the client.
Interpersonal style	The therapeutic mode or set of modes typically used when interacting with a client.
Mindful empathy	An objective mode of observation in which the therapist comes to feel and understand a client's underlying emotions, needs, and motives, while at the same time maintaining an objective viewpoint.

(table continues on page 144)

Table 10.4 **Terms of the Model continued**

Mode shift	A conscious change in one's way of relating to a client.
Ongoing critical awareness	A constant mindfulness about what one is communicating verbally, nonverbally, and emotionally.
Situational characteristics	Aspects of a client's acute emotional reaction to a specific situation.
Therapeutic mode	A specific way of relating to a client.
Therapeutic relationship	A socially defined and personally interpreted interactive process between a therapist and client.

SUMMARY: THE INTENTIONAL RELATIONSHIP MODEL

✦ The intentional relationship model explains how the relationship between client and therapist affects the overall process of occupational therapy and how that relationship can be used to enhance occupational therapy outcomes

Theory

✦ IRM views the therapeutic relationship as being composed of:
  • The client
  • The interpersonal events that occur during therapy
  • The therapist
  • The occupation

✦ IRM emphasizes that it is the therapist's responsibility to develop a positive relationship with the client

✦ In order to develop this relationship and respond appropriately to the client, a therapist must work to understand the client's situational and enduring interpersonal characteristics.

✦ An interpersonal event occurs naturally during therapy and has the potential to detract from or strengthen the therapeutic relationship

✦ When optimally responded to, interpersonal events are opportunities for positive client learning or change and for solidifying the therapeutic relationship

✦ The therapist is responsible for making every reasonable effort to make the relationship work. The therapist brings three main interpersonal capacities into the relationship:
  • An interpersonal skill base
  • Therapeutic modes (or interpersonal styles)
  • Capacity for interpersonal reasoning

✦ The desired occupation refers to the task or activity that the therapist and the client have selected for therapy

✦ The therapeutic relationship functions as:
  • A support to occupational engagement
  • A place where the emotional and coping processes associated with the client's impairment and its implications for occupational performance are addressed

✦ This relationship can be viewed at two different levels or scales:
  • Macro-level (i.e., the ongoing enduring rapport and patterns of interaction between client and therapist)
  • Micro-level (i.e., the moment-by-moment therapeutic relationship as influenced by interpersonal events of therapy that have the potential to challenge or enrich the relationship)

✦ IRM underscores that the occupational therapist must assume the ultimate responsibility for the relationship

✦ Failure to respond adequately to interpersonal events may negatively affect occupational engagement and weaken the therapeutic relationship

✦ Ten fundamental principles underlie this model:
  • Critical self-awareness is key to the intentional use of self
  • Interpersonal self-discipline is fundamental to effective use of self
  • It is necessary to keep head before heart
  • Mindful empathy is required to know your client
  • Grow your interpersonal knowledge base
  • Provided that they are purely and flexibly applied, a wide range of therapeutic modes can work and be utilized interchangeably in occupational therapy
  • The client defines a successful relationship
  • Activity focusing must be balanced with interpersonal focusing
  • Application of the model must be informed by core values and ethics
  • Cultural competency is central to practice

Practice Resources

✦ The resources of the model are focused on helping therapists better understand both their clients' and their own interpersonal characteristics and on helping therapists become more able to monitor and respond to the inevitable interpersonal events of therapy. They include:
  • Materials and procedures for better understanding and monitoring clients' interpersonal characteristics
  • Resources for identifying inevitable interpersonal events in therapy
  • A format for applying interpersonal reasoning
  • Guidelines and materials for developing one's interpersonal skill base (conflict resolution)

✦ Actively seeking to know and understand each client's interpersonal characteristics (client emotions, behaviors, and reactions that occur in interactions between the client and therapist) is essential to an intentional

and tailored relationship in which the client feels comfortable

✦ IRM identifies 12 categories of interpersonal characteristics
  • Communication style
  • Capacity for trust
  • Need for control
  • Capacity to assert needs
  • Response to change and challenge
  • Affect
  • Predisposition to giving feedback
  • Capacity to receive feedback
  • Response to human diversity
  • Orientation toward relating
  • Preference for touch
  • Capacity for reciprocity

✦ In addition to being aware of a client's tendency to display certain interpersonal characteristics, therapists must also be vigilant during therapy to:
  • Recognize a client's emotion, reaction, or behavior
  • Understand its source
  • Consciously and reflectively consider options for how to act
  • Monitor the client's response

✦ Self-knowledge and self-discipline are key to becoming an intentional and interpersonally effective therapist

✦ The ideal is a multi-modal therapist whose use of modes reflects a vigilant understanding of the client's unfolding needs rather than one's personal comfort zone

✦ Interpersonal events are distinguished from other therapy events in that they are emotionally charged and ripe with both threat and opportunity

✦ If ignored, they can lead to difficulties in the therapeutic relationship and negatively affect occupational engagement. If addressed appropriately these events may lead to positive outcomes that involve feelings such as gratification, fulfillment, satisfaction, or intimacy

✦ Interpersonal reasoning is "the process by which a therapist monitors the interpersonal events of therapy, the client's unique interpersonal characteristics, and her or his own behavior in a reflective way to maximize the likelihood that the therapeutic relationship will be successful and supportive of the client's engagement in occupation"

✦ Interpersonal reasoning involves six steps:
  • Anticipate interpersonal events or client behaviors that may test, challenge, or threaten the therapeutic relationship
  • Accurately identify interpersonal events and coping
  • Determine if a mode shift is required
  • Choose a response mode or a sequence of modes
  • Draw upon any relevant interpersonal skills associated with the mode(s) in responding
  • Gather feedback and strive toward mutual understanding if the client does not feel the event has been adequately resolved

✦ A therapist's ability to effectively draw upon his or her interpersonal skills during therapist-client interactions can enhance the therapeutic alliance and help ensure more positive therapy outcomes

REFERENCES

Allison, H., & Strong, J. (1994). Verbal strategies used by occupational therapists in direct client encounters. *Occupational Therapy Journal of Research, 14*, 112–29.

American Occupational Therapy Association. (1993). Core values and attitudes of occupational therapy practice. *American Journal of Occupational Therapy, 47,* 1085–1086.

American Occupational Therapy Association. (2005). Occupational therapy code of ethics. *American Journal of Occupational Therapy, 59,* 639–642.

Cole, B., & McLean, V. (2003). Therapeutic relationships re-defined. *Occupational Therapy in Mental Health, 19*(2), 33–56.

Eklund, M., & Hallberg, I. (2001). Psychiatric occupational therapists' verbal interaction with their clients. *Occupational Therapy International, 8*(1), 1–16.

Palmadottir, G. (2006). Client-therapist relationships: Experiences of occupational therapy clients in rehabilitation. *British Journal of Occupational Therapy, 69,* 394–401.

Taylor, R. (2008). *The intentional relationship: Occupational therapy and use of self.* Philadelphia: F.A. Davis.

Taylor, R., Lee, S.W., Kielhofner, G., & Ketkar, M. (in press). The therapeutic relationship: A nationwide survey of practitioners' attitudes and experiences. *American Journal of Occupational Therapy.*

CHAPTER 11

The Model of Human Occupation

A client works in a café that is operated to provide work training and experience for persons with mental health problems. With the support and guidance of an occupational therapist, the client has opportunities to develop a sense of competence and satisfaction in working. He will also develop the habits and skills necessary for success in the workplace. Importantly, the program also allows the client to take on the role of worker in a real life context where the ordinary demands and expecta-

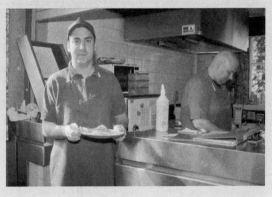

tions, as well as the social identity of the role, are present. Like other programs based on the model of human occupation, this one emphasizes engagement in meaningful occupations to address multiple personal and environmental factors that influence occupational adaptation.

Katie Fortier is helping 9-year-old Victoria, who has diagnoses of bipolar disorder and attention-deficit hyperactivity disorder, work on a range of factors that influence her performance in school. Victoria was referred to occupational therapy due to behavioral outbursts, difficulty with social-ization, and problems at school involving following rules and paying attention. Katie has carefully assessed Victoria in order to understand what her interests are and how she feels about her ability to do the kinds of things that are required in school. By guiding Victoria to participate in person-ally motivating activities, Katie is helping

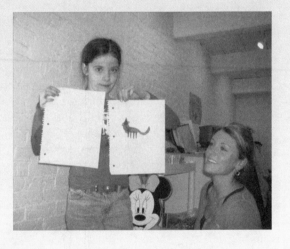

Victoria develop necessary skills (e.g., following directions, problem-solving). The intervention also reinforces positive habits that support Victoria's role as a student. Katie provides a safe and supportive environment for Victoria and serves as a positive role model for involvement in therapeutic activities. Overall, Katie's approach is holistic, in that it considers multiple factors that influence Victoria's success as a student, and client-centered, in that it reflects a thorough understanding of Katie's thoughts, feelings, and desires as well as her unique challenges.

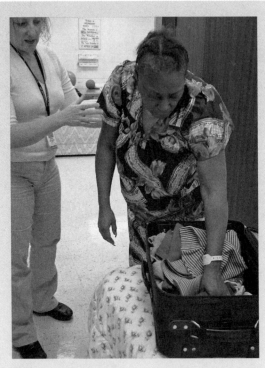

Following a subarachnoid hemorrhage, Magnolia underwent a craniotomy and clipping of three aneurysms. She subsequently experienced residual left-sided weakness and inattention. Her treatment goals for occupational therapy included increasing her independence as well as improving the use of her affected side. Magnolia was very determined to return to her prior level of function. However, her immediate occupational goal was to be able to attend a previously planned family trip to Las Vegas, which was scheduled for one week after her discharge from rehabilitation. Given the importance of this goal to Magnolia, Erica Mauldin, her occupational therapist, organized treatment sessions to address the various tasks that Magnolia would need to perform to make the trip. Packing, transporting, and unpacking a suitcase allowed Magnolia to practice these activities prior to her trip. At the same time, these activities that reflected Magnolia's priorities allowed her to develop a sense of confidence as well as improve her endurance and use of her left side.

T hese three scenarios are characteristic of interventions based on the model of human occupation (MOHO). Work on MOHO began in the 1970s when the contemporary paradigm and its emphasis on occupation were emerging. In addition to its focus on occupation, MOHO also emphasized the importance of client-centered practice that reflected clients' values and desires. At that time, occupational therapy practice still focused mainly on understanding and reducing impairment. MOHO recognized that many factors beyond motor, cognitive, and sensory impairments contribute to difficulties in everyday occupation. These included problems or challenges in relation to:

• The motivation for occupation
• Maintaining positive involvement in life roles and routines
• Skilled performance of necessary life tasks
• The influence of physical and social environment (Kielhofner & Burke, 1980)

MOHO focuses on these factors. Because this model addresses broad issues faced by clients with a variety of impairments and throughout the life course, it is used in many types of intervention settings and with a wide range of populations. MOHO has also been used with clients at quite different levels of functioning. This includes both people with severe disabilities and those without disabilities who have received wellness-based services based on MOHO.

Theory

MOHO is ultimately concerned with individuals' participation and adaptation in life occupations (see Fig. 11.1). The model postulates that:

• A person's characteristics and the external environment are linked together into a dynamic whole
• Occupation reflects the influence of both the person's characteristics and the environment
• A person's inner characteristics (i.e., capacities, motives, and patterns of performance) are maintained and changed through engaging in occupations

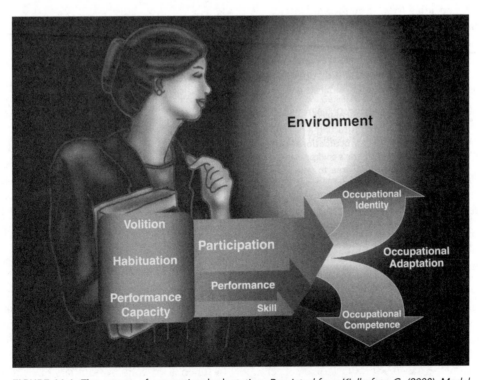

FIGURE 11.1 The process of occupational adaptation. *Reprinted from Kielhofner, G. (2008). Model of human occupation: Theory and application (4th ed.). Baltimore: Lippincott Williams & Wilkins.*

Concepts Related to the Person's Characteristics

MOHO conceptualizes the person's inner characteristics as three interacting elements: volition, habituation, and performance capacity (Kielhofner, 2008). Volition refers to the person's motivation for occupation. Habituation refers to how the person organizes performance into roles and routines. Performance capacity refers to the person's abilities for performance. Each of these concepts is explained further.

Volition

Volition is the process by which people are motivated toward and choose the activities they do. It begins with the universal human desire to do things and is shaped by life experiences. Volition consists of thoughts and feelings that occur in a cycle of:

* Anticipating possibilities for doing (e.g., looking forward to a weekend outing, worrying about an upcoming exam, feeling challenged and excited about a new job assignment)
* Choosing what to do (e.g., starting a new hobby, deciding to work in the yard after work, deciding to spend another hour studying for an exam in order to be better prepared)
* Experiencing what one does (e.g., enjoying a favorite pastime, feeling confident about how one completed a work task)
* Subsequent interpretation of the experience (e.g., reflecting on how well one performed during an activity or recalling how enjoyable it was to do an activity)

The thoughts and feelings that make up volition are referred to as personal causation, values, and interests; they concern, respectively:

* How capable and effective one feels
* What one holds as important or meaningful
* What one finds enjoyable and satisfying

Personal causation refers to the thoughts and feelings about personal capacities and effectiveness that people have as they do everyday activities. These include, for example, recognizing strengths and weaknesses, feeling confident or anxious when faced with a task, and reflecting on how well one did following performance.

Values are beliefs and commitments about what is good, right, and important to do. They reflect one's beliefs about what is worth doing, how to perform, and what goals or aspirations deserve commitment. People experience a sense of worth and belonging when they engage in activities that enact their values.

Interests are generated through the experience of pleasure and satisfaction in occupation. They begin with natural dispositions (e.g., the tendency to enjoy physical or intellectual activity). They further develop through the experience of pleasure and satisfaction derived from occupational engagement. Therefore, the development of interests depends on available opportunities to engage in occupations.

Volition (i.e., the cycle of thoughts and feelings that reflect one's personal causation, values, and interests) has a pervasive influence on occupational life (Kielhofner, 2008). It shapes:

* How people see the opportunities and challenges in their environment
* What people choose to do
* How they experience and make sense of what they have done

How people experience life and regard themselves and their world is largely a function of their volition. Importantly, when people experience impairments, their volition can be severely affected. People may experience themselves as losing capacities and being unable to perform as they feel is important. They may not develop or no longer enjoy activities of interest.

When volition is negatively impacted, people may make decisions that worsen or amplify the impact of their impairments. For instance, feelings of helplessness and hopelessness may lead them to avoid activities that could build their confidence and abilities. Such volitional decisions may also contribute to further loss of skills. Thus, occupational therapy based on MOHO often involves identifying and addressing clients' volitional problems. MOHO emphasizes that volition is also central to occupational therapy since the therapy process requires clients to make choices to do things. Finally, how clients experience what they do in therapy (a function of volition) to a large extent determines therapy outcomes (Kielhofner, 2008).

Habituation

Habituation is a process whereby people organize their actions into patterns and routines. Through repeated action within specific contexts, people establish habituated patterns of doing. These patterns of action are governed by habits and roles. Together, they shape how people go about the routine aspects of their lives. Because of roles and habits, most routines of daily life unfold automatically and predictably.

Habits involve learned ways of doing things that unfold automatically. They operate in cooperation with context, using and incorporating the environment as a resource for doing familiar things. They influence how people perform routine activities, use time, and behave. For instance, habits shape how one intuitively goes about self-care each morning. One's weekly routine is largely a function of habits. Even the way one completes a familiar activity is influenced by habits.

Roles give people an identity and a sense of the obligations that go with that identity. People may see themselves as students, workers, or volunteers and know how they should behave in order to fulfill those roles. Much of what people do is guided by the roles they inhabit. Roles are defined by the social system of which the role is a part (e.g., school, workplace, family, community) and by the expectations of others in that system. For instance, a child entering the role of student in grade school learns what it means to be a student from expectations given by teachers as well as attitudes and behaviors displayed by other students. The same process occurs for worker, family, volunteer, and other roles.

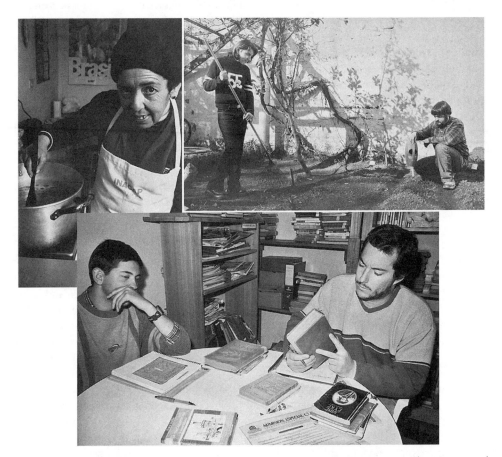

In a community rehabilitation center in Chile, clients engage in preparing a noon meal, maintaining the center's library, and clearing the grounds. This program provides these, and other real life occupations, as a means of enhancing clients' skills, habits, roles, and sense of meaning and efficacy in doing things.

Learning a new role involves internalizing an identity, an outlook, and an expected way of behaving.

The habits and roles that make up habituation guide how people interact with their physical, temporal, and social environments. When habituation is challenged by impairments or environmental circumstances, people can lose a great deal of what has given life familiarity, consistency, and relative ease. For example, a serious impairment such as a spinal cord injury may eliminate or interrupt all of one's occupational roles and may require one to learn a whole new set of everyday habits. Chronic conditions such as serious mental illness may interfere with developing normal roles and with establishing a functional routine guided by habits. One of the major tasks of therapy is to construct or reconstruct habits and roles so that the person can more readily participate in everyday occupations.

Performance Capacity

Performance capacity refers to underlying mental and physical abilities and how they are used and experienced in performance. The capacity for performance is affected by the status of musculoskeletal, neurological, cardiopulmonary, and other bodily systems that are called on when a person does things. Performance also calls on mental or cognitive abilities such as memory. Consequently, the biomechanical, motor control, cognitive, and sensory integration models that are discussed in this book are necessary for addressing this aspect of performance capacity. MOHO recognizes the importance of these models for addressing physical and mental capacities for performance and is typically used in conjunction with such models.

At the same time, MOHO stresses the importance of attending to the experience of performance and, in particular, the experience of having limitations in performance. It asserts that therapists should pay careful attention to how people experience impairments (e.g., paying attention to how people's bodies feel to them and how they perceive the world when they have impairments). For example, people with a variety of physical impairments frequently report feeling alienated from their bodies. According to MOHO, occupational therapy can support people to reclaim their bodies experientially and to integrate their bodies into new ways of doing things.

MOHO Concepts Concerning the Environment

MOHO stresses that occupation results from an interaction of the inner characteristics of the person (volition, habituation, and performance capacity) with the environment (Kielhofner, 2008). The **environment** includes the particular physical, social, cultural, economic, and political features within a person's context that influence the motivation, organization, and performance of occupation. Several dimensions of the environment may have an impact on occupation. These include physical spaces, objects, and people, as well as expectations and opportunities for doing things. Moreover, culture, economic conditions, and political factors also have an influence. Accordingly, the environment includes:

- The objects that people use when they do things
- The spaces within which people do things
- The occupational forms or tasks that are available, expected, and/or required of people in a given context
- The social groups (e.g., family, friends, coworkers, neighbors) that make up the context
- The surrounding culture; political and economic forces

For example, political and economic conditions determine what resources people have for doing things and culture shapes beliefs about how one should perform and what is worth doing. Further, the demands of a task can determine the extent to which a person feels confident or anxious. How well objects and spaces are suited to capacity of the individual influences how the person performs. In these and many other ways, the environment influences what people do and how they think and feel about their doing. In turn, people also may choose and modify their environments. For instance, people select environments that match and allow them to realize their values and interests.

Dimensions of Doing

As Figure 11.1 shows, MOHO identifies three levels for examining what a person does:

- Occupational participation
- Occupational performance
- Occupational skill (Kielhofner, 2008)

Occupational participation refers to engaging in work, play, or activities of daily living that are part of one's sociocultural context and that are desired and/or necessary to one's well-being. Examples of occupational participation are working in a full- or part-time job, pursuing a hobby, doing routine self-care, maintaining one's home, and attending school. Each area of occupational participation involves a cluster of related activities. For example, maintaining one's home may include such things as paying the rent, doing repairs, and cleaning. The process of doing such occupational forms or tasks is referred to as **occupational performance**. Moreover, this occupational performance requires discrete purposeful actions. For example, making a sandwich is a culturally recognizable occupational form or task in many cultures. To do so, one *gathers* together bread and other ingredients such as meat, cheese, lettuce, and condiments; one *handles* these materials; and one *sequences* the steps necessary to construct the sandwich. These discrete actions (gathering, handling, and sequencing) along with other such actions that make up occupational performance are referred to as skills.

Skills are goal-directed actions that a person uses while performing (Fisher, 1998; Fisher & Kielhofner, 1995; Forsyth, Salamy, Simon, & Kielhofner, 1998). In contrast to performance capacity, which refers to underlying ability (e.g., range of motion and strength), skill refers to the purposeful actions that make up occupational performance. There are three categories of skills: motor skills, process skills, and communication and interaction skills. Definitions and examples of each category of skill are shown in Table 11.1.

Occupational Identity, Competence, and Adaptation

Over time, people create their own **occupational identity,** the cumulative sense of who they are and wish to become as occupational beings. The degree to which people are able to sustain a pattern of doing that enacts their occupational identity is referred to as **occupational competence.** As Figure 11.1 shows, **occupational adaptation** refers to the process of creating and enacting a positive occupational identity.

People achieve coherence and meaning in their occupational identity through narratives. An **occupational narrative** is a story (both told and enacted) that integrates across time one's unfolding volition, habituation, performance

Table 11.1   **Definitions and Examples of Skill Categories**

Skill Category	Definition	Examples
Motor	Moving self or task objects (Fisher, 1999).	Stabilizing and bending one's body and manipulating, lifting, and transporting objects.
Process	Logically sequencing actions over time, selecting and using appropriate tools and materials, and adapting performance when encountering problems (Fisher, 1999).	Choosing and organizing objects in space as well as initiating and terminating steps in performance.
Communication and Interaction	Conveying intentions and needs and coordinating social action to act together with people (Forsyth et al., 1998; Forsyth, Lai, & Kielhofner, 1999).	Gesturing, physically contacting others, speaking, engaging and collaborating with others, and asserting oneself.

capacity, and environments and that sums up and assigns meaning to these elements. Occupational narratives can either impede or focus occupational adaptation. For example, if someone's narrative portrays life as a tragedy, there is little reason to work toward goals. On the other hand, if someone's narrative portrays life as getting better, he or she will likely be motivated to work hard toward that outcome. Research has shown that occupational narratives predict future adaptation of occupational therapy clients (Kielhofner, Braveman, et al., 2004; Kielhofner, Braveman, Fogg, & Levin, 2008).

There are situations in which one is unable to enact the life story one envisions and desires. There is evidence that following onset of disability, many persons may initially experience a gap between the identity reflected in their narratives and what they are able to enact (Kielhofner, Mallinson, Forsyth, & Lai, 2001; Mallinson, Mahaffey, & Kielhofner, 1998). These same studies also suggest that one cannot have competence without an intact identity. Occupational adaptation begins with what one imagines in the occupational narrative. In the end the occupational narrative determines the meaning people assign to occupational life and guides how they seek to enact occupational life.

> **MOHO conceptualizes occupational therapy as a process in which clients engage in occupations that shape their abilities, routine ways of doing things, and thoughts and feelings about themselves.**

Change and the Process of Therapy

MOHO asserts that all change in occupational therapy is driven by clients' **occupational engagement** (i.e., clients' doing, thinking, and feeling under certain environmental conditions in the midst of therapy or as a planned consequence of therapy). Thus, MOHO conceptualizes occupational therapy as a process in which clients engage in occupations that shape their abilities, routine ways of doing things, and thoughts and feelings about themselves. Moreover, when clients engage in occupations, volition, habituation, and performance capacity are all involved in some way. For example, in any moment of therapy, a client may be:

- Practicing skills necessary for occupational performance
- Learning new habits that shape how the occupational performance is done
- Enacting a new role
- Experiencing satisfaction and enjoyment
- Valuing the accomplishment
- Feeling competent at performance

Each of these aspects of what the client does, thinks, and feels is essential to the process of therapy. For this reason, therapists using MOHO concepts are mindful of their clients' volition, habituation, performance capacity, and environmental conditions. Therapists monitor how these elements interact as therapy unfolds. To help therapists think about the process of occupational engagement, MOHO identifies the nine dimensions of occupational engagement shown in Table 11.2. They provide a basic structure for thinking about how clients achieve change and for planning how therapy goals will be achieved.

Practice Resources

Extensive resources have been developed for this model. They include a therapeutic reasoning process, a wide range of assessments, standardized programs and intervention protocols, and a large number of case examples.

Therapeutic Reasoning

Therapeutic reasoning is a process for MOHO concepts and resources to understand and address clients' needs. Therapeutic reasoning involves six steps:

- Generating questions about the client
- Gathering information on, from, and with the client
- Using the information gathered to create an explanation of the client's situation
- Generating goals and strategies for therapy
- Implementing and monitoring therapy
- Determining outcomes of therapy

Table 11.2   Definitions and Examples of the Dimensions of Client Occupational Engagement

Dimension	Definition	Examples
Choose/decide	Anticipate and select from alternatives for action.	Decide whether to role-play a job interview or work on a resume during a vocationally oriented therapy session.
Commit	Decide to undertake a course of action to accomplish a goal, fulfill a role, or establish a new habit.	Decide to enroll in a training program to develop skills for a particular job.
Explore	Investigate new objects, spaces, social groups, and/or occupational forms/tasks; do things with altered performance capacity; try out new ways of doing things; examine possibilities for occupational participation in one's context.	Play with a new toy; try out a new motorized wheelchair.
Identify	Locate novel information, alternatives for action, and new feelings that provide solutions for and/or give meaning to occupational performance and participation.	Recognize how one's values result in decisions to engage in occupations beyond one's capacity, leading to failure.
Negotiate	Engage in a give-and-take with others that creates mutually agreed-upon perspectives and/or finds a middle group between different expectations, plans, or desires.	Mutually decide upon treatment goals with the occupational therapist.
Plan	Establish an action agenda for performance or participation.	Determine what steps are necessary to complete a task or achieve a goal.
Practice	Repeat a certain performance or consistently participate in an occupation with the intent of increasing skill, ease, and effectiveness of performance.	Work toward learning to transfer from a wheelchair to bed by repeating it with supervision from an occupational therapist.
Reexamine	Critically appraise and consider alternatives to previously held beliefs, attitudes, feelings, habits, or roles.	Rethink ways that one can still enjoy leisure activities involving sports, following an injury that limits capacity to do the activities.
Sustain	Persist in occupational performance or participation despite uncertainty or difficulty.	Continue working toward learning a skill despite anxiety associated with performance.

MOHO emphasizes that therapeutic reasoning must be client-centered in that:

• The process reflects a deep appreciation for the client's circumstances
• The client is involved in the process to the extent possible

Therapists may move back and forth between the steps of therapeutic reasoning, which are

briefly described here. The box featuring a young client named Drew and the case at the end of the chapter also illustrate this therapeutic reasoning process.

Generating Questions

Therapists must understand their clients before planning therapy. This understanding begins

---

Box 11.1 An Example of the Process of Therapeutic Reasoning

Drew is a first grader who has difficulty keeping his attention focused in the classroom and when doing homework. His parents have reported that he had been increasingly dreading going to school. Drew has been having particular difficulty with his homework assignments. Recently he started ignoring some of his homework assignments altogether. Drew's occupational therapist agreed to evaluate this difficulty with homework and develop a therapy plan. In doing so, she followed the therapeutic reasoning process.

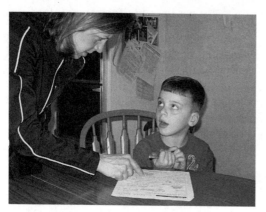

Drew's mother supports him in completing his homework.

Generating Questions: The therapist began by generating questions to guide her approach to Drew. Since making decisions about doing one's homework is a function of volition, the occupational therapist began with questions about Drew's volition: Does he value school? What are his feelings about his ability to do schoolwork (especially homework)?

Gathering Information: The therapist gathered information from the teacher and from Drew's parents using brief interviews. She also briefly observed Drew in the classroom and then met with him to discuss how he approaches his homework. The

therapist learned that Drew's parents highly value school performance and that Drew very much wants to please his parents. The therapist observed in the classroom that Drew was having difficulty organizing his school materials. When she asked Drew about homework, he admitted that while he sometimes found homework difficult, he also sometimes lost his homework assignments or forgot they were in his backpack. After missing several homework assignments he admitted that he "kind of gave up."

Creating a Theory-Based Explanation: Based on the information she gathered, the therapist arrived at a theory-based understanding of Drew's homework difficulties. She reasoned that while Drew has positive values about school and wants to do well, he has a poor sense of efficacy (i.e., he believes he will fail to get his homework assignments completed because of past failures). Drew's feelings of inefficacy have led him to choose to avoid homework (in Drew's words, "giving up") that, in turn, leads to further failure and a poorer sense of efficacy. She also noted that Drew's feelings are based on a genuine difficulty organizing his school materials.

Therapy Goals and Strategies: Thus she generated the following therapy goals:

• Drew's sense of efficacy for completing homework will increase
• Drew will consistently make choices to do homework

In order to achieve these goals, the therapist came up with the following plan for Drew's occupational engagement. She decided that Drew would create and learn to use a system of organizing with a homework folder. She felt it was important that Drew be a partner with her in coming up with how he could use the folder to be more organized. She also decided that she would validate Drew's feelings, collaborate with him to get the folder labeled,

Box 11.1   **An Example of the Process of Therapeutic Reasoning** continued

and develop a plan to use it. She also decided to let Drew's teacher and parents know about the folder and how Drew planned to use it, so that they could also support him.

Monitoring and Determining Outcomes: Drew's therapist planned to monitor's Drew's reaction as

they worked on the folder and also to check in with his teacher and parents to see if he was able to more successfully follow through on doing his homework.

---

with asking questions about each client. MOHO concepts provide a framework for generating these questions. For example, therapists using MOHO ask what their clients' thoughts and feelings are in relation to personal causation, values, and interests. Moreover, they ask about their clients' roles and habits and how these things affect the clients' routines. Such questions are, of course, tailored to the clients' circumstances (e.g., age and impairment).

Gathering Information

Therapists must gather information on, from, and with the client in order to answer the questions they have generated about the client. Such information gathering may take advantage of informal, naturally occurring opportunities. For example, a therapist might learn about a client's personal causation by observing the client's behavior when facing a challenging new task or by engaging in a conversation about the client's concerns over some future task or role.

Therapists also use structured MOHO assessments. Some of these assessments focus on specific factors such as interests and roles while others capture comprehensive information on several aspects of the person and the environment. A wide range of MOHO-based assessments have been developed; they are summarized in Table 11.3. All of these assessments may be obtained free of charge or purchased on the MOHO website (http://www.moho.uic.edu/).

Creating a Theory-Based Understanding of Clients

Information that therapists gather to answer questions about their clients is used to create a theory-based understanding of those clients. To

this end, therapists use MOHO theory as a framework for creating a conceptualization or explanation of each particular client's situation. As part of creating a conceptualization of clients' circumstances, therapists identify problems or challenges to address as well as strengths that can be built upon in therapy.

Generating Therapy Goals and Strategies

The theory-based understanding of clients is used to:

- Generate therapy goals (i.e., identify what will change as a result of therapy)
- Decide what kinds of occupational engagement will enable the client to change
- Determine what types of therapeutic strategies will be needed to support the client to change

Change is required when the client's characteristics and/or environment are contributing to occupational problems or challenges. For instance, if a client's personal causation is characterized by feelings of ineffectiveness, therapy would seek to enable the client to feel more effective, or if a client has too few or no roles, therapy would seek to enable the client to choose and enact new roles. In this way, identifying challenges or problems in the third step allows one to select the goals in the fourth step.

The next element in this step is to identify how the goals will be achieved. This involves indicating what occupation(s) the client will engage in to achieve the goals. It also involves consideration of how the therapist will support the client during this occupational engagement.

To support the steps of therapeutic reasoning, a therapeutic reasoning table has been developed and can be found in *Model of*

(text continues on page 161)

Table 11.3 **MOHO Assessment Summary Table**

MOHO Assessment	Method of Administration	Description
Assessment of Communication and Interaction Skills (ACIS)	Observation	Gathers information about the communication and interaction skills that a person displays while engaged in an occupation across the domains of physicality, information exchange, and relations. Used to generate goals for therapy related to communication/interaction skills and to assess outcomes/changes in skill.
Assessment of Motor and Process Skills (AMPS)	Observation	Gathers information about the motor and process skills that a person displays while engaged in an occupation. Used to generate goals for therapy related to motor and process skills and to assess outcomes/changes in skill.
Assessment of Occupational Functioning- Collaborative Version (AOF-CV)	Interview and/or client self-report	Yields qualitative information and a quantitative profile of the impact of a client's personal causation, values, roles, habits, and skills on occupational participation. Used to inform intervention.
Child Occupational Self Assessment (COSA)	Client self-report	Children and youths rate their occupational competence for engaging in 25 everyday activities in the home, school, and community and the importance of those activities. Used to generate goals and assess outcomes/changes in competence and values.
Interest Checklist	Client self-report	Checklist that indicates strength of interest and past, present, and future engagement in 68 activities. Used to inform intervention.
Model of Human Occupational Screening Tool (MOHOST)	Observation, interview(s), and/or chart review	Information gathered assesses impact of volition, habituation, skills, and environment on client's occupational participation. Used to generate goals and assess outcomes/changes in participation.

MOHO Assessment	Method of Administration	Description
NIH Activity Record	Client self-report	Self-report "log" records information in half-hour intervals throughout the day on perceptions of competence, value, enjoyment, difficulty, and pain experienced when engaging in various occupations in that time period. Used to inform intervention and assess outcomes/changes in participation.
Occupational Circumstances Assessment-Interview and Rating Scale (OCAIRS)	Interview	Interview yields information to assess values, goals, personal causation, interests, habits, roles, skills, readiness for change, and environmental impact on participation. Used to generate goals and assess outcomes/changes in participation.
Occupational Performance History Interview-II (OPHI-II)	Interview	Detailed life history interview that yields (1) scales measuring competence, identity, and environmental impact, and (2) a narrative representation/analysis of the life history. Used as an in-depth, comprehensive assessment to generate goals, inform intervention, and build the therapeutic relationship.
Occupational Questionnaire (OQ)	Client self-report	Self-report "log" records information in half-hour intervals throughout the day on perceptions of competence, value, and enjoyment experienced when engaging in various occupations in that time period. Used to inform intervention and assess outcomes/changes in participation.
Occupational Self Assessment (OSA)	Client self-report	Clients rate their occupational competence for engaging in 21 everyday activities and the importance of those activities. Allows clients to set priorities for change. Used to generate goals and assess outcomes/changes in competence and values.

(table continues on page 160)

Table 11.3 **MOHO Assessment Summary Table continued**

MOHO Assessment	Method of Administration	Description
Pediatric Interest Profiles (PIP)	Client self-report	Assessment includes three age-appropriate scales (some with line drawings) for children and adolescents to indicate participation, interest, and perceived competence in a variety of play and leisure activities. Used to generate goals and assess outcomes/changes in participation.
Pediatric Volitional Questionnaire (PVQ)	Observation	Guides a systematic observation of a child across multiple environments to assess volition and the impact of the environment on volition. Used as an in-depth assessment of volition to generate goals and assess outcomes/changes in volition.
Role Checklist	Client self-report	Checklist provides information on past, present, and future role participation and the perceived value of those roles. Used to inform intervention and assess outcomes/changes in role performance.
Short Child Occupational Profile (SCOPE)	Observation, interview(s), and/or chart review	Information gathered assesses impact of volition, habituation, skills, and environment on child's/adolescent's occupational participation. Used to generate goals and assess outcomes/changes in participation.
School Setting Interview (SSI)	Interview	Interview works with students to gather information on student-environment fit and identify need for accommodations. Used to generate goals, inform intervention, and assess outcomes/changes in student-environment fit.
Volitional Questionnaire (VQ)	Observation	Guides a systematic observation of a client across multiple environments to assess volition and the impact of the environment on volition. Used as an in-depth assessment of volition to generate goals and assess outcomes/changes in volition.

MOHO Assessment	Method of Administration	Description
Worker Role Interview (WRI)	Interview	Interview yields information to rate the impact that volition, habitation, and perceptions of the environment have on psychosocial readiness for the worker role/return to work. Used to generate goals and assess outcomes/changes in psychosocial readiness for work.
Work Environment Impact Scale (WEIS)	Interview	Interview works with client to assess environmental impact on participation in the worker role and to identify needed accommodations. Used to generate goals and inform intervention.

Human Occupation: Theory and Application, 4th edition (Kielhofner, 2008). This table identifies a wide range of problems and challenges that correspond to the concepts of MOHO along with types of changes that

Box 11.2 **Therapeutic Strategies Identified by MOHO**

* *Validating:* Attending to and acknowledging the client's experience.
* *Identifying:* Locating and sharing a range of personal, procedural, and/or environmental factors that can facilitate occupational performance.
* *Giving Feedback:* Sharing one's understanding of the client's situation or ongoing action.
* *Advising:* Recommending intervention goals/strategies.
* *Negotiating:* Engaging in a give-and-take with the client.
* *Structuring:* Establishing parameters for choice and performance by offering a client alternatives, setting limits, and establishing ground rules.
* *Coaching:* Instructing, demonstrating, guiding, verbally, and/or physically prompting.
* *Encouraging:* Providing emotional support and reassurance in relation to engagement in an occupation.
* *Physical Support:* Using one's body to provide support for a client to complete an occupational form/task.

would be warranted. The table also indicates what types of occupational engagement could contribute to achieving those changes and what type of support from the therapist could facilitate change. Table 11.4 shows a small section from this therapeutic reasoning table related to personal causation.

Implementing and Monitoring Therapy

Monitoring how the therapy process unfolds may confirm the therapist's conceptualization of the client's situation or it may require the therapist to rethink the client's situation. The monitoring process may confirm the utility of the planned client occupational engagement and therapist strategies. On the other hand, it may require the therapist to change the therapy plan. When things do not turn out as expected, the therapist returns to earlier steps of generating questions, selecting methods to gather information, conceptualizing the client's situation, setting goals, and establishing plans.

Collecting Information to Assess Outcomes

Determining therapy outcomes is an important final step in the therapy process. Typically, therapy outcomes are documented by:

* Examining the extent to which goals have been achieved

Table 11.4   **Excerpt From the Therapeutic Reasoning Table Showing a Problem/Challenge Related to Personal Causation and Corresponding Intervention Goals and Strategies**

Problem/Challenge	Goal	Client Occupational Engagement	Therapeutic Strategies to Support the Client
• Feelings of lack of control over occupational performance leading to anxiety (fear of failure) within occupations.	• Reduce client's anxiety and fear of failure in occupational performance (e.g., "The client will complete a simple three-step meal in 20 minutes without verbalizing anxiety or concern"). • Build up confidence to face occupational performance demands (e.g., "The client will identify and participate in three new leisure activities with minimal support in one week").	• *Reexamine* anxieties and fears in the light of new performance experiences. • *Choose* to do relevant and meaningful things that are within performance capacity. • *Sustain* performance in occupational forms despite anxiety.	• *Validate* how difficult it can be to do things that provoke anxiety. • *Identify* client's strengths and weaknesses in occupational performance. • Give *feedback* to client about match/mismatch between choice of occupational forms/tasks and performance capacity. • Give *feedback* to support a positive reinterpretation of their experience of engaging in an occupation. • *Advise* client to do relevant and meaningful things that match performance capacity.

Source: Kielhofner (2008).

• Readministering structured assessments to determine whether the client's scores have improved

Both approaches are valuable means of determining whether positive outcomes have been achieved; they are sometimes used in combination.

Standardized Programs and Intervention Protocols

A large number of MOHO-based programs and standardized protocols for intervention have been developed and published. Two examples are the Remotivation Process and the Enabling Self-Determination Program.

Remotivation Process

The Remotivation Process is a standardized intervention developed for clients of any diagnosis who have significant volitional (i.e., motivational) problems (de las Heras, Llerena, & Kielhofner, 2003). This intervention was developed based on research about volition and a long process of experimentation in practice with clients who had severe motivational problems. The Remotivation Process involves three levels of intervention (see Table 11.5). The level that one begins with depends on the severity of the volitional problem. Within each level there are specific steps and strategies for working with clients to support occupational engagement that will enhance volition. A manual details how to undertake this intervention protocol; it includes specific assessment guidelines, explanations and examples of the stages, steps, and strategies of the intervention, and case examples of clients receiving Remotivation services (de las Heras et al., 2003). This manual may be obtained online at http://www.moho.uic.edu/programs.html.

Enabling Self-Determination (ESD) Program

The ESD program was developed to enhance productivity and participation in persons facing substantial personal and environmental challenges (Kielhofner et al., 2008). This program

Table 11.5   **Modules, Goals, Stages, and Strategies of the Remotivation Process**

Modules	Goals	Stages and (Strategies)
Exploration	• Facilitate a client's sense of personal significance • Facilitate a client's basic sense of capacity • Facilitate a sense of security with the environment	• Validation (significant greeting; introduction of meaningful elements into the individual's personal space; participation in activities of interest to the individual; generating interaction) • Environmental exploration (introduce change to allow for exploration; keep a familiar routine for sense of security amid novelty) • Choice-making (increase novelty [new settings, people, etc.]; increase invitations for participation) • Pleasure and efficacy in action (facilitate participation in collaborative projects; incorporate feedback; facilitate a sense of life story)
Competency	• Increase emerging sense of efficacy • Begin looking at experiences as they relate to meeting goals • Develop a sense of responsibility with personal and collective projects	• Internalized sense of self-efficacy (provide physical or emotional "accompaniment" in new and challenging situations; facilitate skill learning when appropriate; introduce the counseling process and use of feedback) • Living and telling one's story (allow for "moments of reflection" or disorder in change process; continue counseling process to further insight through more in-depth analysis and questions)
Achievement	• Autonomy in a variety of settings • Striving for personal goals; making occupational choices • Seeking new challenges in relevant occupational environments • Continued learning of critical skills and new strategies/tools for seeking and confronting challenges	(Advise client; give feedback; provide information and resources; step back)

was originally developed and tested with persons who had combinations of HIV/AIDS, mental illness, and substance abuse histories. It consists of group and individual interventions designed to enhance volition and to support the development of routines, habits, and skills for new productive occupational roles. The program helps clients examine their own volition, lifestyle, and skills and begin a process of identifying personal goals for enhanced productivity.

Development of the program was guided by a prior three-year research and development project (Kielhofner, Braveman, et al., 2004) and focus groups with consumers for whom the program was designed (Paul-Ward, Braveman, Kielhofner, & Levin, 2005). A control group study provided evidence of the effectiveness of the program in helping clients achieve more productive lives (Kielhofner et al., 2008). This program is described in a detailed manual, which may be downloaded from the MOHO Clearinghouse website (http://www.moho.uic.edu/mohorelatedrsrcs.html#OtherInstrumentsBasedon MOHO).

Case Examples

MOHO emphasizes an individualized, client-centered approach to intervention based on thorough understanding of the client's unique characteristics. For this reason, using MOHO requires therapists to assess carefully and come to understand a client and then to develop, implement, and monitor a plan of therapy that addresses the client's specific needs, desires, and challenges. Because this therapeutic reasoning process is individualized, therapists can benefit from case examples that illustrate the process. A large number of case examples have been published. Some of these can be found in the text, *Model of Human Occupation: Theory and Application*, 4th edition (Kielhofner, 2008); others are in individual articles and chapters. Citations for these resources can be found at the MOHO clearinghouse website (http://www.moho.uic.edu/referencelists.html).

> Using MOHO requires therapists to assess carefully and come to understand a client and then to develop, implement, and monitor a plan of therapy that addresses the client's specific needs, desires, and challenges.

Research and Evidence Base

Since MOHO was first published nearly 30 years ago, more than 400 articles and chapters based on MOHO have been published and these include well over 100 studies. This model's developers have emphasized conducting research with practice relevance (Forsyth, Melton, & Mann, 2005; Kielhofner, 2005a, 2005b) and many of the studies represent partnerships between researchers, therapists, and clients.

Resources are available to help practitioners access and use the MOHO body of evidence. First, the MOHO Clearinghouse website (http://www.moho.uic.edu/evidence_based_practice.php#Search) includes an evidence-based search engine that enables practitioners to locate citations relevant to practice topics. Citations of studies have links to *Evidence Briefs* that summarize the research and discuss its implications for practice. These can be printed directly from the website.

There are also publications that synthesize the evidence related to this model. For instance, Kramer, Bowyer, and Kielhofner (2008) have organized available evidence to answer the following practice-relevant questions:

- What does MOHO research tell us about the occupational lives and needs of people with disabilities?
- What evidence exists for the dependability and utility of MOHO-based assessments?
- What does practice based on MOHO looked like?
- What evidence is there that MOHO-based service produces positive outcomes?
- What do clients have to say about MOHO-based services?

Another example is a paper by Lee and Kielhofner (2009) that locates and synthesizes evidence related to the vocational rehabilitation practice area; evidence is organized according to common practice questions that arise when making decisions about program design and service delivery.

Discussion

MOHO was introduced in 1980 by three practitioners seeking to articulate an approach to occupation-based intervention (Kielhofner, 1980a, 1980b; Kielhofner & Burke, 1980; Kielhofner, Burke, & Heard, 1980). Evidence indicates that MOHO is widely used in practice worldwide (Haglund, Ekbladh, Thorell, & Hallberg, 2000; Law & McColl, 1989; National Board for Certification in Occupational Therapy, 2004; Wilkeby, Pierre, & Archenholtz, 2006). A national study of occupational therapists in the United States (Lee, Taylor, Kielhofner, & Fisher, 2008) indicated that 75.7% of therapists make use of MOHO in their practice. These therapists reported that MOHO allows them to have an occupation-focused practice and a clearer professional identity. They also reported that MOHO provides a holistic view of clients, supports client-centered practice, and provides a useful structure for intervention planning.

Box 11.3

Model of Human Occupation Case Example: MARISOL

Introduction and the Process of Generating Questions

Marisol is a 45-year-old woman and the older of two sisters. She was recently diagnosed with schizophrenia. Marisol recently entered Senderos Foundation, the community center in Santiago, Chile. Andrea Girardi, her occupational therapist, knew that Marisol had a long period of poor occupational functioning prior to admission. Thus she generated the following questions about Marisol:

- What is Marisol's occupational identity and how is it reflected in her occupational narrative? To what extent has she been able to enact that identity (occupational competence)?
- What is the state of Marisol's volition? (Does she have interests? Does she feel effective? What is important to her? Does she make choices for activities based on her own volition?)
- What is her history of involvement in roles?
- What is her typical routine?
- What is her current performance capacity?
- What is her environment and how does it influence her occupational life?

Evaluation Process

In order to answer these questions, Andrea began the evaluation process, using the Occupational Performance History Interview-Second Version (OPHI-II) (Kielhofner, Mallinson, et al., 2004). This interview gathers information on clients' occupational identity, competence, and environment. It is an historical interview that ascertains the occupational narrative of the client. In the interview, Marisol described her childhood as positive and filled with family and social activities. In preadolescence, she began to experience difficulties in her student role. During this period, Marisol experienced an abusive relationship with her stepfather and became depressed. She dropped out of school and subsequently was in a relationship with an abusive partner. She has attempted and failed to re-enter the student role and has failed in attempts to enter the worker role.

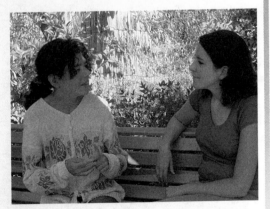

Marisol discusses her life history with Andrea.

(box continues on page 166)

Box 11.3 (continued)

Most recently, two years ago, she attempted once again to return to school to study tourism but had to drop out. Following that she attempted to work as a janitor in a fast-food restaurant. With the stress of the job, her auditory hallucinations increased and she began to have conflicts with some of her coworkers. Due to both these factors Marisol quit her job.

The one activity she has been able to maintain with some consistency over a 10-year period is participation in yoga classes, which her mother teaches. The last 20 years of her life were characterized by a lack of roles and the absence of productive occupation; this was the case despite Marisol's desire for roles and her attempts to be a student or to work continuously in something. Her previous routine consisted of participating in yoga classes that her mother directed, helping in tasks of the home, and occasionally preparing lunch and listening to music.

Marisol's scores on the OPHI-II rating scales (Fig. 11.2) indicated that she had difficulty in the area of occupational identity. While she had struggled in most areas of occupational identity her primary strength was that she took responsibility for her own life and was committed to trying to achieve a more productive and satisfying occupational life. Her major problems have been in enacting that identity through sustaining roles, working toward her own goals, and performing in the way she believes she should.

The narrative slope that emerged from the OPHI-II is shown in Figure 11.3. While the lowest point in her occupational narrative was during her childhood abuse and her abusive relationship with her partner, her recent job and school failures coupled with her diagnosis represented a new low point. In spite of the difficulties that she had faced in her life, Marisol felt there was a possibility of overcoming her challenges and was able to articulate some hope for the future.

Andrea decided to further evaluate Marisol by observing her as she began to participate in occupational therapy groups. Informal observation revealed that her movements were very slow and rigid and she appeared unkempt. As a side effect of her medication, she also experienced sleepiness that interfered with her process skills and made it difficult for her to maintain an

Occupational Identity Scale	1	2	3	4
Has personal goals and projects		X		
Identifies a desired occupational lifestyle		X		
Expects success		X		
Accepts responsibility			X	
Appraises abilities and limitations		X		
Has commitments and values		X		
Recognizes identity and obligations		X		
Has interests		X		
Felt effective (past)		X		
Found meaning and satisfaction in lifestyle (past)			X	
Made occupational choices (past)		X		
Occupational Competence Scale				
Maintains satisfying lifestyle	X			
Fulfills role expectations		X		
Works toward goals	X			
Meets personal performance standards	X			
Organizes time for responsibilities		X		
Participates in interests		X		
Fulfilled roles (past)	X			
Maintained habits (past)		X		
Achieved satisfaction (past)	X			
Occupational Settings (Environment) Scale				
Home life occupational forms		X		
Major productive role occupational forms	Not applicable			
Leisure occupational forms	X			
Home life social group		X		
Major productive role social group	Not applicable			
Leisure social group		X		
Home spaces, objects, and resources			X	
Major productive role spaces, objects, and resources	Not applicable			
Leisure spaces, objects, and resources		X		

Key:

1=Extreme occupational functioning problems
2=Some occupational functioning problems
3=Appropriate satisfactory occupational functioning
4=Exceptionally competent occupational functioning

FIGURE 11.2 Marisol's Scores on the OPHI-II Scales.

Box 11.3 (continued)

appropriate pace during any task. Marisol's therapist reported the pharmaceutical side effects to her psychiatrist who decided to modify her medication.

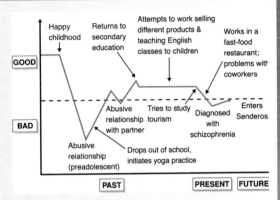

The therapist also observed that Marisol always tended to agree with everything that was proposed, without discriminating what she was interested in or what she wanted for herself and without considering her own preferences and opinions. Andrea initially planned to use the Interest Checklist (Matsutsuyu, 1969) to help Marisol reflect on her interests. However, because Marisol had difficulty identifying which occupations were of greater interest to her, the therapist also decided to further evaluate her volition through use of the

FIGURE 11.3 Marisol's Narrative Slope from the OPHI-II.

Volitional Questionnaire (a short rating scale that can be quickly competed following observation of a client in an activity) (de las Heras, Geist, Kielhofner, & Li, 2007). She completed the Volitional Questionnaire several times following observations of Marisol in various activities and groups offered in the setting. The Volitional Questionnaire confirmed that Marisol's volition was quite low and that she needed support to exhibit the most basic, exploratory level of motivation. Andrea also identified that Marisol expressed her highest motivation while playing tennis, in secretarial tasks, and when participating in English classes.

An Explanation of Marisol's Situation

Andrea created the following explanation of Marisol's situation:

> Marisol has a history of personal trauma and a psychiatric illness that both have interfered with her ability to develop and enact a positive occupational identity. Her volition is a major area of weakness as she has difficulty identifying and choosing the things that are of interest and have significance for her. At the same time, she has a very strong value that she should be productive but does not know how to go about this. Her actual performance capacity is unknown (and cannot be fully ascertained until she is stabilized on medication).

Goals, Strategies, and Implementation of Therapy

Andrea's goals for Marisol were:

- Increase her volition (i.e., development of her interests, identification of significant activities, and realistic belief in her abilities)
- Explore her performance in order to more clearly understand what skills she has

In order to address Marisol's low volition, Andrea decided to use the Remotivation Process (de las Heras et al., 2003) beginning with exploratory level intervention. Because the Remotivation Process requires cooperation of many people in the client's environment, Andrea presented this treatment strategy to the interdisciplinary team of Senderos. The team agreed with this recommendation and basic strategies for the validation process (step one of Remotivation) were outlined for the interdisciplinary staff.

Andrea began the Remotivation Process at the exploratory level. She worked to create a safe environment with opportunities for Marisol to engage in occupations that could promote her

(box continues on page 168)

Box 11.3 (continued)

basic sense of capacity and of pleasure in doing. As Marisol was able to do activities with some success, Andrea coached Marisol on how to be more aware of her own experience of engaging in occupation. She also helped her to interpret and reflect upon her experiences of doing things. During their discussions, Marisol indicated three possible long-term goals: to return to study tourism, to teach English classes to children, or to work with older adults. The therapist validated these goals and committed to Marisol that they would find opportunities for her to try out these areas of work.

During the second, competence, stage of the Remotivation Process, Marisol began to assume small tasks and take on roles in the community of Senderos. She agreed to work as an assistant supporting the English teacher in her classes. She also began to volunteer doing some secretarial work in Senderos. After trying out this role she became very motivated to try to learn how to use a computer. She began to spontaneously greet others in Senderos and to smile at her own achievements.

During this time, she also chose to take tennis classes that were taught by an instructor from the community. At first, she had difficulty even hitting the tennis ball. Her movements were so slow that by the time she was able to raise the racket, the ball was already past her. In spite of her feelings of incapability, she tried it again and again. Despite her difficulties Marisol really wanted to learn to play. So Andrea decided to meet with the tennis instructor in order to provide him an introduction to the Remotivation Process so that he would know what strategies to use when teaching Marisol to play tennis. Andrea also gave the tennis instructor guidance in how to grade the demands of the instruction to Marisol's level of motor skills.

As Marisol progressed (i.e., began to show increasing pleasure and a greater sense of efficacy in doing things, ability to commit herself to learning new skills, solving problems, and other behaviors indicative of the competence level of volition), Andrea decided to introduce strategies from the achievement level of the Remotivation Process. Andrea and Marisol together decided to work toward the goal of Marisol working as a tour guide. At first, Marisol indicated an interest in writing articles related to local areas of interest for a newsletter published in the center. She also began to explore the role of tour guide during outings with other members of Senderos. With support from Andrea, she researched and prepared material for giving tours on planned outings.

Andrea also worked with Marisol to reconstruct her occupational narrative focusing on where she wanted her life story to go in the future. Marisol's family also participated actively in Marisol's therapy process. They attended family counseling provided by the occupational therapist. In these counseling sessions the therapist explained the Remotivation Process to members of the family and demonstrated how they could best support Marisol as she passed through the three modules of the Remotivation Process.

Six months into her involvement in the center, the female participants of Senderos decided to

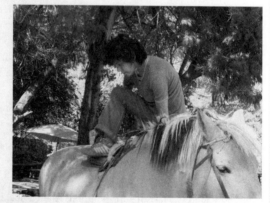

Marisol tries horseback riding during a group outing.

create a special space for women (a beauty salon). Marisol proved to be very interested in it and decided to take part in the creation of the salon. Through her participation, she discovered that she had a lot of knowledge to contribute and began to see herself as more attractive and to take an interest in keeping herself well groomed. She also received validation from other members of the female group concerning her much improved appearance.

At this time Marisol started to teach in the elementary English course offered in the setting. This experience allowed her to investigate what it meant to be a teacher, how to prepare

Box 11.3 (continued)

the classes, how to adapt the methodology to her pupils, and how to prepare didactic material. To support Marisol, Andrea graded the various teaching related activities that Marisol undertook.

Marisol also decided to begin volunteer work with elderly people in order to build her sense of capacity, practice maintaining a work routine, and grow more comfortable around other people. Together, Andrea and Marisol began to look for institutions and make telephone calls. Andrea accompanied Marisol to potential volunteer settings for interviews. Marisol was accepted as a volunteer in one nursing home for the elderly and began working there. Her job was initially to accompany the elderly and to give help to the nursing personnel when feeding and bathing elderly residents. The personnel in the institution value Marisol's work and the elderly residents have grown to know Marisol and feel comforted by her presence. Marisol has worked in the nursing home for four months and mostly goes there on her own. Andrea accompanies her occasionally when she takes on new challenges such as organizing games for small groups of elderly residents.

While participating in this volunteer work, Marisol took advantage of the opportunity to participate in courses related to teaching offered in the local community. In counseling, Andrea had introduced the possibility of taking some courses related to her goals and Marisol decided that she felt prepared to take courses that would qualify her as a preschool assistant. As she took on the student role, she was able to dress and groom herself appropriately and she showed up to classes with notebooks and materials to take notes. She successfully completed the necessary courses to qualify as a teaching assistant.

Now, Marisol is looking for a place to do her practicum experience in a classroom with children. Through the Remotivation Process, Marisol has been able to develop a sense of efficacy to explore and identify her own interests and to sort out what is important to her. She has also successfully sustained a productive routine and succeeded in several roles. Most importantly, Marisol reports that now she feels much happier than at any other time in her life.

Table 11.6   **Terms of the Model**

Environment	The particular physical, social, cultural, economic, and political features within a person's context that have an impact on the motivation, organization, and performance of occupation.
Habits	Acquired tendencies to respond automatically and perform in certain, consistent ways in familiar environments or situations.
Habituation	An internalized readiness to exhibit consistent patterns of behavior guided by our habits and roles and fitted to the characteristics of routine temporal, physical, and social environments.
Interests	What one finds enjoyable or satisfying to do.
Occupational adaptation	Constructing a positive occupational identity and achieving occupational competence over time in the context of one's environment.
Occupational competence	Degree to which one is able to sustain a pattern of occupational participation that reflects one's occupational identity.

(table continues on page 170)

Table 11.6 **Terms of the Model** continued

Occupational engagement	Clients' doing, thinking, and feeling under certain environmental conditions in the midst of or as a planned consequence of therapy.
Occupational identity	Composite sense of who one is and wishes to become as an occupational being generated from one's history of occupational participation.
Occupational narrative	A person's story (both told and enacted) that integrates across time one's unfolding volition, habituation, performance capacity, and environments and that sums up and assigns meaning to these elements.
Occupational participation	Engagement in work, play, or activities of daily living that are part of one's sociocultural context and that are desired and/or necessary to one's well-being.
Occupational performance	Doing an occupational form.
Performance capacity	Ability for doing things provided by the status of underlying objective physical and mental components and corresponding subjective experience.
Personal causation	One's sense of competence and effectiveness.
Role	The incorporation of a socially and/or personally defined status and a related cluster of attitudes and actions.
Skills	Observable, goal-directed actions that a person uses while performing.
Therapeutic reasoning	A six-step process used to understand and address clients' needs.
Values	What one finds important and meaningful to do.
Volition	Pattern of thoughts and feelings about oneself as an actor in one's world, which occurs as one anticipates, chooses, experiences, and interprets what one does.

SUMMARY

+ MOHO became the first client-centered model by looking beyond impairment to other client-related factors affecting occupational performance

Theory

+ MOHO is ultimately concerned with individuals' participation and adaptation in life occupations

+ Volition is the process by which people are motivated toward and choose the activities they do. It begins with the universal human desire to do things and is shaped by life experiences. Volition consists of thoughts and feelings that occur in a cycle of:
• Anticipating possibilities for doing
• Choosing what to do

- Experiencing what one does
- Subsequent interpretation of the experience

+ The thoughts and feelings that make up volition are referred to as personal causation, values, and interests
  - Personal causation refers to the thoughts and feelings about personal capacities and effectiveness that people have as they do everyday activities
  - Values are beliefs and commitments about what is good, right, and important to do
  - Interests are generated through the experience of pleasure and satisfaction in occupation

+ Volition has a pervasive influence on occupational life. It shapes:
  - How people see the opportunities and challenges in their environment
  - What people choose to do
  - How they experience and make sense of what they have done

+ Occupational therapy based on MOHO often involves identifying and addressing clients' volitional problems

+ Habituation is a process whereby people organize their actions into patterns and routines

+ Habits involve learned ways of doing things that unfold automatically

+ Roles give people an identity and a sense of the obligations that go with that identity

+ Learning a new role involves internalizing an identity, an outlook, and an expected way of behaving

+ One of the major tasks of therapy is to construct or reconstruct habits and roles so that the person can more readily participate in everyday occupations

+ Performance capacity refers to underlying mental and physical abilities and how they are used and experienced in performance

+ The capacity for performance is affected by the status of musculoskeletal, neurological, cardiopulmonary, and other bodily systems that are called on when a person does things

+ Performance also calls on mental or cognitive abilities such as memory

+ MOHO stresses the importance of also attending to the experience of performance and, in particular, the experience of having limitations in performance

+ MOHO stresses that occupation results from an interaction of the inner characteristics of the person (volition, habituation, and performance capacity) with the environment

+ The environment includes the particular physical, social, cultural, economic, and political features within a person's context that influence the motivation, organization, and performance of occupation

+ The environment includes:
  - The objects that people use when they do things
  - The spaces within which people do things
  - The occupational forms or tasks that are available, expected, and/or required of people in a given context
  - The social groups that make up the context
  - The surrounding culture, political, and economic forces

+ MOHO identifies three levels for examining what a person does:
  - Occupational participation refers to engaging in work, play, or activities of daily living that are part of one's sociocultural context and that are desired and/or necessary to one's well-being
  - Occupational performance is the process of doing such occupational forms or tasks
  - Occupational skills are the purposeful actions that make up occupational performance. Skills are goal-directed actions that a person uses while performing
    - Categories of skills include motor, process, and communication and interaction skills

+ Occupational identity is a person's cumulative sense of who they are and wish to become as occupational beings

+ The degree to which people are able to sustain a pattern of doing that enacts their occupational identity is referred to as occupational competence

✦ Occupational adaptation refers to the process of creating and enacting a positive occupational identity

✦ An occupational narrative is a person's story that integrates across time one's unfolding volition, habituation, performance capacity, and environments and that sums up and assigns meaning to these elements

✦ Research has shown that occupational narratives predict future adaptation of occupational therapy clients

✦ MOHO asserts that all change in occupational therapy is driven by clients' occupational engagement (i.e., clients' doing, thinking, and feeling under certain environmental conditions in the midst of therapy or as a planned consequence of therapy)

✦ Each of these aspects of what the client does, thinks, and feels is essential to the process of therapy

Practice Resources

✦ Therapeutic reasoning is a process for MOHO concepts and resources to understand and address clients' needs. Therapeutic reasoning involves six steps:
  • Generating questions about the client
    ▪ Therapists must understand their clients before planning therapy
    ▪ This understanding begins with asking questions about each client derived from MOHO concepts
  • Gathering information on, from, and with the client
    ▪ Therapists must gather information on, from, and with the client in order to answer the questions they have generated about the client
    ▪ Such information gathering may take advantage of informal, naturally occurring opportunities
    ▪ Therapists also use structured MOHO assessments
  • Using the information gathered to create an explanation of the client's situation

    ▪ Information that therapists gather to answer questions about their clients is used to create a theory-based understanding of those client
    ▪ As part of creating a conceptualization of clients' circumstances, therapists identify problems or challenges to address as well as strengths that can be built upon in therapy
  • Generating goals and strategies for therapy
    ▪ The theory-based understanding of clients is used to generate therapy goals, decide what kinds of occupational engagement will enable the client to change, and determine what kind of therapeutic strategies will be needed to support the client to change
    ▪ Change is required when the client's characteristics and/or environment are contributing to occupational problems or challenges
    ▪ The next element in this step is to identify how the goals will be achieved
  • Implementing and monitoring therapy
    ▪ Monitoring how the therapy process unfolds may confirm the therapist's conceptualization of the client's situation or it may require the therapist to rethink the client's situation
    ▪ The monitoring process may confirm the utility of the planned client occupational engagement and therapist strategies or it may require the therapist to change the therapy plan
    ▪ When things do not turn out as expected, the therapist returns to earlier steps of generating questions, selecting methods to gather information, conceptualizing the client's situation, setting goals, and establishing plans.
  • Determining outcomes of therapy
    ▪ Typically, therapy outcomes are documented by examining the extent to which goals have been achieved and readministering structured assessments to determine whether the client's scores have improved

✦ Therapeutic reasoning must be client-centered

- The process reflects a deep appreciation for the client's circumstances
- The client is involved in the process to the extent possible

+ Therapists may move back and forth between the steps of therapeutic reasoning

Intervention

+ A large number of MOHO-based programs and standardized protocols for intervention have been developed and published

+ The Remotivation Process is a standardized intervention developed for clients of any diagnosis who have significant volitional problems

+ The Remotivation Process involves three levels of intervention (exploration, competence, and achievement); the level that one begins with depends on the severity of the volitional problem

+ A manual details how to undertake this intervention protocol; it includes specific assessment guidelines, explanations and examples of the stages, steps and strategies of the intervention, and case examples of clients receiving Remotivation services

+ The Enabling Self-Determination Program was developed to enhance productivity and participation in persons facing substantial personal and environmental challenges

+ The program helps clients examine their own volition, lifestyle, and skills and begin a process of identifying personal goals for enhanced productivity

+ Because the therapeutic reasoning process is individualized, therapists can benefit from case examples that illustrate the process

+ A large number of MOHO case examples have been published

REFERENCES

de las Heras, C.G., Geist, R., Kielhofner, G., & Li, Y. (2007). *The volitional questionnaire (VQ)* (version 4.1). Chicago: Department of Occupational Therapy, University of Illinois at Chicago.

de las Heras, C.G., Llerena, V., & Kielhofner, G. (2003). *Remotivation process: Progressive intervention for individuals with severe volitional challenges* (version 1.0). Chicago: Department of Occupational Therapy, University of Illinois at Chicago.

Fisher, A. (1998). Uniting practice and theory in an occupational framework. *American Journal of Occupational Therapy, 52,* 509–520.

Fisher, A.G. (1999). *The assessment of motor and process skills (AMPS)* (3rd ed.). Ft. Collins, CO: Three Stars Press.

Fisher, A., & Kielhofner, G. (1995). Skill in occupational performance. In G. Kielhofner (1995), *A model of human occupation: Theory and application* (2nd ed., pp. 113–137). Baltimore: Lippincott Williams & Wilkins.

Forsyth, K., Lai, J., & Kielhofner, G. (1999). The Assessment of Communication and Interaction Skills (ACIS): Measurement properties. *British Journal of Occupational Therapy, 62,* 69–74.

Forsyth, K., Melton, J., & Mann, L.S. (2005). Achieving evidence-based practice: A process of

continuing education through practitioner-academic partnership. In P. Crist & G. Kielhofner (Eds.), *The scholarship of practice: Academic-practice collaborations for promoting occupational therapy* (pp. 211–227). New York: The Haworth Press.

Forsyth, K., Salamy, M., Simon, S., & Kielhofner, G. (1998). *Assessment of communication and interaction skills* (version 4.0). Chicago: Department of Occupational Therapy, University of Illinois at Chicago.

Haglund, L., Ekbladh, E., Thorell, L., & Hallberg, I.R. (2000). Practice models in Swedish psychiatric occupational therapy. *Scandinavian Journal of Occupational Therapy, 7*(3), 107–113.

Kielhofner, G. (1980a). A model of human occupation, part 2. Ontogenesis from the perspective of temporal adaptation. *American Journal of Occupational Therapy, 34,* 657–663.

Kielhofner, G. (1980b). A model of human occupation, part 3. Benign and vicious cycles. *American Journal of Occupational Therapy, 34,* 731–737.

Kielhofner, G. (2005a). Scholarship and practice: Bridging the divide. *American Journal of Occupational Therapy, 59,* 231–239.

Kielhofner, G. (2005b). A scholarship of practice: Creating discourse between theory, research, and practice. *Occupational Therapy in Health Care, 19*, 7–17.

Kielhofner, G. (2008). *Model of human occupation: Theory and application* (4th ed.). Baltimore: Lippincott Williams & Wilkins.

Kielhofner, G., Braveman, B., Finlayson, M., Paul-Ward, A., Goldbaum, L., & Goldstein, K. (2004). Outcomes of a vocational program for persons with AIDS. *American Journal of Occupational Therapy, 58*, 64–72.

Kielhofner, G., Braveman, B., Fogg, L., & Levin, M. (2008). A control study of services to enhance productive participation among persons with HIV/AIDS. *American Journal of Occupational Therapy, 62*, 36–45.

Kielhofner, G., & Burke, J. (1980). A model of human occupation, part 1. Conceptual framework and content. *American Journal of Occupational Therapy, 34*, 572–581.

Kielhofner, G., Burke, J., & Heard, I.C. (1980). A model of human occupation, part 4. Assessment and intervention. *American Journal of Occupational Therapy, 34*, 777–788.

Kielhofner, G., Mallinson, T., Crawford, C., Nowak, M., Rugby, M., Henry, A., & Walens, D. (2004). *Occupational performance history interview II* (OPHI-II) (version 2.1). Chicago: Department of Occupational Therapy, University of Illinois at Chicago.

Kielhofner, G., Mallinson, T., Forsyth, K., & Lai, J. (2001). Psychometric properties of the second version of the Occupational Performance History Interview (OPHI-II). *American Journal of Occupational Therapy, 55*, 260-267.

Kramer, J., Bowyer, P., & Kielhofner, G. (2008). Evidence for practice from the model of human occupation. In G. Kielhofner, *Model of human occupation: Theory and application* (4th edition, pp. 466–505). Baltimore: Lippincott Williams & Wilkins.

Law, M., & McColl, M.A. (1989). Knowledge and use of theory among occupational therapists: A Canadian survey. *Canadian Journal of Occupational Therapy, 56*, 198–204.

Lee, J., & Kielhofner, G. (2009). *Vocational intervention based on the model of human occupation: A synthesis of evidence.* Manuscript submitted for publication.

Lee, S.W., Taylor, R.R., Kielhofner, G., & Fisher, G. (2008). Theory use in practice: A national survey of therapists who use the model of human occupation. *American Journal of Occupational Therapy, 62*, 106–117.

Mallinson, T., Mahaffey, L., & Kielhofner, G. (1998). The Occupational Performance History Interview: Evidence for three underlying constructs of occupational adaptation. *Canadian Journal of Occupational Therapy, 65*, 219–228.

Matsutsuyu, J. (1969). The interest checklist. *American Journal of Occupational Therapy, 23*, 323–328.

National Board for the Certification in Occupational Therapy. (2004). A practice analysis study of entry-level occupational therapist registered and certified occupational therapy assistant practice. *Occupational Therapy Journal of Research: Occupation, Participation and Health, 24* (Suppl. 1), s1–s31.

Paul-Ward, A., Braveman, B., Kielhofner, G., & Levin, M. (2005). Developing employment services for individuals with HIV/AIDS: Participatory action strategies at work. *Journal of Vocational Rehabilitation, 22*, 85–93.

Wilkeby, M., Pierre, B.L., & Archenholtz, B. (2006) Occupational therapists' reflection on practice within psychiatric care: A Delphi Study. *Scandinavian Journal of Occupational Therapy, 13*, 151-159.

CHAPTER 12

The Motor Control Model

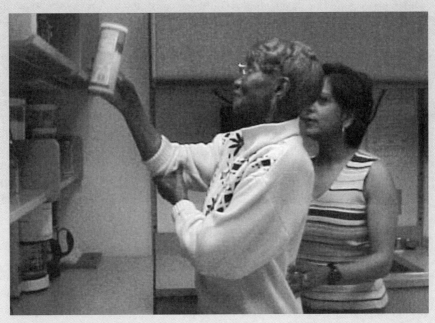

A client is engaged in a cooking activity. As the client does the various tasks required (e.g., reaching for ingredients on a shelf), the occupational therapist carefully observes her motor actions, at the same time giving her physical support to stabilize her standing. The therapist will facilitate the client's discovery of the most functional way she can go about accomplishing this necessary everyday activity while also noting how modifications in the physical environment and the way the client does the cooking tasks can increase her client's effectiveness. This combination of strategies for enabling the client to successfully complete a meal is reflective of the motor control model as it is practiced today.

Occupational therapists have been concerned with difficulties with the control of movement following brain trauma through much of the profession's history. The term **motor control** refers to the ability to use one's body effectively while performing an occupation (Giuffrida, 2003; Radomski & Trombly Latham, 2008). Motor control includes such functions as generating and coordinating movement patterns of the head, limbs, and trunk, and maintaining balance during occupational performance.

Approaches to addressing motor control impairments have evolved with changes in the understanding of how movement is controlled. Theories about how people learn and manage to control movement come from neurophysiology, neuropsychology, human development, psychology, and human movement science (Shumway-Cook & Woollacott, 2007). Early motor control interventions in occupational therapy reflected the understanding of the nervous system that existed at the time. As the limitations of these early motor control theories became apparent through research and new theories were proposed to explain motor control, changes in the occupational therapy intervention approaches similarly evolved.

Understanding of how movement is controlled (and of the nature of motor control impairments) has been cumulative. That is, older theories of movement have not been completely rejected but rather modified and incorporated into newer theories. The same is true of motor control interventions. While it is understood that older approaches were incomplete and not optimally effective, some of the concepts and techniques are still in use alongside more contemporary approaches.

Traditional and Contemporary Motor Control Approaches

Four traditional treatment approaches of similar origin and with similar concepts and techniques have been used in occupational therapy for persons with brain trauma resulting in difficulty controlling movement. These are:

* The Rood approach
* Bobaths' neurodevelopmental treatment

* Brunnstrom's movement therapy
* Proprioceptive neuromuscular facilitation

These approaches share similar concepts and techniques (Trombly & Radomski, 2002). They are referred to collectively as neurodevelopmental approaches because they are based on a view of the nervous system that emphasizes its developmental nature. All four of these neurodevelopmental approaches share the goal of improving motor control. Consequently, this chapter will provide an overview of earlier motor control concepts and approaches before going on to discuss the contemporary motor control approach.

As a group, these approaches sought to explain motor impairment and to specify strategies of intervention aimed at improving motor control. These approaches address motor problems that occur as a result of damage to the central nervous system (CNS). With CNS damage, neural communication to muscles is often preserved but impaired because of the insult to central processing components of the brain. The neurodevelopmental approaches are often taught and used together not only because they share concepts, but also because they draw upon much of the same knowledge about the control of movement.

More recently, conceptualizations of how humans achieve motor control have changed dramatically (Giuffrida, 2003; Mathiowetz & Bass-Haugen, 1994; Radomski & Trombly Latham, 2008). As a consequence, occupational therapists have developed a new conceptualization of motor control. It is typically referred to as the contemporary motor control approach.

Because both the traditional neurodevelopmental approaches and the new motor control model are in use in practice, this chapter covers both. The organization of the chapter is as follows. In keeping with other chapters there is an overall discussion of theory. This discussion of theory focuses on concepts concerning the control of movement. It begins with an examination of the traditional views of motor control followed by contemporary motor control concepts. Then the chapter presents the four neurodevelopmental approaches in terms of how they view motor control problems, their rationale for intervention, and their resources for intervention. Finally, the chapter presents the contemporary motor control approach. It discusses the contemporary view of motor problems, rationale for intervention, and resources for intervention.

Theory

Traditional Concepts of Motor Control

The earliest theory, dating to the beginning of the 20th century, asserted that movement was controlled by reflexes based on "genetically wired configurations of neurons" (Trombly, 1989, p. 78). **Reflexes** are biologically encoded movements that occur in response to sensory stimuli. Different reflex patterns emerge as the nervous system matures in the course of normal development. Movement patterns associated with the spinal cord and lower brain centers appear first, followed by those associated with higher brain centers. It was hypothesized that complex movement was the result of many reflexes being chained together. Thus, this theory hypothesized that complex movement was achieved through collective action of multiple reflexes (Mathiowetz & Bass-Haugen, 1994, 2002; Shumway-Cook & Woollacott, 2007).

Later research and concepts showed the reflex model to be insufficient to explain motor control. For instance, it was recognized that much of complex movement is under voluntary control and happens in the absence of sensory stimuli while reflexes require a sensory stimulus and are involuntary.

Recognition of the limitations of the reflex explanation of motor control led to the concept of **hierarchical control**, which argued that movements are controlled from the top down (Shumway-Cook & Woollacott, 2007). According to this argument, higher centers in the nervous system exert control over lower-level parts of the nervous system (Mathiowetz & Bass-Haugen, 1994, 2002).

The higher centers acquire and store motor programs that act as instructions for movement. The **motor program** is a set of neurologically wired instructions (sometimes called a central pattern generator) for accomplishing a complex movement (Shumway-Cook & Woollacott, 2007). It can be initiated either by voluntary control or by a sensory stimulus.

For example, the motor program concept holds that the instructions for the pattern of movement required for reaching to grasp an object is stored in a CNS motor program. The program is acquired from previous experiences of reaching and grasping. This program, an abstract representation of the sequence, duration, speed, and direction of movements, is used in each instance of reaching to effect the appropriate motion and postural adjustments.

According to the hierarchical and motor program explanations, reflex patterns are integrated into more complex movement and, therefore, come under higher-level control. Both the emergence of reflexes and their eventual integration into hierarchically controlled patterns of movement are considered to be the result of ongoing development and reorganization in the CNS. As the nervous system is considered the highest executive system involved in motor control, all abilities for and problems of motor control were considered to emanate from problems in the CNS.

Other important early concepts were related to development (Mathiowetz & Bass-Haugen, 1995). Neurodevelopmental concepts stress that there is an invariant sequence of development. Motor control develops from head to foot **(cephalocaudal)** and from the middle of the body to the distant limbs **(proximodistal)**. This sequence of development was believed to be driven by maturation of the CNS and to represent the gradual development of control of higher centers over lower centers. In this conceptualization, the environment did not have a direct role in influencing motor control. Rather, the organization of the CNS determined movement patterns, and changes in the CNS produced changes in motor performance.

A final concept common to all four neurodevelopmental approaches is the **plasticity** of the nervous system. The neurodevelopmental approaches all assume that the CNS is a flexible system with potential for organization and reorganization as the result of experience. Drawing upon the concept of neuroplasticity, the neurodevelopmental approaches argue that, because the experience of controlling movement is necessary to brain organization, such experience can be utilized in therapy to achieve organization or reorganization of the brain.

Contemporary Concepts of Motor Control

While the concepts of hierarchical control and motor programs represented an advance over the reflex model of motor control, they were also eventually shown to have limitations (Kamm, Thelen, & Jensen, 1990; Mathiowetz & Bass-Haugen, 1994, 2002; Shumway-Cook & Woollacott, 2007). One important limitation of the idea of hierarchical control of movement is that it would require an almost infinite number of motor programs to specify the necessary detail for even a simple task to be performed.

Briefly stated, the argument goes as follows. The various muscles and joints involved in motion can be used and combined in a very large number of ways (these possibilities are referred to as degrees of freedom). The degrees of freedom problem is further complicated by the fact that humans perform in an almost infinite variety of circumstances. This contextual variability means that each and every instance of a particular movement is unique. No two instances of performing the same action (e.g., signing one's name, hammering a nail, reaching for a cup, putting on one's clothes, typing out a word) are exactly the same. Thus the idea of pre-set instructions cannot account for the variability in performance (Turvey, 1990).

Another limitation of the motor program concept is that identical commands for movement will produce quite different results depending on a number of factors (Shumway-Cook & Woollacott, 2007). For example, the position of the body when a movement is generated will determine how gravity is acting on the body part that is moved. Different gravitational forces will result in different movements even when the same command is given. Another example is the state of muscles when the movement is initiated. The same command will produce different results when the muscles involved are rested than when they are fatigued. Hence, hierarchical conceptualization of motor control by a central motor program does not fully explain how movement is accomplished in real life conditions.

Heterarchical Control, Emergence, and Control Parameters

A number of new concepts based on systems theory are now used to more fully understand motor control (Kamm et al., 1990; Mathiowetz & Bass-Haugen, 1994, 2002). The first concept rejects the older idea of top-down, hierarchical control of movement. This new concept, **heterarchical control,** explains that movement is the result of several factors interacting together. That is, movement is understood to result from the interaction of:

• Personal factors (including the central nervous and musculoskeletal systems)
• The nature of the task being performed
• Conditions in the environment

In this new explanation, no single factor is viewed as controlling the others. Rather, each of these factors contributes something toward a dynamic whole, out of which the motor behavior emerges.

Another important and related concept in contemporary understanding of how movement is controlled is **emergence.** In motor control theory this concept refers to the spontaneous occurrence of complex motor actions that come out of the interactions of person, task, and environment rather than being controlled top down by a motor program (Clark 1997; Haken, 1987). Thus, the control of movement is understood to be distributed among the three components of person, task, and environment. Moreover, a change in one of these components can result in a change in the movement pattern. Such a change that shifts or alters the pattern of motor action is considered a **control parameter.** The feature box in this section illustrates the concepts of emergence and control parameters through an example.

When persons perform routine tasks they use certain preferred movement patterns out of the many patterns that are possible for accomplishing that particular task. These preferred patterns of doing a task, such as reaching for an object, are conceptualized as **attractor states.** These attractor states do not require centralized instructions (i.e., motor programs), which have pre-coded all the necessary movement patterns.

Box 12.1   Emergence and Control Parameters

The following is an example of an emergent motor behavior that is easily demonstrated. It involves reaching bilaterally (i.e., with both hands) at the same time for two different objects (for instance, the left hand reaching for a nearer object and the right hand for a more distant object). If anyone attempts this task by moving both hands at the same time, the same solution will always emerge (you might want to try the task yourself before reading on).

That is, the two reaches become linked together in a specific way. Both hands terminate at their target objects at the same time. To accomplish this, the hand reaching for the more distant object travels at a higher speed than the other hand reaching for the nearer object. What feels most natural or effortless is to move one's arms in such a way that the two different movements are functionally linked by a simple relationship. That is, the relative distance each must travel always defines the ratio of one hand's speed of travel to the other. The task can be varied by placing the two objects at different distances from each hand; in each instance the emergent behavior will follow the same formula (i.e., the hand moving to the more distant object moving at faster speed that is determined by how much greater a distance it must travel).

This movement pattern is not hard-wired. Rather, it emerges out of the interaction of the person, the task (bilateral reaching for two different objects), and the environment (where the objects are placed in

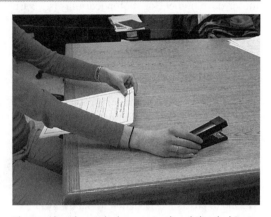

The two hands reach the proximal and distal objects at the same time.

front of the person). Using this example, one can see how the environment, the person, or the task can become a control parameter. Change the position of the objects and the movement pattern will change. Change the task by instructing the person to pick up one object at a time and the movement pattern will change. Finally, of course, a change in the CNS (such as that which occurs following brain damage) or musculoskeletal system (e.g., muscle weakness) would change how the person would move. Whenever one of these person, environmental, or task factors changes, it becomes a control parameter that shifts the movement into a different pattern.

Rather, these preferred patterns of movement emerge from the dynamic interaction of the person, the task, and the environment.

Hence, contemporary motor control theory does not view the CNS as the central executor of movement and eliminates the need for precoded instructions that specify all the details of movement ahead of time. Rather than depending on a motor program that contains all the necessary information for movement, the control of movement depends on the interaction of the person, task, and environment (Mathiowetz & Bass-Haugen, 1994, 2002).

Contemporary motor control concepts not only explain normal movement but also allow abnormal patterns of movement to be understood and addressed in a more accurate way than they

were by the traditional concepts of motor control. That is, traditional motor control concepts understood dysfunctional movement patterns to be the result of the disturbance of hierarchical control and the dominance or re-emergence of primitive reflex patterns. The contemporary concepts of motor control acknowledge that multiple factors may contribute to the abnormal movement. Moreover, these concepts allow practitioners to consider which factor(s) might be changed in order to make the movement pattern more functional. This idea will be discussed more in the contemporary motor control approach.

Contemporary motor control concepts also emphasize that development is influenced not only by changes in the CNS but also by changes in all the elements involved in motor control (e.g., environment, task, and person). Rather than being a fixed sequence of motor changes, motor development or motor learning is a variable process of finding individual optimal solutions to motor challenges such as learning to reach out and grasp an object (Mathiowetz & Bass-Haugen, 1994, 2002). The second feature box of this chapter illustrates how the contemporary motor control model provides a more comprehensive explanation of movement.

The Traditional Neurodevelopmental Approaches

This section highlights the four neurodevelopmental treatment approaches. While these approaches overlap somewhat, they are discussed separately since they have different emphases and somewhat different arguments about movement problems and recovery of motor control.

Box 12.2   How Are the Movements for Grasping a Glass of Water Controlled?

The motor program explanation for how humans reach out and grasp a glass went something like the following. Complex instructions for reaching and grasping are encoded in the brain. These instructions, containing all the necessary information about the finely tuned movements required to grasp a glass, are retrieved and used to send biochemical effector signals that travel down the spinal cord and through peripheral nerves to stimulate very specific muscle contractions. This precise stimulation of muscles to contract produces just the right amount and combinations of tension across the joints to effect the exact movements needed to reach for and grasp the glass. Therefore, a strict causal chain unfolds in which biochemical signals cause muscle contractions, and the latter cause movements of the bones that bring the body into the proper alignment.

However, grasping a glass is not completely dependent on instructions for how to configure the fingers to effectively get hold of the glass. Configuring fingers to grasp the contours of a glass is, in part, accomplished when the fingers meet the glass. Once the hand is in position to grasp the object, the CNS only needs to increase muscle tension. The fingers will flex until they reach the glass's surface, which brakes the fingers in the appropriate spot. In fact, the most delicate adjustments are made in the rubber-like pads of the fingers, which take on the shape of the glass. All of this fine-tuning of the grasp is accomplished without the brain having to specify all the details. Consequently, much less information is needed in the brain to grasp a glass than was supposed by the motor program explanation.

Details of the action are worked out in the interaction between the person and the object being grasped (Clark, 1997; Thelen & Ulrich, 1991; Turvey, 1990). The fine-tuning of grasp depends on hand-glass interaction. Correct movements are generated in the midst of the interaction.

So, let us apply the concepts of heterarchy and emergence to the problem of reaching and grasping a glass. Something is contributed by each of the following elements:

- Intention to pick up the glass for a drink of water
- Working instructions in the brain for moving groups of muscles
- Kinetic dynamics arising out of the biomechanical organization of the shoulder and arm (i.e., how bones and muscles are connected and the movement possibilities they provide)
- Size, shape, weight, and texture of the glass

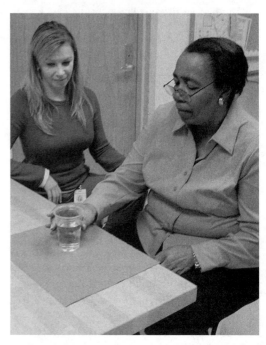

Tunde Koncz watches as her client, who experienced a stroke, reaches for a glass of water using her affected upper extremity.

Intention, neurological organization, biomechanics, and the object to be grasped become a functional heterarchy, linked together in reaching and grasping. The actual movements for reaching and grasping emerge out of their total dynamics. In this heterarchy, each element has some influence on both what gets done and how it gets done. No single element completely controls or determines what happens. Rather, the elements of the human being and environment cooperate together, each contributing something toward the total dynamics and the outcome (Kelso & Tuller, 1984).

Since the overall dynamics account for the emergent action, any difference in one of these elements that changes the total dynamics can alter the

emergent action. For example, each of the following would change how one reaches and grasps a glass:

- One is reaching for a drink nervously at a formal reception versus having a relaxed glass of tea at home
- The glass is large, heavy, and full versus small, light, and nearly empty
- The glass is sitting on a table versus someone is handing it over

In sum, the contemporary motor control theory provides a comprehensive explanation of how a simple movement such as reaching for a glass of water is accomplished.

The Rood Approach

This approach is named for its originator, Margaret Rood, an occupational therapist and physical therapist. She originally developed this approach for the treatment of persons with cerebral palsy, but it has since been applied to a wide variety of motor control problems.

Rood based her approach on the traditional view that normal motor control emerges from the use of reflex patterns present at birth. As these reflex patterns are used and generate sensory stimuli in purposeful activities, they support voluntary control at a conscious (cortical) level. However, the reflex patterns remain under unconscious (subcortical) control. Hence, basic movement patterns do not require conscious attention, which instead can be directed to the goal or purpose of the task. This subconscious organization of motor control makes for efficiency in motor tasks.

An additional observation of this approach is that different muscles have different responsibilities in the body; that is, they perform different kinds of work. Accordingly, Rood classified muscles into light-work muscles (muscles whose function is primarily movement) and heavy-work muscles (those whose function is primarily stabilization). These two types of muscles are under different types of nervous system control (i.e., heavy-work muscles tend to

be more reflexively controlled while light-work muscles are more voluntarily controlled), and they respond differently to sensory stimulation.

Rood's View of Motor Problems
Rood (1956) observed that, with CNS damage, the normal sequence of reflex development and learned voluntary motor control did not occur. Moreover, abnormal muscle tone was often present. **Muscle tone** refers to the state of stiffness or tension in muscle. Muscle tension is necessary to maintain postural states. A muscle that is sufficiently stiff is ready to be called on to contract appropriately when required. Muscle tone is maintained by the CNS in response to ongoing sensory information. When the CNS is impaired, muscles may not be adequately tense (hypotonic) or may be too tense (hypertonic).

Rood's Approach to Therapeutic Intervention
Underlying this approach is the hypothesis that appropriate sensory stimulation can elicit specific motor responses (McCormack & Feuchter, 1996). The therapeutic approach includes four strategies:

- Normalizing muscle tone by using sensory stimuli to evoke an appropriate muscle response
- Beginning with the person's current developmental level and progressing through the normal sequence of motor development

- Focusing attention on the goal or purpose of an activity
- Providing opportunities for repetition to reinforce learning

Much of Rood's technique centers on providing appropriate sensory inputs to evoke muscle responses (Rood, 1956). Sensory stimuli (e.g., applying ice, brushing, stroking the area over muscles) and proprioceptive stimuli (e.g., manual joint compression, quick stretching, tapping, pressure applied by the therapist, resistance to movement) are used to facilitate muscles. Sensory stimuli such as slow rhythmic movement, neutral warmth, and maintained stretching are used by the therapist to inhibit muscles. Olfactory, gustatory, auditory, and visual stimuli are also used to facilitate or inhibit responses. These latter sensory stimuli are used when voluntary control is minimal and where abnormal tone and reflexes are present.

Treatment progresses sequentially, from evoking muscle response with sensory stimuli to using obtained responses in developmentally appropriate patterns of movement to purposeful use of the movements in activities. Rood identified a normal developmental sequence of motor behavior to be followed in treatment. Ideally, the various techniques of sensory stimulation are used in occupational therapy to assist the client to move voluntarily and to prepare the client for active participation in purposeful activities (McCormack & Feuchter, 1996).

Practice Resources for Rood's Approach

Within the Rood approach, therapists first identify the highest developmental motor pattern that the person can manage with ease. Treatment then begins with the next level, at which the person must struggle. Sensory stimulation and manual assistance may be used to help the person perform the movement until the person is able to achieve satisfactory voluntary control of the movement.

Rood's work initiated interest in occupational therapy concerning the role of sensory stimulation in recovery of motor control. However, information from neuroscience suggests that the way in which sensory stimulation affects motor responses is more complex than the approach suggested (Brunnstrom, 1970). For example, there is evidence that the physical response to sensory stimulation is mediated or modulated by psychological factors, such as the individual's emotional state and the perceived significance of sensory stimulation (e.g., touch). Hence, the relationship between sensory stimulation and motor response is not a simple linear one as assumed in the traditional therapeutic use of sensory stimulation.

Bobaths' Neurodevelopmental Treatment

The Bobaths, a neurologist and physiotherapist team, originally developed the neurodevelopmental treatment (NDT) approach for persons with cerebral palsy (Bobath, 1978). This approach is also believed to be effective for any person with abnormal movement due to a CNS deficit. For example, this approach is frequently included in the treatment of adult hemiplegia (Trombly & Radomski, 2002).

NDT is based on the following premises:

- Motor control involves learning the sensations of movement (not the movement per se)
- Basic postural movements are learned first, later elaborated on, and integrated into functional skills
- Every activity has postural control as its underlying foundation

Bobaths' View of Motor Problems

Motor problems following brain damage involve abnormal muscle tone (e.g., spasticity) and abnormal patterns of posture and movement that interfere with everyday functional activity. Moreover, when posture and movement are abnormal, the individual's sensation reflects these abnormal patterns and provides incorrect information to the CNS. Therefore, the person is unable to experience and learn or relearn normal movement.

Bobaths' Approach to Therapeutic Intervention

Treatment requires that abnormal patterns be inhibited and replaced with the normal movement patterns that will provide appropriate sensory information for motor learning. Abnormal patterns are inhibited and normal ones are elicited by providing appropriate sensory stimuli. When persons are enabled to perform correct patterns of movement, the sensory information about movement that they generate for themselves enables the learning of motor control. Thus, the basis of this approach is for the client to learn how appropriate movement feels.

Practice Resources for Bobaths' Approach
Evaluation consists of determining the highest developmental level at which the person can consistently perform. Evaluation also aims to describe muscle tone when the body is in various developmental positions and how tone changes in response to external stimulation or voluntary effort. The evaluation identifies, for example, whether a person is arrested at a particular developmental level of motor control or whether motor abilities are scattered across developmental levels with gaps in between. Thus, the evaluation provides an individualized picture of the person's development of motor control.

Treatment follows the developmental progression and emphasizes the correct **handling** of the person to inhibit abnormal distribution of tone or postures while stimulating and encouraging active motor performance at the next developmental level. Handling is based on the principle that there are key points of control for movement (usually, but not always, proximal areas, such as the shoulder girdle). The therapist handles these points to inhibit abnormal movement and facilitate normal movement (Trombly & Radomski, 2002). Handling can take place in association with voluntary efforts of the client; its aim is to facilitate more normal movement.

Sensory stimulation, such as physically tapping muscles, may also be used. Once normal responses are elicited, they are repeated, and the person is given the opportunity to practice the movement in purposeful tasks. The thrust of therapy is to encourage voluntary control over normal responses. The underlying belief of the NDT approach is that once a person is able to control a particular developmental motor pattern voluntarily, that person will be able to integrate it into skilled activities. The goal of treatment is to prepare the person for functional performance. However, direct involvement in tasks that significantly challenge capacities are considered

contraindicated because they may elicit and reinforce maladaptive muscle tone and motor patterns.

The NDT approach has been used in occupational therapy to support and facilitate normal movement in the context of purposeful activities (Trombly & Radomski, 2002). Therapeutic activities can be adapted for clients with hemiplegia to follow the principles of this approach. Additionally, principles are incorporated into training adults with hemiplegia to perform daily living activities (e.g., teaching a person to inhibit abnormal muscle tone in his or her own body when such tone would otherwise interfere with dressing) (Trombly & Radomski, 2002).

Brunnstrom's Movement Therapy

Brunnstrom developed movement therapy as an approach to the treatment of motor control problems in persons with hemiplegia following cerebrovascular accident (Brunnstrom, 1970).

The view of organization is based on the observation that normal development involves progression of reflex development. Moreover, reflexes are modified, and their components are rearranged into purposeful movement. This is accomplished as higher centers in the brain take over.

Brunnstrom's View of Motor Problems
Brunnstrom observed that persons who experienced cerebrovascular accidents exhibited lower levels of motor function (i.e., reflex behavior) (Brunnstrom, 1970). She identified and categorized stereotypical limb movement patterns that occur sequentially in recovery from hemiplegia. She referred to these patterns as limb synergies. These synergies are patterned flexion or extension movements of the entire limb that are evoked by attempts to move the limb voluntarily, by efforts to move the unaffected limb, and/or by other sensory stimuli. Brunnstrom reasoned that because each of these reflex patterns was normal at some stage in the course of development, they could be considered normal when they appeared in persons with hemiplegia resulting from brain damage. The occurrence of these patterns was simply evidence that the function of the damaged CNS had reverted to an earlier developmental stage.

Brunnstrom's Approach to Therapeutic Intervention

Brunnstrom's therapeutic approach begins with eliciting reflex synergies and using them as the basis for progressively learning more mature voluntary movement, much as it is learned in normal development. This approach stresses using the motor patterns that are available to the client in order to progress through the recovery stages (Pedretti & Zoltan, 2001).

Practice Resources for Brunnstrom's Approach

In this approach, evaluation involves determining the person's sensory status (since the ability to sense and recognize patterns of movement is important to treatment), which reflexes are present, and the current level of recovery. Brunnstrom (1970) identified six levels of recovery from hemiplegia:

1. Flaccidity with no voluntary movement
2. Movement synergies beginning to appear
3. Voluntary control of synergies
4. Voluntary movements deviating from synergies
5. Voluntary independence from basic synergies
6. Voluntary isolated joint movements with near-normal coordination

Treatment is based on the following principles:

• Using the developmental recovery sequence
• Facilitating movement through sensory stimulation when no voluntary movement is present
• Encouraging volitional control over stimulated movements
• Reinforcing emerging synergies by asking the client to hold positions and move voluntarily
• Employing synergies that are under control in functional activities

The occupational therapy application of this approach centers on the use of controlled movements in purposeful activities. In stages three and four of recovery, when the client has some voluntary control, activities can be adapted to make use of these motor behaviors. Sometimes this involves using the affected extremity to stabilize objects while the unaffected arm is used in the task. Activities can be adapted to promote the use of existing synergies and to elicit motor behaviors that break out of, or combine, synergies and thus accomplish even greater volitional control of movement (Pedretti & Zoltan, 2001).

Brunnstrom's approach differs from the Bobath approach. The Bobaths maintained that motor patterns appearing after brain damage should not be used in retraining motor control. However, Brunnstrom argued that in the early stages of recovery, when only reflex activity is present, such activity must be used. Brunnstrom did agree, however, that reflex activity should be inhibited in the later stages of recovery.

Proprioceptive Neuromuscular Facilitation

Proprioceptive neuromuscular facilitation (PNF) is defined as "a method of promoting or hastening the response of the neuromuscular mechanism through stimulation of the proprioceptor" (Voss, Ionta, & Meyers, 1985, p. xvii). This approach is somewhat broader and more eclectic than the other three.

Several principles define the organization held by this approach (Meyers, 1995). According to this view, normal motor development proceeds cephalocaudally and proximodistally. Reflexes dominate early motor behavior and, with maturity, are integrated into voluntary motor behavior. Motor behavior is cyclic (alternating between flexion and extension phases). Normal goal-directed behavior is made up of reversing movements (e.g., flexing then extending) and depends on a balance between antagonistic muscles (e.g., flexors and extensors). Motor behavior develops in an orderly sequence of total movement patterns. This development is not stepwise; instead, there is overlap between successive stages of motor development.

Increases in motor abilities require learning. This learning often involves acquiring a chain or series of steps and later integrating them into the task. Frequent stimulation and motor repetition support retention of learned motor abilities. A final important principle is that motor learning requires multisensory information. Auditory, visual, and tactile systems provide sensory data along with proprioceptive information to program the learning of movement.

PNF View of Motor Problems

In terms of this approach, impairment is any difficulty with motor control. PNF was originally developed for the treatment of persons with cerebral palsy and multiple sclerosis, but it has found application with a wide range of clients, including persons whose motor limitations are not of CNS origin.

PNF Approach to Therapeutic Intervention

The therapeutic approach of PNF is multisensory. The kinds of sensory stimulation used include physical contact by the therapist, visual cues, and verbal commands. The central feature of treatment is the use of diagonal patterns of movement (i.e., moving extremities in a plane diagonal to the body midline) for recovery of motor function. Diagonal patterns are considered the treatment of choice because they involve natural movements that are part of normal development and require integration of both sides of the body.

Practice Resources for PNF

Evaluation is broad-based and may include determination of the developmental postures and movement patterns of which the individual is capable and of the person's ability to use these capacities in functional activities. The goal of evaluation is to gather a comprehensive picture of the strengths and challenges of the client's capacity for movement and to identify these in sufficient detail so that appropriate techniques for intervention can be selected.

Several techniques are used to encourage the client's engaging in natural diagonal patterns of movement. One method is irradiation, which seeks to facilitate specific muscle action by using stronger muscle groups to stimulate activity of weaker groups. Another technique, successive induction, aims to facilitate one voluntary motion by using another. A third technique, reciprocal innervation, uses voluntary motion to inhibit reflexes. Other techniques include appropriate positioning, use of manual contact for positioning or stimulation, and verbal commands and instructions for movement. Other methods of sensory stimulation, such as stretching muscles and providing resistance to movement, are also employed. Goal-directed movements combined with facilitation techniques are believed to be the most effective means of treatment.

Summary of the Neurodevelopmental Approaches

Although the previous discussion illustrates the different emphases of the four neurodevelopmental approaches, they share the following view of motor control (Mathiowetz & Bass-Haugen, 1994, 2002). They assert that the CNS is hierarchically organized (i.e., higher centers control lower centers) and that movement is controlled by sensory input to lower centers and through the encoded motor programs of higher centers. They assert that development and learning occur because of maturational or experientially driven changes in the CNS.

According to the neurodevelopmental approaches, motor control occurs because the human being learns to master movements and then uses those movements to accomplish tasks. Fixed sequences of motor learning and development are viewed as necessary consequences of how the system hierarchically builds on and modifies lower-level movement patterns (e.g., voluntary movement builds on reflex-driven postural control).

Understanding Motor Problems

According to the neurodevelopmental approaches, abnormal patterns of movement result directly from disorganization in the CNS. Damage to the CNS disrupts or interferes with sensory/perceptual inputs, motor programs, and the normal hierarchical organization of motor control. This, in turn, produces abnormal muscle tone, reflexes, and movement patterns.

Therapeutic Intervention

The neurodevelopmental approaches focus exclusively on understanding and remediating motor control deficits that are believed to result directly from the nature of damage to or disorganization in the CNS. The most basic concepts underlying the approach to intervention focus on:

- Inhibiting with sensory stimuli abnormal muscle tone, reflexes, and movement patterns
- Facilitating with sensory stimuli normal muscle tone and movement patterns

Underlying this focus is the assumption that all observed changes in the dynamics of muscle and movement are directly related to changes achieved in CNS organization.

The neurodevelopmental approaches emphasize learning through task repetition with constant assistance (e.g., handling, positioning, instructions) and feedback from the therapist. They also emphasize a developmental progression from learning parts of a task to proceeding to combine the parts into a whole.

Recovery and treatment are expected to follow normal developmental sequences from reflex to voluntary control, from gross to discrete movements, and from proximal to distal control. Consequently, these approaches emphasize using movements that are normal or that follow recovery sequences. The perceived importance of these sequences is based on the assumption that they are "hard-wired" in the CNS.

Practice Resources

In the neurodevelopmental approaches, evaluation focuses on:

- Determining the status of muscle tone, sensation and perception, and postural control
- Identifying abnormal reflexes and movement patterns
- Ascertaining the developmental level of existing motor control patterns

The technology for treatment relies heavily on the use of external sensory stimulation and handling to elicit correct patterns of movement. Moreover, these approaches emphasize practicing and mastering movement patterns with the assumption that, once normal movement patterns are mastered, they will generalize to functional motor control in occupational performance.

Participation in occupation is not emphasized. When occupations are used, they are chosen because they are thought to elicit the appropriate movement patterns. Sometimes the use of occupational activities has been discouraged because they are seen as developing isolated splinter skills. Such splinter skills are viewed as specific to the task performed and hence not

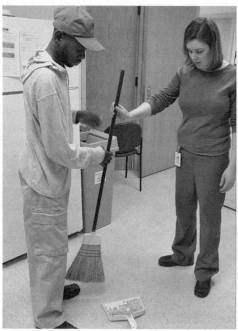 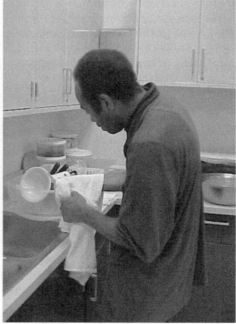

Everyday tasks are used as a context for evaluation and intervention in the model of motor control.

generalizable to other areas of performance. In general, occupation does not play a central role in the remediation of motor control deficits in the neurodevelopmental approaches.

Theory and Practice Resources of the Contemporary Motor Control Approach

The contemporary motor control approach has been articulated in occupational therapy (Bass-Haugen, Mathiowetz, & Flinn, 2008; Mathiowetz & Bass-Haugen, 1994, 1995, 2002; Radomski & Trombly Latham, 2008).

Theory

Motor control is viewed as emerging from the interaction of the human (including motivational, cognitive, CNS, and musculoskeletal components) with environmental and task variables. Movement is understood to be a self-organizing phenomenon that depends on this dynamic interaction. Importantly, in this approach movement is understood not to depend solely on the CNS. Rather, the control of movement is multivariate; that is, it is controlled by the interaction of person, task, and environmental factors. This idea of the control of movement reflects the concepts of heterarchy and emergence discussed earlier.

In the contemporary motor control approach the CNS is viewed as a heterarchically organized system with higher and lower centers interacting cooperatively with each other and with the musculoskeletal system. Moreover, movement patterns are understood not as invariant sequences "pre-wired" into the CNS but as stable (or preferred) ways to accomplish occupational performance, given the unique characteristics of the human being and certain environmental conditions. This view reflects the concepts of attractor states discussed earlier. These preferred patterns of movement can be perturbed by changes in any of the participating systems or in the environment (i.e., by variables that become control parameters).

According to the contemporary motor control approach, motor control is learned through a process in which the person seeks optimal solutions for accomplishing an occupation. Hence, learning is dependent on the characteristics of the performer, the context, and the task being performed. When patterns of movement are practiced, they become attractor states. When they are practiced under a wider range of conditions, they are more stable than when learned under narrow conditions.

Changes in the environmental conditions, the task, or the person can result in a disintegration or a qualitative shift in the preferred pattern of movement. Thus, control parameters that change motor behavior may be within the CNS or musculoskeletal system, within the task, or within the environment. For example, changes in strength, CNS maturation, size or weight of an object being handled, or the speed of action required for the task can be control parameters that change motor behavior patterns.

The contemporary model of motor control in occupational therapy emphasizes the role of the occupation being performed and the occupational context in which it is performed. The task being performed is recognized as having an important influence on all motor control. Within this model, motor control is viewed as behavior that self-organizes specifically in the context of performing a given task (Lin, Wu, & Trombly, 1998; Trombly, 1995; Wu, Trombly, & Lin, 1994).

Finally, the contemporary motor control model does not emphasize a fixed developmental or motor learning sequence. Rather the sequence of motor change or learning depends both on the unique characteristics of the individual and on variations in the environment in which motor control is learned.

Understanding Motor Problems

When persons have CNS damage, problems of motor behavior result from the attempt to compensate for the damage while performing a specific occupational form in a given context. If the occupation or the environment in which the person is performing changes, the kind of motor behavior the person exhibits may also change (Mathiowetz & Bass-Haugen, 1994, 1995; Trombly, 1995). Hence, while impairment of movement is related to deficits in the CNS, it is not directly caused by those deficits. Rather, movement patterns are a consequence of the dynamics that occur between a person with specific abilities and limitations (as represented in both the CNS and the musculoskeletal system), the task being performed, and the environmental conditions in which performance takes place. Thus, for example, an abnormal movement pattern may be jointly influenced by CNS impairment and muscle weakness but may be present only under certain occupational and environmental conditions.

Therapeutic Intervention

A central premise of the task-oriented approach is that "functional tasks help organize behavior" (Mathiowetz & Bass-Haugen, 2002, p. 139). According to Mathiowetz and Bass-Haugen, therapy begins by identifying those tasks that are difficult to perform and by noting the preferred movement patterns the person uses for those tasks. The therapist then determines the personal and environmental systems that either support optimal performance or contribute to ineffective performance. This provides an identification of the supporting and limiting factors in motor control and serves as a basis for determining intervention.

> The contemporary motor control approach stresses learning the entire task rather than discrete parts.

The therapist also seeks to determine the stability or instability of motor behaviors across occupational and environmental conditions. In this way, the range of conditions in which functional and impaired movement patterns are manifest can be determined. This reveals how strong an attractor state a particular movement pattern is and, therefore, how easily it can be disturbed or shifted to another pattern.

Depending on what evaluation reveals, intervention can differ. For example, if a person's motor behavior is unstable, the therapist may help the client find the optimal motor solution and practice it so that it becomes more stable. If the client is using a motor control strategy that accomplishes the goal of the task but that is not the most efficient or safe, the therapist may help the client to find and stabilize different strategies of movement.

The contemporary motor control approach stresses learning the entire task rather than discrete parts. This approach also emphasizes

allowing persons to find their own optimal solutions to motor problems rather than relying on instructions and constant feedback. Persons are allowed to experiment and problem-solve in the context of occupational performance. Feedback on the overall consequences of performance is considered more useful than discrete feedback about parts of the performance.

The goals of treatment in this approach focus on:

- Accomplishing necessary and desired tasks in the most efficient way, given the client's characteristics
- Allowing the person to practice in varying and natural contexts so the learned motor behaviors are more stable
- Maximizing personal and environmental characteristics that enhance performance
- Enhancing problem-solving abilities of clients so they will more readily find solutions to challenges encountered in new environments beyond the treatment setting

Overall, this approach stresses a collaborative and client-centered approach that considers the client's roles and motives.

Practice Resources

The approach to evaluation is client-centered and task-oriented, emphasizing the observation of a person's attempts to perform meaningful tasks in context as illustrated in the example featuring Mariela, a young woman who experienced a stroke (see Box 12.4). Evaluation methods incorporate both quantitative and qualitative data-gathering that examines how motor control varies in different occupational forms and contexts (Mathiowetz & Bass-Haugen, 2002; Trombly, 1995). Evaluation begins with observation of occupational performance and proceeds to examine underlying systems only when further understanding of how those systems are constraining performance is needed.

For example, the therapist would not begin with evaluation of reflexes and muscle tone. Rather, the therapist would begin with examination of whether and how the person performed

Box 12.3 **Task-Oriented Treatment**

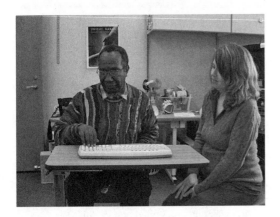

In this picture, Heidi Fischer and a client are involved in motor control treatment that focuses on massed practice of movements in a task-oriented context. The client pictured here was an engineer who often used the computer and played the piano before his stroke. He is practicing several repetitions of finger extension and abduction during a keyboarding task. Another motor control strategy used with this client is shaping to enhance movement. For example, the client practices opening the fingers to grasp a cup with the wrist extended for several repetitions before picking it up.

necessary occupational forms. Then, when difficulties are noted, the therapist might proceed to identify whether and how muscle tone and abnormal reflexes contribute (along with the environment and the occupational form) to difficulties in performance. Consequently, the focus of evaluation is on occupational performance, not on the underlying general motor abilities.

This also means that the therapist begins by learning what tasks are necessary for the role performance of the client. When therapists examine human systems to determine how they are contributing to difficulties in performance, the CNS is recognized as important but only as one among several factors that co-determine performance. There are not yet validated standard methods of evaluation. However, principles of assessment and ways of incorporating existing assessments into the approach have been identified (Mathiowetz & Bass-Haugen, 2002).

Because this model emphasizes the use of client-centered occupational forms, natural environments, and a process of active experimentation for optimal motor solutions, its techniques cannot be as readily specified as those of the neurodevelopmental approaches. These traditional approaches assumed that motor control was driven by a single system, the CNS. Hence, techniques were quite specific.

The contemporary approach identifies multiple factors that influence motor control and argues that their relative importance and influence on a client's performance are situationally dependent. Hence, the actual techniques used in therapy require an individualized understanding of the client's situation across many dimensions. For those accustomed to the much more standardized approaches of the neurodevelopmental approaches, the motor control approach may, at first, appear much less prescriptive and specific. Bass-Haugen et al. (2008) outline a number of principles of this approach. For example, under the general approach using an occupation-based focus, they note that the therapist should:

- Use functional tasks as the focus in treatment
- Select tasks that are meaningful and important in the client's roles
- Analyze the characteristics of the tasks selected for treatment
- Describe the movements used for the task performance
- Determine whether the movement patterns are stable or in transition
- Analyze the movement patterns and functional outcomes of task performance

Mastos, Miller, Elliasson, and Imms (2007) have introduced a goal-directed training approach based on contemporary motor control theory. They stress the importance of goal setting in ensuring that meaningful task goals are selected. This intervention also stresses analyzing how the task and environment can be modified to support performance along with involving the client in a process of problem-solving to achieve strategies that optimize functional capacity.

Davis (2006) describes task selection and environmental enrichment intervention for persons with stroke that uses the contemporary motor control approach. This approach stresses

Box 12.4

Case Example: Using the Contemporary Motor Control Approach

Tunde Koncz works with patients who have experienced neurological damage resulting in difficulty with occupational performance. Tunde has been working with Mariela, a 21-year-old woman recovering from a stroke, for almost a year. Mariela's hemorrhagic stroke at age 20 left her with a right upper extremity that had almost no movement. When she entered occupational therapy, Mariela's right hand and arm were completely nonfunctional and she had no use of them in her daily life. Since her stroke, Mariela had favored her unaffected left side and had adjusted her daily activities around use of this side.

Tunde chose to consider Mariela's case from a motor control perspective because of the damage to her central nervous system and Mariela's difficulty with movement and limited use of her hemiplegic side. Tunde began her assessment by observing Mariela's occupational performance and noting that Mariela was not using her right hand in any activity. Tunde conducted observations of Mariela's performance in upper body dressing, self-feeding, and grooming activities like combing her hair. Mariela's difficulty incorporating her right side into tasks indicated that decreased strength and range of motion were control parameters that prevented any significant use of her affected arm and hand.

Mariela came to occupational therapy hoping to incorporate her formerly dominant right hand into activities like dressing, feeding herself, and tub transfers. She wanted to be able to use her right side to increase her independence in her daily life. Mariela also hoped to be able to use both hands to play with her dog as she had in the past.

Tunde collaborated with Mariela to set short-term goals of improving Mariela's strength and active range of motion. They also agreed on the long-term goals of Mariela becoming independent in ADL activities and using her right hand to assist in two-handed tasks. Early in Mariela's treatment, Tunde incorporated various exercises that would be used to increase Mariela's range of motion and strength on her affected side.

Once Mariela's strength and range of motion had improved enough for her to have some functional capacity, Tunde began to incorporate more task-oriented approaches in her occupational therapy intervention to enhance Mariela's motor skills. For instance, Mariela used her right hand to reach for a comb that she then used to comb her hair and she reached for a water bottle to take a drink. Repetition of appropriate movements in therapy was used to help Mariela relearn these motor tasks. Asking Mariela to practice reaching in different contexts made it more likely that the movement learned by her affected side would be able to be applied later.

Other activities that Tunde and Mariela frequently worked on in therapy included cooking, cleaning, turning lights on and off, handling money, bathing, dressing, and feeding. Tunde had Mariela complete all of these activities with assistance from her affected side to improve function. These functional approaches were chosen with the intention of retraining Mariela's movement through repetition in varied contexts.

Since beginning her occupational therapy treatment, many of Mariela's range of motion

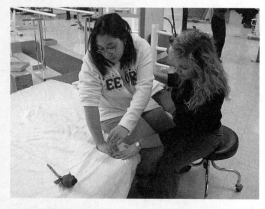

Mariela reaches for a pen that she will use to sign her name.

measurements have entered into normal ranges and her grip strength has improved. She is able to use her right hand to assist in some daily tasks. Mariela has made improvements and continues to work toward her long-term goals. Tunde continues to work with Mariela toward her goals of becoming completely independent in ADLs and improving her ability to incorporate her right hand into her daily tasks.

the use of real life tasks that are motivating to the client and careful selection of environmental factors that elicit the most desirable movements and that increase functioning. The approach involves a number of principles such as careful positioning of the person and task objects, incorporating the involved extremity into all tasks, and selecting tasks well matched to the person's impairments.

Additionally, Flinn (1995, 1999), Sabari (1991), and Tse and Spaulding (1998) have outlined the implications of this approach for treatment of persons with specific impairments such as hemiplegia and Parkinson's disease. Finally, one of the most recent treatment approaches to emanate from the contemporary motor control approach is constraint-induced therapy. This approach combines constraining use of the unaffected or less affected limb with practice of functional tasks using the affected or more affected extremity (Morris, Crago, DeLuca, Pidikiti, & Taub, 1997; Roberts, Vegher, Gilewski, Bender & Riggs, 2005; Stevenson & Thalman, 2007).

Summary and Comparison of the Neurodevelopmental and the Contemporary Motor Control Approaches

The previous sections overviewed the traditional neurodevelopmental and the contemporary motor control approaches. In general, the contemporary motor control approach offers a more dynamic and holistic explanation of movement than the traditional neurodevelopmental approaches. In contrast to the neurodevelopmental approaches, which de-emphasized the role of the environment and of the task in motor control and in the remediation of motor control deficits, the contemporary model places a great deal of emphasis on both of these elements.

Research and Evidence Base

The Bobath NDT approach is the most studied of the four neurodevelopmental approaches, although the studies tend to be methodologically weak (Levit, 2002). Research does not clearly show that NDT therapy is an effective treatment. For example, one study suggested that nonspecific play activities were as effective as NDT in producing motor behavior gain (Levit, 2002). There are no published studies of the effectiveness of NDT with persons who have hemiplegia. Research concerning the PNF approach is limited and focuses primarily on normal populations (Trombly & Radomski, 2002). Usually, each of these studies examined an isolated aspect of PNF, and the results from these studies are mixed. Overall, no systematic body of occupational therapy research has accumulated on the neurodevelopmental approaches.

While the contemporary motor control approach is relatively new, studies (Eastridge & Rice, 2004; Fasoli, Trombly, Tickle-Degnen, & Verfaellie, 2002; Mathiowetz & Bass-Haugen, 1994; Wu et al., 1994) have begun to provide support for the theory and efficacy of this model. In summary of research, Ma and Trombly (2002) and Trombly and Ma (2002) note that 15 studies have examined the impact of occupational therapy on coordinated movement. Those studies concluded that among factors associated with positive outcomes are the use of meaningful objects and goal-oriented activities. These studies provide some support for the new motor control model, but it is noted that more research is needed. Dickson (2002) also reviewed evidence concerning motor control interventions for persons with stroke and concluded that there is little evidence for the traditional neurodevelopmental approaches. She also noted that, while there is more evidence for the contemporary motor control approach, more evidence needs to be forthcoming.

Both the traditional neurodevelopmental and contemporary motor control approaches are heavily based on movement science research. Clearly, there is strong evidence that contradicts many traditional concepts of motor control. Moreover, a robust research literature supports the contemporary approach. Hence, this body of research strongly suggests that the traditional neurodevelopmental approaches need to be reconsidered and incorporated into the contemporary motor control approach.

Discussion

In the transition from traditional neurodevelopmental approaches to a contemporary motor control approach, consideration will need to be given to which concepts and techniques from the traditional approach are still valid and useful in a contemporary framework. Moreover, further work to develop resources for application of the contemporary motor control model is needed.

The use of traditional neurodevelopmental approaches is still widespread and characterized by strong allegiance of therapists to one or more approaches. Thus, there are disagreements between those who espouse traditional neurodevelopmental methods and those promoting the contemporary motor control approach and its explicit criticism of the traditional neurodevelopmental approaches (Cammisa et al., 1995; Mathiowetz & Bass-Haugen, 1995). Nonetheless, the kinds of changes in conceptualization and application that are called for by the contemporary motor control approach are very promising. They reaffirm many traditional occupational therapy ideas that emphasize the importance of occupation in learning motor skills and restoring motor capacity.

The neurodevelopmental approaches were founded in the paradigm of inner mechanisms described in Chapter 4. The reorganization of these approaches into a more contemporary motor control model signals the transformation of practice that emanated from that older paradigm to practice consistent with the current paradigm of occupational therapy.

Box 12.5

Motor Control Model Case Example: JIM

Jim is 71 years old. A stroke 10 years ago affected the left side of his body. Jim's occupational therapist, Heidi Fischer, did an informal interview with Jim to learn more about his goals for treatment, what he finds enjoyable or meaningful, and what motivates him. Her assessment also included a comprehensive evaluation of his motor performance.

Jim has regained the ability to walk without a cane. He is independent with his self-care but needs assistance with certain bimanual tasks due to decreased hand function and weakness on his left side. Specifically, he has decreased finger extension, fine motor coordination, and grip and pinch strength. He is unable to grasp with his left hand and has difficulty performing tasks that require the use of individual fingers. He has increased muscle tone throughout his left side limiting his ability to fully extend his elbow and perform shoulder movements. He has no proprioception in his left upper extremity (i.e., no sense of where his arm is in space). When performing tasks, especially if strenuous, his muscle tone increases, making it more difficult to complete the task.

Overall, Jim is very independent and able to do most things he wants to do with extra time. His main concern is to be able to use his hand more effectively to make some tasks less frustrating and difficult including buttoning, tying laces, tying a tie, putting gloves on, and using some of his tools for woodworking and home projects.

Jim is a retired electrician and lives with his wife. He is responsible for managing his lawn and various other projects around their two homes. He enjoys fishing, cooking, woodworking, driving his convertible, watching movies, playing cards, going to dinner, and spending time with his family. He volunteers for research studies (such as the one in which he is currently participating) to help researchers learn about strokes as well as to improve his function. He is a hard worker and very competitive.

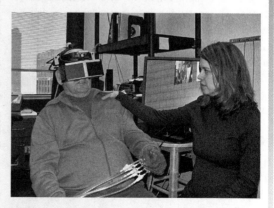

Jim practices virtual object grasp and release.

Box 12.5 (continued)

Jim's main goal is to increase his finger extension and improve his overall hand function to make tasks easier to accomplish. Jim enjoys games and competition and finds this challenge motivating during therapy. Jim's treatment is part of a research protocol to improve hand function using virtual reality and a pneumatic orthosis that assists with finger extension.

Jim participated in six weeks of therapy that occurred three times per week for one hour each day. During each session, he practiced grasp and release of virtual objects with the pneumatic glove during a game for 30 minutes for a total of 120 repetitions. He then practiced actual functional tasks with the pneumatic glove and real objects. He was able to choose these tasks according to what goals were meaningful to him. For example, he wanted to improve his ability to use his tools and to manage nails and screws with his left hand so some of his sessions focused on improving these skills. Many of the sessions focused on increasing coordination and his ability to extend his fingers during tasks, such as playing cards. He also worked on trying to increase control of his left upper extremity by relaxing between tasks and decreasing overrecruitment of muscles during difficult tasks to increase efficiency.

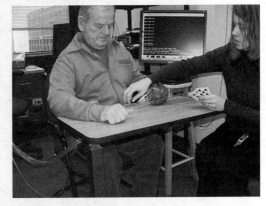

Heidi and Jim play cards to allow him to practice finger extension.

Jim showed improvement during the first few weeks of therapy by increasing muscle control and learning to calibrate force during grasp and release tasks. By repetitively practicing finger extension and shaping his movement during functional tasks, he was able to achieve success. At the beginning of treatment, Jim was only able to grasp and release five virtual objects successfully. By the end of treatment, he was able to grasp and release all 60 virtual objects. His grip and pinch strength improved and he was now able to perform a palmar grasp. He demonstrated increased shoulder abduction, shoulder flexion, forearm pronation, wrist extension, circumduction, and pincer grasp, as well as increased smoothness of upper extremity movement. For example, with the development of a pincer grasp, he is now able to hold nails when hammering in order to complete a woodworking project.

Table 12.1 **Terms of the Model**

Attractor states	Preferred movement patterns that emerge from the dynamic interaction of the person with the environment without centralized instructions.
Cephalocaudal	Refers to sequence of motor development from the head downward.
Control parameter	A variable whose change can shift a pattern of motor behavior into another pattern.
Emergence	The spontaneous occurrence of complex motor actions that come out of the interactions of person, task, and environment rather than being controlled top down by a motor program.
Handling	Therapist's manipulation of the client's body.

(table continues on page 194)

Table 12.1 **Terms of the Model** continued

Heterarchical control	Conceptualization that argues that movements are controlled by systems cooperating toward the production of movement but without central executive control.
Hierarchical control	Conceptualization that argues that movements are controlled from the top down (i.e., higher brain centers control lower ones).
Motor control	The ability to use one's body effectively in interacting with the environment.
Motor program	A set of neurologically wired instructions (sometimes called a central pattern generator) for accomplishing a complex movement.
Muscle tone	The state of stiffness or tension in muscle.
Plasticity	The nervous system's potential for organization and reorganization as the result of experience.
Proximodistal	Refers to the sequence of motor development from the middle of the body to the distant limbs.
Reflex	A biologically determined movement pattern not under volitional control.

Table 12.2 **Motor Control Model**

FOCUS
- Concerned with problems of movement following brain damage
- Consists of four traditional treatment approaches and a contemporary motor control model

INTERDISCIPLINARY BASE
- Concepts from neurophysiology, neuropsychology, cognitive psychology, and movement science

COMPARISION OF EACH OF THE MOTOR CONTROL APPROACHES

The Rood Approach	Bobaths' Neurodevelopmental Treatment	Brunnstrom's Movement Therapy	Proprioceptive Neuromuscular Facilitation
Organization Normal motor control emerges from the use of subcortically controlled reflex patterns present at birth; they support voluntary control at a conscious (cortical) level.	Motor control involves learning the sensations of movement. Basic postural movements are learned first, later elaborated, and integrated into functional skills.	Normal development involves a progression of reflexes that are modified and components of which are rearranged into purposeful movement as higher centers in the brain take over.	Development of motor behavior is cyclic—that is, made up of reversing movements (e.g., flexing then extending) and depends on a balance between "antagonistic" muscles (e.g., flexors and extensors).

The Rood Approach	Bobaths' Neurodevelopmental Treatment	Brunnstrom's Movement Therapy	Proprioceptive Neuromuscular Facilitation
Light-work muscles primarily provide movement and are more voluntarily controlled. Heavy-work muscles primarily stabilize and are more reflexively controlled.			Motor behavior develops in an orderly sequence of total movement patterns with overlap between successive stages of motor development. Motor learning involves acquiring a chain or series of steps and later integrating them into the task through stimulation and motor repetition. Motor learning requires multisensory information (i.e., auditory, visual, tactile, and proprioceptive).

Problems and Challenges

With CNS damage the normal sequence of reflex development and learning of voluntary motor control are impaired, and abnormal muscle tone is often present.	Brain damage results in spasticity and abnormal patterns of posture and movement that interfere with everyday functional activity. When posture and movement are abnormal, sensation provides incorrect information to the CNS, preventing learning or relearning of normal movement.	Cerebrovascular accident (and other brain damage) leads to regression to lower levels of motor function (i.e., reflex behavior). Stereotypical limb flexion or extension movement patterns occur sequentially in recovery from hemiplegia (limb synergies).	CNS damage and orthopedic problems can interfere with normal patterns of movement, reducing capacity for functional activity.

Therapeutic Intervention

Progress from appropriate sensory inputs to evoke muscle response when voluntary control is minimal and abnormal	Abnormal patterns are inhibited and normal ones elicited by sensory stimuli. When persons perform normal patterns	Reflex patterns (normal at various stages in the course of development) elicited by brain damage	Multisensory stimulation (including physical contact, verbal commands, and visual cues).

(table continues on page 196)

Table 12.2   **Motor Control Model continued**

The Rood Approach	Bobaths' Neurodevelopmental Treatment	Brunnstrom's Movement Therapy	Proprioceptive Neuromuscular Facilitation
tone and reflexes are present, to using obtained responses in developmentally appropriate patterns of movement, to purposeful use of the movements in activities.	of movement, sensory information about movement allows learning of motor control.	can be built upon for relearning of motor control (thus, they should be initially facilitated and later inhibited).	Employment of natural diagonal patterns of movement (i.e., moving extremities in a plane diagonal to the body midline).

Technology for Application

Identify the highest developmental motor pattern that the person can do with ease. Use sensory stimuli to normalize muscle tone. Begin with current developmental level and progress through normal sequence of motor development. Focus attention on the goal or purpose of an activity. Provide opportunities for repetition to reinforce learning.	Determine the highest developmental level at which the person can consistently perform, distribution of muscle tone when the body is in various developmental positions, and how tone changes in response to external stimulation or voluntary effort. Abnormal patterns stopped (inhibited through sensory stimuli) and replaced with normal movement patterns (elicited through sensory stimuli) to provide appropriate sensory information for motor learning in developmental sequence. Handling of the person to inhibit abnormal distribution of tone or postures while stimulating and encouraging active motor performance at the next developmental level.	Identify person's sensory status (sensation to recognize patterns of movement is important to treatment). Identify which reflexes are present and determine level of recovery as manifest in reflex synergies of movement. Elicit reflex synergies of movement and use them as the basis for learning progressively more mature voluntary movement. Employment of developmental recovery sequence: Facilitate movement through sensory stimulation. Encourage volitional control over stimulated movements. Reinforce emerging synergies through voluntary use in functional activities.	Determine available developmental postures and movement patterns and ability to use them in functional activities to generate a comprehensive picture of capacity for movement. Stimulate diagonal patterns for recovery of motor function through: Facilitating specific muscle action by using stronger muscle groups to stimulate activity of weaker groups (irradiation). Facilitating one voluntary motion by using another (successive induction) and inhibiting reflexes by voluntary motion (reciprocal innervation). Appropriate positioning, using manual contact to position or stimulate the individual.

The Rood Approach	Bobaths' Neurodevelopmental Treatment	Brunnstrom's Movement Therapy	Proprioceptive Neuromuscular Facilitation
	Practice new abilities in purposeful tasks to encourage voluntary control over normal responses in purposeful activities.	Elicit motor behaviors in purposeful tasks that break out of, or combine, synergies for greater volitional control of movement.	Giving verbal commands and instructions for movement. Sensory stimulation such as stretching muscles and providing resistance to movement. Goal-directed activities combined with facilitation techniques.

COMPARISON OF NEURODEVELOPMENTAL APPROACHES AND MOTOR CONTROL APPROACHES

Traditional Neurodevelopmental Approaches (Common Features)	Contemporary Motor Control Approach
Organization CNS is hierarchically organized (i.e., higher centers control lower centers). Movement is controlled by sensory input to lower centers and through the encoded motor programs of higher centers. Development and learning result from changes in the CNS. Fixed sequences of motor learning and development.	Motor control is a self-organizing phenomenon that emerges from the interaction of the human system (CNS and musculoskeletal components) with environmental and occupational variables. CNS is a heterarchically organized system with higher and lower centers interacting cooperatively and with the musculoskeletal system. Movement patterns are stable/preferred ways to accomplish occupational performance (attractor states) given the unique characteristics of the human being and environmental conditions. Motor control is learned when the person seeks optimal solutions for accomplishing an occupation and depends on the characteristics of the performer, the context, and the goal of the occupation being performed. Developmental pathways depend on unique characteristics of the individual and on variations in the environment.
Problems and Challenges Abnormal muscle tone, reflexes, and patterns of movement result directly from disorganization in the CNS.	Motor impairment is a consequence of the dynamics that occur between a person with specific abilities and limitations (as represented in both the CNS and the musculoskeletal system) and the occupational and environmental demands faced in trying to perform.

(table continues on page 198)

Table 12.2   **Motor Control Model** continued

Traditional Neurodevelopmental Approaches (Common Features)	Contemporary Motor Control Approach
Therapeutic Intervention Inhibition of abnormal muscle tone, reflexes, and movement patterns with sensory stimuli. Facilitation of normal muscle tone and movement patterns with sensory stimuli. Learning through task repetition with constant assistance (e.g., handling, positioning, instructions) and feedback from the therapist. Progression from learning parts of a task to combining the parts into a whole. Progression of recovery and treatment through developmental sequence (reflex to voluntary control, gross to discrete movements, and proximal to distal control). Using movements that are normal or that follow recovery sequences.	Emphasizes person's attempts to perform meaningful occupational tasks in context. Intervention depends on: Identification of those tasks that are difficult to perform, noting the preferred movement patterns for these tasks and their degree of stability/ instability. Determination of personal and environmental systems that either support optimal performance or contribute to ineffective performance. Emphasizes: Learning the entire occupation rather than discrete parts. Allowing persons to find their own optimal solutions to motor problems.
Technology for Application Determine status of muscle tone, sensation and perception, and postural control. Identifying abnormal reflexes and movement patterns. Ascertaining the developmental level of existing motor control patterns. External sensory stimulation and handling to elicit correct patterns of movement. Practicing and mastering movement patterns. Participation in occupational forms is not emphasized.	Examines occupational performance and proceeds to examine underlying systems when further understanding of how those systems are constraining performance is needed. Emphasizes the use of client-centered occupational forms, natural environments, and a process of active experimentation for optimal motor solutions. Techniques used in therapy require an individualized understanding of the client's situation across many dimensions.
Research Research on neurodevelopmental approaches is limited.	Preliminary studies have begun to provide support for the theory of contemporary motor control approach.

SUMMARY OF THE CONTEMPORARY MOTOR CONTROL MODEL

Theory

+ Motor control is viewed as emerging from the interaction of the human (including motivational, cognitive, CNS, and musculoskeletal components) with environmental and task variables

+ In this approach, movement is understood not to depend solely on the CNS

+ The CNS is viewed as a heterarchically organized system with higher and lower centers interacting cooperatively with each other and with the musculoskeletal system

+ Movement patterns are understood not as invariant sequences "pre-wired" into the CNS but as stable ways to accomplish occupational performance, given the unique characteristics of the human being and certain environmental conditions

+ Motor control is learned through a process in which the person seeks optimal solutions for accomplishing an occupation

+ When patterns of movement are practiced, they become attractor states

+ Changes in the environmental conditions, the task, or the person can result in a disintegration or a qualitative shift in the preferred pattern of movement

+ The contemporary model of motor control in occupational therapy emphasizes the role of the occupation being performed and the occupational context in which it is performed

+ Within this model, motor control is viewed as behavior that self-organizes specifically in the context of performing a given task

+ The sequence of motor change or learning depends both on the unique characteristics of the individual and on variations in the environment in which motor control is learned

Understanding Motor Problems

+ When persons have CNS damage, problems of motor behavior result from the attempt to compensate for the damage while performing a specific occupational form in a given context

+ Movement patterns are a consequence of the dynamics that occur between a person with specific abilities and limitations, the task being performed, and the environmental conditions in which performance takes place

Therapeutic Intervention

+ Therapy begins by identifying those tasks that are difficult to perform and by noting the preferred movement patterns the person uses for those tasks

+ The therapist then determines the personal and environmental systems that either support optimal performance or contribute to ineffective performance

+ The therapist also seeks to determine the stability or instability of motor behaviors across occupational and environmental conditions

+ This reveals how strong an attractor state a particular movement pattern is and, therefore, how easily it can be disturbed or shifted to another pattern

+ The contemporary motor control approach stresses learning the entire task rather than discrete parts

+ This approach also emphasizes allowing persons to find their own optimal solutions to motor problems rather than relying on instructions and constant feedback

+ The goals of treatment in this approach focus on:
  • Accomplishing necessary and desired tasks in the most efficient way, given the client's characteristics
  • Allowing the person to practice in varying and natural contexts so the learned motor behaviors are more stable
  • Maximizing personal and environmental characteristics that enhance performance
  • Enhancing problem-solving abilities of clients so they will more readily find solutions to challenges encountered in new environments beyond the treatment setting

Practice Resources

+ The approach to evaluation is client-centered and task-oriented, emphasizing the observation of a person's attempts to perform meaningful tasks in context

+ Evaluation methods incorporate both quantitative and qualitative data-gathering

+ Evaluation begins with observation of occupational performance and proceeds to examine underlying systems only when further understanding of how those systems are constraining performance is needed

+ The therapist begins by learning what tasks are necessary for the role performance of the client

+ There are not yet validated standard methods of evaluation. However, principles of assessment and ways of incorporating existing assessments into the approach have been identified

+ Because this model emphasizes the use of client-centered occupational forms, natural environments, and a process of active

experimentation for optimal motor solutions, its techniques cannot be as readily specified as those of the neurodevelopmental approaches

+ The contemporary approach identifies multiple factors that influence motor control and argues that their relative importance and influence on a client's performance are situationally dependent

+ The actual techniques used in therapy require an individualized understanding of the client's situation across many dimensions. It has been suggested that therapists should:
  • Use functional tasks as the focus in treatment
  • Select tasks that are meaningful and important in the client's roles
  • Analyze the characteristics of the tasks selected for treatment
  • Describe the movements used for the task performance
  • Determine whether the movement patterns are stable or in transition
  • Analyze the movement patterns and functional outcomes of task performance

REFERENCES

Bass-Haugen, J., Mathiowetz, V., & Flinn, F. (2008). Optimizing motor behavior using the occupational therapy task-oriented approach. In M.V. Radomski & C.A. Trombly Latham (Eds.), *Occupational therapy for physical dysfunction* (6th ed., pp. 598–617). Philadelphia: Lippincott Williams & Wilkins.

Bobath, B. (1978). *Adult hemiplegia: Evaluation and treatment* (2nd ed.). London: William Heinnemann Medical Books.

Brunnstrom, S. (1970). *Movement therapy in hemiplegia.* New York: Harper & Row.

Cammisa, K., Calabrese, D., Myers, M., Tupper, G., Moser, K., Crawford, K., et al. (1995). NDT theory has been updated. *American Journal of Occupational Therapy, 49,* 176.

Clark, A. (1997). *Being there: Putting brain, body and world together again.* Cambridge, MA: MIT Press.

Davis, J.Z. (2006). Task selection and enriched environments: A functional upper extremity training program for stroke survivors. *Topics in Stroke Rehabilitation, Summer,* 1–11.

Dickson, M. (2002). Rehabilitation of motor control following stroke: Searching the evidence. *British Journal of Occupational Therapy, 65,* 269–274.

Eastridge, K.M., & Rice, M.S. (2004). The effect of task goal on cross-transfer in a supination and pronation task. *Scandinavian Journal of Occupational Therapy, 11,* 128–135.

Fasoli, S.E., Trombly, C.A., Tickle-Degnen, L., & Verfaellie, M.H. (2002). Context and goal-directed movement: The effect of materials-based occupation. *Occupational Therapy Journal of Research: Occupation, Participation and Health, 22,* 119–128.

Flinn, N. (1995). A task-oriented approach to the treatment of a client with hemiplegia. *American Journal of Occupational Therapy, 49,* 560–569.

Flinn, N. (1999). Clinical interpretation of "Effect of rehabilitation tasks on organization of movement after stroke." *American Journal of Occupational Therapy, 53,* 345–347.

Giuffrida, C. (2003). Motor control theories and models guiding occupational performance interventions: Principles and assumptions. In

E.B. Crepeau, E.S. Cohn, & B.A.B. Schell (Eds.), *Willard and Spackman's occupational therapy* (10th ed., pp. 587–594). Philadelphia: Lippincott Williams & Wilkins.

Haken, H. (1987). Synergetics: An approach to self-organization. In F.E. Yates (Ed.), *Self-organizing systems: The emergence of order.* New York: Plenum.

Kamm, K., Thelen, E., & Jensen, J.L. (1990). A dynamical systems approach to motor development. *Physical Therapy, 70,* 763–775.

Kelso, J.A.S., & Tuller, B. (1984). A dynamical basis for action systems. In M.S. Gazzaniga (Ed.), *Handbook of cognitive neuroscience.* New York: Plenum.

Levit, K. (2002). Optimizing motor behavior using the Bobath approach. In C.A. Trombly & M.V. Radomski (Eds.), *Occupational therapy for physical dysfunction,* (5th ed., pp. 521–541). Philadelphia: Lippincott Williams & Wilkins.

Lin, K., Wu, C., & Trombly, C.A. (1998). Effects of task goal on movement kinematics and line bisection performance in adults without disabilities. *American Journal of Occupational Therapy, 52,* 179–187.

Ma, H., & Trombly, C.A. (2002). A synthesis of the effects of occupational therapy for persons with stroke, part II: Remediation of impairments. *American Journal of Occupational Therapy, 56,* 260–274.

Mastos, M., Miller, K., Elliasson, A.C., & Imms, C. (2007). Goal-directed training: Linking theories of treatment to clinical practice for improved functional activities in daily life. *Clinical Rehabilitation, 21,* 47–55.

Mathiowetz, V., & Bass-Haugen, J. (1994). Motor behavior research: Implications for therapeutic approaches to central nervous system dysfunction. *American Journal of Occupational Therapy, 48,* 733–745.

Mathiowetz, V., & Bass-Haugen, J. (1995). Authors' response (to NDT theory has been updated). *American Journal of Occupational Therapy, 49,* 176.

Mathiowetz, V., & Bass-Haugen, J. (2002). Assessing abilities and capacities: Motor behavior. In C.A. Trombly & M.V. Radomski (Eds.), *Occupational therapy for physical dysfunction* (5th ed., pp. 137–159). Philadelphia: Lippincott Williams & Wilkins.

McCormack, G.L., & Feuchter, F. (1996). Neurophysiology of sensorimotor approaches to treatment. In L.W. Pedretti (Ed.), *Occupational therapy: Practice skills for physical dysfunction* (4th ed., pp. 351–376). St. Louis: C.V. Mosby.

Meyers, B.J. (1995). Proprioceptive neuromuscular facilitation (PNF) approach. In K. Trombly (Ed.), *Occupational therapy for physical dysfunction* (4th ed., pp. 474–498). Baltimore: Williams & Wilkins.

Morris, D.M., Crago, J.E., DeLuca, S.C., Pidikiti, R.D., & Taub, E. (1997). Constraint-induced movement therapy for motor recovery after stroke. *Neurorehabilitation, 9,* 29–43.

Pedretti, L.W., & Zoltan, B. (Eds.). (2001). *Occupational therapy practice skills for physical dysfunction* (5th ed.). St Louis: C.V. Mosby.

Radomski, M.V., & Trombly Latham, C.A. (Eds.). (2008). *Occupation therapy for physical dysfunction* (6th ed.). Philadelphia: Lippincott Williams & Wilkins.

Roberts, P.S., Vegher, J.A., Gilewski, M., Bender A., & Riggs, R.V. (2005). Client-centered occupational therapy using constraint-induced therapy. *Journal of Stroke and Cerebrovascular Diseases, 14*(3), 115–121.

Rood, M. (1956). Neurophysiological mechanisms utilized in the treatment of neuromuscular dysfunction. *American Journal of Occupational Therapy, 10,* 220–224.

Sabari, J.S. (1991). Motor learning concepts applied to activity-based intervention with adults with hemiplegia. *American Journal of Occupational Therapy, 45,* 523–530.

Shumway-Cook, A., & Woollacott, M.H. (2007). *Motor control: Translating research into clinical practice* (3rd ed.). Philadelphia: Lippincott Williams & Wilkins.

Stevenson, T., & Thalman, L. (2007). A modified constraint-induced movement therapy regimen for individuals with upper extremity hemiplegia. *Canadian Journal of Occupational Therapy, 74,* 115–124.

Thelen, E., & Ulrich, B.D. (1991). Hidden skills: A dynamic systems analysis of treadmill stepping during the first year. *Monographs of the Society for Research in Child Development, 56* (1, Serial No. 223).

Trombly, C.A. (1989). Motor control therapy. In C.A. Trombly (Ed.), *Occupational therapy for physical dysfunction* (3rd ed., pp. 72–95). Baltimore: Williams & Wilkins.

Trombly, C.A. (1995). Occupation: Purposefulness and meaningfulness as therapeutic mechanisms. *American Journal of Occupational Therapy, 49,* 960–972.

Trombly, C.A., & Ma, H. (2002). A synthesis of the effects of occupational therapy for persons with stroke, part I: Restoration of roles, tasks, and activities. *American Journal of Occupational Therapy, 56,* 250–259.

Trombly, C.A., & Radomski, M. (Eds.). (2002). *Occupation therapy for physical dysfunction* (5th ed.). Philadelphia: Lippincott Williams & Wilkins.

Tse, D., & Spaulding, S. (1998). Review of motor control and motor learning: Implications for occupational therapy with individuals with Parkinson's disease. *Physical & Occupational Therapy in Geriatrics, 15*(3), 19–38.

Turvey, M.T. (1990). Coordination. *American Psychologist, 45*, 938–953.

Voss, D.E., Ionta, M.K., & Meyers, B.J. (1985). *Proprioceptive neuromuscular facilitation: Patterns and techniques* (3rd ed.). New York: Harper & Row.

Wu, C-Y., Trombly, C., & Lin, K-C. (1994). The relationship between occupational form and occupational performance: A kinematic perspective. *American Journal of Occupational Therapy, 48*, 679–687.

CHAPTER 13

The Sensory Integration Model

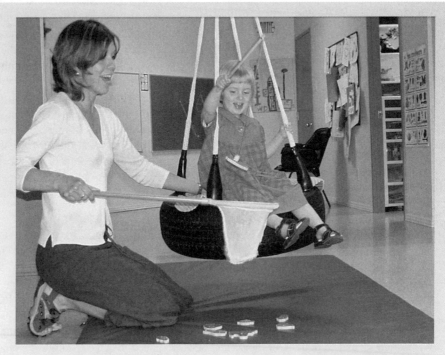

An occupational therapist engages a young client in a pretend game of fishing as the client sits on a suspended swing. While on the surface the activity looks simply like play, the occupational therapist has carefully selected the activity to give the child the opportunity to develop better control of her posture and arm movements while dealing with the various sensations of moving her body, feeling the sway of the swing, and watching her targets. This kind of experience, which emphasizes helping a client integrate and use a number of sources of sensory information in the midst of accomplishing a meaningful pleasurable task, is typical of the sensory integration model.

The sensory integration model was originated by A. Jean Ayres as she studied the relationship between children's learning disabilities and their problems in interpreting sensation from the body and environment. Ayres published two books, *Sensory Integration and Learning Disabilities* (Ayres, 1972) and *Sensory Integration and the Child* (Ayres, 1979). Numerous publications by other authors have presented clinical application and research related to this model of practice. The most recent texts concerning this model are the first and second editions of *Sensory Integration: Theory and Practice* (Bundy, Lane, & Murray, 2002; Fisher, Murray, & Bundy, 1991). These texts provide comprehensive reviews of concepts, research, and clinical applications of this model. Another recent text, *Sensory Integration and Self-Regulation in Infants and Toddlers* (Williamson & Anzalone, 2001) also provides resources for applying this model to children ages one to three years.

This model grew out of Ayres' observation that a subgroup of children with learning disabilities had difficulty interpreting **sensory information** from their bodies and the environment. She also observed that sensory processing problems were often related to deficits in motor and academic learning. Sensory integration is based on a conceptualization of how the brain functions as an organizer and interpreter of sensory information. Sensory integration dysfunction occurs when the brain does not become properly organized for processing and integrating sensory information.

The sensory integration model is generally considered most relevant for persons with mild to moderate problems in learning and behavior who do not have frank neurological damage. The model addresses difficulties in sensory organization in the brain but not outright physical damage to the central nervous system (CNS) such as that which occurs in stroke, cerebral palsy, and spina bifida. Accordingly, sensory integrative impairment is recognized when the brain fails to organize properly in the absence of clear neurological damage to the CNS or peripheral sensory pathways. The model was originally designed for application with children, but it is applied to adults who continue to demonstrate problems that were present in childhood (Bundy & Murray, 2002).

Ayres believed that children with learning disabilities and sensory issues were not a homogeneous group. Rather, she suspected that they would manifest different types of sensory integrative problems. To pursue this line of reasoning, she constructed tests to study the behavioral manifestations of sensory processing problems. Findings from a series of studies comparing typical children and children with sensory integrative problems were analyzed to identify patterns of sensory integrative impairment. The identified patterns were interpreted in light of what was known about functional neurology and neuropsychology at the time. Thus, the model provided empirical support for the existence of clusters of problems and the neurological explanations for each of those problems.

Theory

The sensory integration model is based on experimental neuroscience (Bundy & Murray, 2002), on normal development studies, and on investigations with children who have learning disabilities (Clark, Mailloux, Parham, & Bissell, 1989). In its early stages of development, the model was influenced by the neurodevelopmental approaches (see Chapter 12). Since understanding of the brain is central to this model, new information from the neurosciences is incorporated in the model and used to revise its theory. The most recent texts (Bundy et al., 2002; Fisher et al., 1991) introduced systems concepts and concepts related to play from psychology and the social sciences. Sensory integration theory refers to "constructs that discuss how the brain processes sensation and the resulting motor, behavior, emotion, and attention responses" (Miller, Anzalone, Lane, Cermak, & Osten, 2007).

Ayres (1972) defined **sensory integration** as the "neurological process that organizes sensation from one's own body and from the environment and makes it possible to use the body effectively within the environment" (p. 11). Sensory integration theory is based on five assumptions (Bundy et al., 2002). The first assumption is that of **neural plasticity**, which is the ability of the brain to change or be modified as a result of ongoing experiences of sensory processing. The second assumption is that there is a developmental sequence of sensory integrative capacities. This sequence unfolds as a result of the interaction between normal brain maturation and accumulation of sensory experiences. While the brain's developmental sequence is considered to be biologically determined, the brain is also dependent on sensory processing to organize its biological potential in the course of development. The third assumption is that the brain functions as an integrated whole. The fourth assumption is that brain organization and adaptive behavior are interactive; that is, brain organization makes possible adaptive behavior, and adaptive behavior (which involves the processing of sensory information) affects brain organization. The fifth assumption is that persons have an inner drive to participate in sensory motor activities. These assumptions are reflected in the theory of the model.

The model proposes a number of constructs related to sensory processing and identifies and hypothesizes relationships between those constructs.

Organization and Use of Sensory Information

The basic view of sensory integration, concerning how persons normally come to organize and use sensory information, is centered on the belief that:

Learning is dependent on the ability to take in and process sensation from movement and the environment and to use it to plan and organize behavior. (Bundy et al., 2002, p. 5)

The model proposes that this ability to organize sensory information and to use it to learn and perform develops as the child interacts with normal environmental challenges. The processing of sensory information in the brain results in development of new neural interconnections that allow sensory information to flow through appropriate channels and be interrelated with other sensory data. Sensory integration results in formation of a meaningful picture of self and the world, which guides performance. For example, learning new motor skills, such as riding a bicycle, involves the generation of an image of

one's own body as well as a sense of the body's movements in relation to the bicycle, to the forces of gravity, and to the changing environment. To be able to ride a bicycle is to have an appreciation of all these factors and to know how it feels to integrate them into the performance. Thus, the integration of sensory data also involves interpreting and making sense of that information (Bundy et al., 2002; Pratt, Florey, & Clark, 1989).

Sensory integration is a process in which **sensory intake**, sensory integration and organization, and adaptive occupational behavior result in a spiral of development (Bundy & Murray, 2002). The child's adaptive use of sensory information in the context of sensory motor activities further develops the sensory integrative capacity of the brain. This enhanced capacity provides the basis for further intake of sensory information in future sensory motor activities. Thus, the spiral continues, with the child building on each new level of brain organization achieved as a result of previous adaptive behavior. According to the model, play is the major arena in which sensory motor behavior takes place, as this is the way that children typically adapt to and learn about their bodies and the world.

The sensory integration model was originally based on an evolutionary view of the brain, which emphasized that "as the brain evolved, higher and newer structures like the cerebral cortex remained dependent on adequate functioning of older structures" (Pratt et al., 1989, p. 45). More recently, the model has stressed that the brain functions as a whole, with important connections between cortical and subcortical functions. The higher cortical processes require that sensory integration occurs at lower subcortical levels. Moreover, lower subcortical levels depend on cortical functions for processing sensory information (Bundy & Murray, 2002). Nonetheless, the focus of sensory integration is on those sensory processes that are mostly subcortical and that profoundly affect higher cortical processes. Because these sensory integrative processes are

> **The model proposes that this ability to organize sensory information and to use it to learn and perform develops as the child interacts with normal environmental challenges.**

so fundamental, they are thought to affect a wide variety of emotional and behavioral aspects of a child's performance as well as the ability to learn academic skills.

Areas of Sensory Functioning

The sensory integration model is concerned with multimodal sensory processing (i.e., integrating at least two sources of sensory information). Most attention has been directed to tactile, vestibular, and proprioceptive sensory information, but auditory and visual sensory information have also been considered (Bundy & Murray, 2002). Ayres, in particular, emphasized **vestibular sensation** (sensory awareness of one's position and head movement in relation to gravity) as a basis for sensory organization in the brain. She indicated that the experience of gravity and the use of the body in relationship to gravity is a ubiquitous feature of human action (Ayres, 1972). For example, the pervasive challenge that infants face in movement is the struggle to rise against gravity.

Proprioception is the perception of joint and body movement and of the position of the body and its segments in space. Proprioception depends on sensory information from the muscles and joints that underlies the development of body awareness. Proprioception also involves information via an important efferent feedback loop. This loop, associated with motor planning, allows sensory data about the position of body parts to be integrated with data about the motor effort exerted to effect placement or movement of the body parts. This feedback allows one to differentiate between active (voluntary) and passive (involuntary) movement and to form an image of the effects of one's efforts in placing and moving body parts (Fisher, 1991).

Together, vestibular and proprioceptive (vestibular-proprioceptive) sensation consists of "inputs derived from active movements of one's own body" (Fisher, 1991, p. 71). Vestibular receptors (located in the inner ear) detect movement of the head and elicit compensatory head, trunk, and limb movements, which correct for any movement of the head, trunk, or limb to help us stay upright against gravity. These receptors are also connected with eye muscles and enable the eyes to move in order to compensate for movement of the head.

The vestibular-proprioceptive system provides a consistent frame of reference from which other sensory data are interpreted. That is, the knowledge of one's position in space and the position of one's body parts provides a constant backdrop of awareness against which other sensory data can be understood. In particular, vestibular-proprioceptive sensory data serve as a reference point for monitoring and controlling movement. Tactile data provide information to the individual concerning physical contact with the external world. Visual and auditory data also provide spatial and temporal information emanating from the external environment. Sensory integration is the process whereby all sensory data are organized and processed in the brain, converted to meaningful information, and used to plan and execute motor behavior.

This process goes on all the time below the level of immediate consciousness. The following is an example of when the process becomes momentarily conscious. Occasionally when in a stopped car, one may misperceive one's car to be moving when, in fact, it is the car next to one's own car that is moving. In this situation, one must use proproprioceptive and tactile input (grab the steering wheel and hit the brakes) to integrate with the visual information in order to perceive what is currently happening. Sensory integration is the process of consistently putting together a variety of sensory inputs into a meaningful whole.

Inner Drive, Play, and Mind-Brain-Body Relations

Ayres argued that children have an inner drive to seek out organizing sensations (Ayres, 1979). This drive is manifest in sensory motor and play activities, and these activities are critical to the development of sensory integration in the child (Bundy, 2002b). It begins with the self-organizing tendency of the brain, which requires the processing of sensory information and is apparent in the subjective urge for exploration and mastery (Pratt et al., 1989).

The model further proposes that the mind and brain are interrelated (Kielhofner & Fisher, 1991). Their interdependence requires that children have positive experiences in using their bodies for the brain to be properly oriented to receive and organize sensory information. In addition, the child must be motivated to seek out appropriate sensory experiences. Thus, experience and motivation are viewed as necessary elements of the process of sensory integration.

In the course of play, children fulfill their needs for action. As Bundy and Koomar (2002) point out, play is the primary medium of sensory integrative experiences. In the occupation of play, the child is properly oriented to generate and process sensory information.

The Spiral Process of Self-Actualization

The various components of the view of order are combined into an overall schema, which the authors (Bundy et al., 2002) refer to as the spiral process of self-actualization. This conceptualization reflects an integration of many ideas developed over the years within the sensory integration model. As Bundy et al. (2002) note, it also reflects an attempt to synthesize sensory integration concepts with the conceptualization of motivation from the model of human occupation (see Chapter 11). Traditionally, sensory integration theory noted that the motivation of the child was important, but the main emphasis

in concepts and arguments was on the neurological structures and processes involved in sensory processing and organization. This conceptualization provides a clearer account of the nature and role of motivation in sensory integration. Figure 13.1 illustrates the process.

As represented in the lower, gray band, the inner drive leads the individual to seek out and engage in sensorimotor activities that provide opportunities for sensory intake (Bundy & Murray, 2002). Through a process of sensory integration, the central nervous system (CNS) must process, organize, and modulate sensory intake from the body and the environment (Bundy & Murray, 2002). Furthermore, the individual must organize and plan adaptive behaviors (which include both postural and motor skills). Neuronal models (i.e., neurologically encoded memories of what to do and how to do it) can be used to plan new and more complex behaviors. This is represented in the second loop (the dark line), which shows neuronal models being generated from sensory integrative experiences and leading to the organization and planning of new adaptive behaviors. Thus, neuronal models develop from sensory feedback generated by the planning,

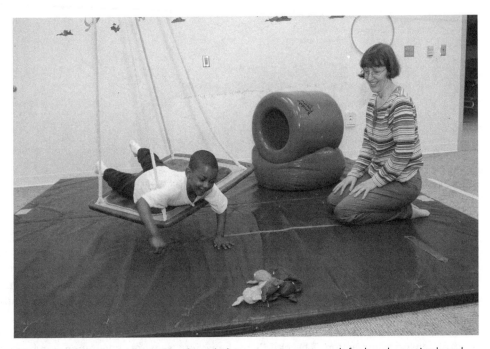

A young boy uses proprioceptive and vestibular sensory input to reach for beanbag animals and help them "find their home" inside the barrel.

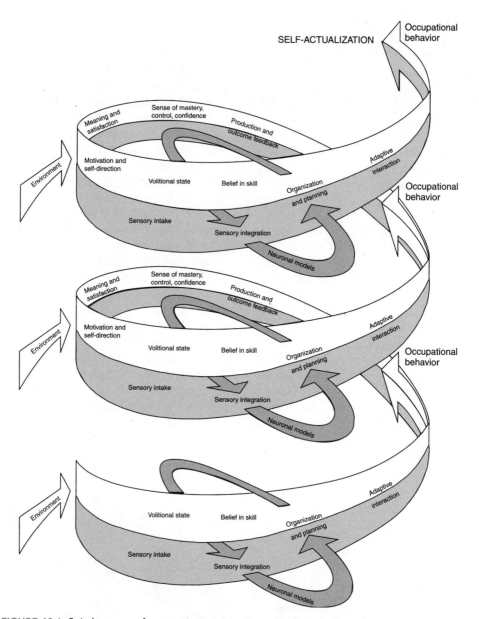

FIGURE 13.1 Spiral process of sensory integration. *From Bundy, A.C., Lane, S.J., & Murray, E.A. (Eds.) (2002). Sensory integration: Theory and practice (2nd ed.). Philadelphia: F.A. Davis with permission.*

active performance, and outcomes of an adaptive behavior (Bundy & Murray, 2002).

The upper white band of the spiral shows how sensory integration is part of the occupational behavior of the child. Volitional state (the innate drive to participate in occupation and the belief in skill) also influences the selection of sensorimotor action. The child's occupational behavior generates feedback on the production and outcome of action. This feedback influences the child's sense of mastery, control, and confidence as well as the experience of meaning and satisfaction in the behavior. This provides the basis for further motivation and self-direction, which in turn influences the ongoing processes of adaptive behavior, sensory integration, and occupational behavior.

Sensory Integrative Problems and Challenges

As noted, an important component of this model has been the identification, through research, of the types of sensory integrative impairments and the explanation of these in light of existing knowledge about nervous system function. The basic view of impairment in the sensory integration model is as follows. When individuals have deficits in processing and integrating sensory inputs, they also experience difficulty in planning and producing behavior that, in turn, interferes with conceptual and motor learning (Bundy et al., 2002). Originally, Ayres proposed and then refined six syndromes of sensory integrative dysfunction (Ayres, 1972, 1979). This delineation of sensory integrative impairments has been discussed in light of new findings. For instance, Bundy and Murray (2002, p. 6) argued that "sensory integrative impairment manifests itself in two major ways: poor modulation and poor praxis."

Recently, Miller, Anzalone, et al. (2007) proposed a new categorization (Fig. 13.2) that identifies three main sensory processing disorders:

• Sensory modulation disorder
• Sensory-based motor disorder
• Sensory discrimination disorder

> **When individuals have deficits in processing and integrating sensory inputs, they also experience difficulty in planning and producing behavior that, in turn, interferes with conceptual and motor learning.**

Sensory Modulation Disorder

A sensory modulation disorder exists when persons have "difficulty responding to sensory input with behavior that is graded relative to the degree, nature, or intensity of the sensory information" (Miller, Anzalone, et al., 2007, p. 136). This disorder includes three subtypes:

• **Sensory overresponsivity,** which is responding with more speed, intensity, or duration than is typical to one or many types of sensory information
• **Sensory underresponsivity,** which is disregarding or not responding to sensory information leading to apathy or lethargy
• **Sensory seeking/craving,** which is having an insatiable desire for and seeking excessive amounts of sensory information or a specific type of sensory information

Sensory-Based Motor Disorder

Sensory-based motor disorders are manifest as difficulties with postural or volitional movement (Miller, Anzalone, et al., 2007). They include:

• Postural disorders
• Dyspraxia

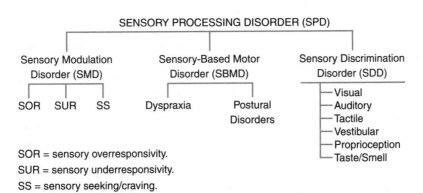

FIGURE 13.2 A proposed new nosology for sensory processing disorder. *From Miller, L.J., Anzalone, M.E., Lane, S.J., Cermak, S.A., & Osten, E.T. (2007). Concept evolution in sensory integration: A proposed nosology for diagnosis. American Journal of Occupational Therapy, 61, 135–140 with permission.*

Postural disorders are difficulties stabilizing during rest or when moving. They are characterized by too high or too low muscle tone and inadequate control of movement or force. This disorder typically occurs in combination with one or more other subtypes of disorders.

Praxis refers to the capacity to plan new actions. **Dyspraxia** is "an impaired ability to conceive of, plan, sequence, or execute novel actions" (Miller, Anzalone, et al., 2007, p. 138). It is manifest in awkwardness or poor coordination and timing with the body in space. Persons with this disorder may be accident-prone, disorganized in their approach to new motor plans, and require extra time and practice to learn motor tasks.

Sensory Discrimination Disorder

Sensory discrimination disorder refers to difficulty interpreting sensory information. Persons with this disorder have difficulty perceiving "similarities and differences among stimuli" (Miller, Anzalone, et al., 2007, p. 138). This disorder can involve problems with visual, auditory, tactile, vestibular, or proprioceptive sensations and with taste/smell. This disorder may manifest as awkward or slow motor performance or as difficulty with learning or language processes, depending on the types of sensations involved.

A great deal of effort and empirical work has gone into documenting and explaining the patterns of sensory processing disorders and the behaviors and emotions often associated with them.

Rationale for Therapeutic Intervention

As noted earlier, the authors view sensory integration as a process in which ongoing experiences of engaging in adaptive behavior result in further brain organization, making possible even more complex adaptive behaviors. When a person's brain fails to organize and process sensory information adequately, a disruption of this normal cycle of sensory integration is recognized.

Therapy based on the sensory integration model traditionally aimed at remediation of the sensory integrative problem. Thus, the goal of sensory integrative therapy has been to improve the ability to integrate sensory information. This

involves changes in the organization of the brain. Sensory integrative approaches are based on the argument that provision of opportunities for enhanced sensory intake, provided within the context of a meaningful activity and the planning and organizing of an adaptive behavior, will improve the ability of the CNS to process and integrate sensory inputs and, through this process, enhance conceptual and motor learning (Fisher & Murray, 1991).

Practice Resources

The sensory integrative model has enjoyed a well-developed technology for application. Assessment and intervention procedures have been thoroughly developed and clearly outlined. Nonetheless, a number of factors including questions about the efficacy of sensory integration treatment, time limitations, and other conditions under which services can be given as well as new views of neuromotor rehabilitation have led to some reformulation of what is considered sensory integration best practice (Bundy & Murray, 2002). This section first discusses the traditional technology for application and then goes on to examine a contemporary perspective on application.

Assessment

Assessment procedures in this model traditionally included the use of a formalized battery of tests, informal observation of performance, and data gathered from caregivers and other sources. Informal data, along with the formal test battery results, are used to arrive at an assessment of whether a person has a sensory integrative impairment and, if possible, to specify the nature of that impairment. Bundy (2002a) offers a comprehensive discussion of assessment that emphasizes the need to begin assessment with a top-down approach that first examines the ability of clients to carry out daily life tasks. Her discussion also recommends alternatives to the more time-consuming formal testing that was traditionally part of sensory integrative assessment.

The Sensory Integration and Praxis Tests (SIPT) are a battery of tests designed to help therapists identify and understand sensory integrative impairments in children four through

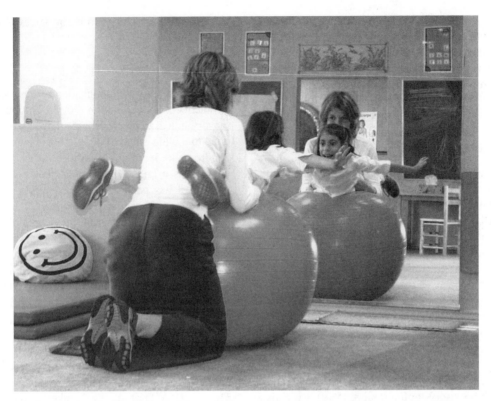

A girl pretends to be an airplane while working on muscle tone and vestibular processing. This activity is used to assess the capacity to take and maintain a position against gravity.

eight years of age (Ayres, 1989). The battery tests the relationships among tactile processing, vestibular-proprioceptive processing, visual perception, and practic (planning) ability. The tests are conceptualized as assessing the major behavioral manifestations of sensory integrative deficits. The tests are grouped in four overlapping areas (Bundy, 2002a):

- Form and space, visual-motor coordination, and constructional ability
- Tactile discrimination
- Praxis
- Vestibular and proprioceptive processing

The SIPT include 17 individually administered tests, which can be completed in about 90 minutes. All of the tasks on the test are performance-oriented. They range from the Finger Identification Test, which asks the child to point to the finger(s) previously touched by an examiner, to the Standing and Walking Balance Test, to Design Copying, a test in which the child is asked to copy designs.

The tests are computer-scored. The company that does the scoring produces a report that includes statistical comparisons between the tested child and those observed in samples of typical and disabled children who were used to develop the tests. The SIPT were developed over nearly three decades, during which clinical experiences and research have been used to determine which testing procedures were the most meaningful to include. Statistical analysis of the items most useful in identifying impairment was used to develop and refine test items and testing procedures. Statistical studies, which have identified patterns of scores that indicate types of impairment, are the basis for interpretation of the test results.

Interpretation of the SIPT scores is based on meaningful clusters of scores. Research has shown that a specific pattern of low scores is indicative of a particular kind of problem. Thus, interpretation begins with examination of test scores to see if any such pattern exists (Bundy, 2002a).

Because the SIPT cannot be used with many clients who receive sensory integrative services (Miller, Anzalone, et al., 2007) and because of the training and time involved in learning and administering the SIPT, other assessment strategies are increasingly used. Bundy (2002a) notes that even when evaluation with the SIPT is done, it should be complemented with the following kinds of information:

• Developmental patterns, intellectual capacity, and diagnoses
• Functional problems in daily life activities
• Observations, especially those of postural responses, use of the eyes with body (eye-hand, eye-foot coordination), bilateral coordination, and efficiency of planning
• Assessment of sensory modulation through observation and history-taking or the use of new assessments such as the Sensory Profile (Dunn, 1999)

Newer assessments developed for use with this model include:

• The Sensory Profile (Dunn, 1999), which is a measure of responses to commonly occurring sensory experiences designed for children aged 3 to 10 years, and the Adolescent/Adult Sensory Profile, which is a self-report (Brown, Tolefson, Dunn, Cromwell, & Filion, 2001)
• The Gravitational Insecurity Assessment (May-Benson & Koomar, 2007), which consists of 15 activities that create fear-inducing situations for children with gravitational insecurity and is used to identify children with this problem
• The Test of Ideational Praxis (May-Benson, 2001; May-Benson & Cermak, 2007), in which children are asked to show the examiner all the things they can think of doing with six standard objects
• The Sensory Processing Measure-School (Miller-Kuhaneck, Henry, Glennon, & Mu, 2007) is a rating scale that captures information on sensory processing, praxis, and participation in school

Since sensory integrative treatment is meant to have a broad impact on behavior, observations of neuromotor status and behavioral organization are also relevant to monitoring progress (Clark et al., 1989).

Treatment Approach

Any discussion of the application of this model in practice must begin with the recognition that sensory integrative procedures have been applied to a wide range of populations beyond the children with learning disabilities for whom the model was originally developed. For example, the model has been applied to adults, persons with frank brain damage, persons with schizophrenia, and individuals with mental retardation (Arendt, MacLean, & Baumeister, 1988; King, 1974). There has been considerable controversy over whether such individuals are appropriate candidates for sensory integrative approaches. Additionally, many persons have been criticized for using techniques from sensory integration without a systematic application of its principles. While they may refer to the resulting therapy as sensory integration, it is in fact not so. The text *Sensory Integration: Theory and Practice* (Bundy et al., 2002) takes a conservative approach, arguing for a clear identification of the presence of sensory integrative problems before the sensory integrative approaches are used. The authors of the text believe that the model has application with adults and may have potential for people with problems other than learning disability. The text outlines the authors' rationales for application of the model.

Traditional Treatment Guidelines

The sensory integrative model provides specific guidelines for the kind of sensory integrative experiences hypothesized to be of most benefit to a child. Intervention planning is based on identification of the child's problems and the underlying reasons for those problems; that is, the particular difficulty with processing sensory information. Understanding the difficulty requires understanding of the structure and function of sensory systems and how they are implicated in sensory integration problems (Lane, 2002).

The vestibular-proprioceptive system provides a good example of the logic of intervention. Knowledge of the anatomy and physiology of the vestibular-proprioceptive system is used

Box 13.1

South Shore Therapies: An Example of a Private Practice Clinic Focused on Sensory Integration

Sensory integration services are often provided in the context of private clinics. One example of a state-of-the-art sensory integration clinic is South Shore Therapies. In this setting, the rooms have been designed to be inviting and safe while affording opportunities for variation and plan-

ning. The floors are covered with mattresses that provide not only a safe landing base but also provide additional sensory feedback that encourages active postural reactions as the child moves across them. Stairs, forts, and slides have been built into the rooms to invite the child to work on functional mobility and play skills. The rooms were named by clients and are themed to encourage imaginative play themes. The playground room has the slide and the zip line while the space mountain room has planet targets on the wall and a blow-up moon walk.

The clinic's goal is to provide an enriched environment for clients to develop the necessary skills for greater independence. Therapists work with a child or adolescent at a level they can un-

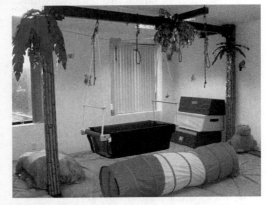

The jungle room at South Shore Therapies.

derstand so that they become involved and invested in their own intervention process. The therapists also work together with families in planning intervention, home programming, and consultation. By educating the whole family to be an integral part of intervention, therapists can better help the child.

When you walk into South Shore Therapies you see children hard at play. There is laughter and a sense of fun. The sensory gyms provide a safe and engaging environment for the child to explore in. The therapists create activities that both support the children's current sensory needs and encourage more complex adaptation. Activities that are relevant and meaningful to the child provide the foundation for change. This may involve simple pretend play such as going to the moon on an expedition to more complex spatial plans like planning and building an above ground road to get from one side of the room to another. Goals developed with the parents address daily functional concerns that impact their daily lives

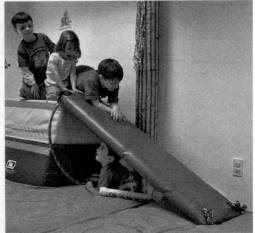

Children on "safari" at South Shore Therapies.

such as the ability to fall asleep, eat a greater variety of foods, get dressed, safely navigate the playground, ride a bicycle, or participate in a social event such as a birthday party. During sensory integration sessions, activities are guided by the child's sensory needs and skill abilities with scaffolding from the therapist to find the right challenge level. This approach promotes feelings of mastery and personal control. The combination of the sensory-rich, playful, and creative treatment space, combined with the artful therapeutic use of self, greatly supports the development of confidence, competence, and coordination.

to determine what kind of sensory experience would most effectively stimulate vestibular organs and proprioceptors and elicit particular **postural reactions.** In this case, understanding neurological structures provides the logic for determining which therapeutic procedures should have particular impacts on the sensory system. The following quote from a discussion of treatment planning for a child, Steven, further illustrates the kind of specificity that can be achieved in choosing appropriate sensory integrative therapy (Bundy, 1991):

> *Sensory integration theory suggests that Steven's difficulties with postural stability and bilateral integration and sequencing of projected limb movements should be addressed by activities that provide opportunities for him to take in enhanced vestibular-proprioceptive information. More specifically, the theory suggests that opportunities to take in linear vestibular-proprioceptive information in the context of activities that demand sustained postural control (in a variety of positions) and coordinated use of both sides of the body will be most appropriate. (p. 342)*

Sensory integration theory does not yet present a complete picture of the various problems children manifest, nor does it explain all the underlying mechanisms. Thus, there are some gaps in information about how best to proceed in therapy. In such cases, the therapist uses all available information about the child to determine a prudent course of therapy.

Play as the Media

This model emphasizes that the child must actively choose and participate in the actions that occur in therapy. In play, the child is given control and the enticement to choose appropriate sensory motor behaviors. Bundy (2002b) emphasizes the importance of play as the vehicle for therapy based on the sensory integrative model. She points out three factors that are critical for maintaining a playful approach to intervention:

• Perception of internal control
• Intrinsic motivation

• Freedom from the constraints of reality (Bundy, 2002b)

Bundy (2002b) also recommends careful assessment of play, using such instruments as the Test of Playfulness (Bundy, 2000). She notes that play can result in improvements in sensory integration and that the most important by-product of therapy may be improving the client's ability to play.

Equipment

Because of the special needs for sensory experiences (especially vestibular), sensory integration treatment has come to be associated with a variety of specially designed suspended equipment (trapezes, hammocks, and swings) and scooter boards. Such equipment, which is commercially available, provides the means of achieving desired sensory experiences in the context of play.

> **This model emphasizes that the child must actively choose and participate in the actions that occur in therapy.**

Contemporary Guidelines for Application of This Model

As noted at the beginning of this chapter, a number of factors have led to some rethinking of how to best deliver sensory integrative therapy. Bundy and Murray (2002) propose a number of principles that reflect current thinking about use of this model in practice. Some of the guidelines, which reflect an appreciation of the more limited time for therapy, include such approaches as setting objectives that can be accomplished in the short term. These objectives should be understandable to both clients and caregivers and should involve clients and caregivers in implementing aspects of intervention. Also related to changes in the context of services is the role of the occupational therapist as a consultant to family members or other professionals. An important component of this role is often to help these persons reframe their understanding of the person with sensory integrative problems (e.g., helping a teacher understand that sitting still may actually interfere with rather than improve a child's ability to pay attention in the classroom).

Box 13.2

Sensory Integration in Practice: SAM

Sam is a four-and-a-half-year-old boy who attends a half-day junior kindergarten program. He lives with his mom and dad and has two older brothers. Sam is a boy who moves quickly and is always "on the run." He is seen to run, jump, and crash at home. Sam frequently bumps into toys, furniture, and people as he is challenged both by how fast he moves and his lack of awareness of his body in space. Mealtime is short and Sam is extremely particular about what he will eat, limiting himself to a few foods. He only likes soft clothes with no tags and will become upset if his mother buys a different brand of underwear. A typical bedtime routine for Sam takes between an hour and an hour-and-a-half. He is difficult to soothe and calm down at bedtime and experiences great difficulties falling asleep. In school, Sam is highly distractible and demonstrates a short attention span. He is fidgety on the rug during circle time and frequently blurts out information. He does not enjoy the fine motor table, particularly when there is play dough or moon sand set out. Sam's fine motor skills lag behind those of his peers and Sam feels frustrated that he cannot write his name like his friends are able to do. Sam has a friend or two but has difficulties reading the nonverbal cues of his peers in the classroom.

Sam was assessed by Rebecca Schatz, his occupational therapist, using various tools to evaluate both motor skill development and sensory processing. Winnie Dunn's Sensory Profile Caregiver Questionnaire (Dunn, 1999) and the Sensory Profile School Companion (Dunn, 2006) were both used to gather information into Sam's sensory processing. These questionnaires, filled out by parents and teachers, help to categorize sensory processing deficits along a continuum. Registration, seeking, sensitivity, and avoiding are the four scored quadrants that provide information on whether the child's behavior is similar to others, whether there is a probable difference between the child's behavior and that of other children, or whether there is a definite difference between the child's behavior and what is typical. With this framework in mind, Sam scored within the definite difference section for registration, seeking, and sensitivity. Collectively, these results demonstrated that Sam was experiencing significant sensory processing challenges, which were interfering with his daily life.

Rebecca recommended to Sam's parents that he receive twice weekly occupational therapy sessions utilizing sensory integration as the form of therapy. Sensory integration would help Sam to be able to effectively interpret and organize the sensory information within his environment that, at the time, was extremely disorganizing and difficult for Sam to process. Sam needed therapy that would focus on the integration of multiple sensory systems including tactile, vestibular, and proprioceptive. This integration needed to be experienced as pleasurable and playful.

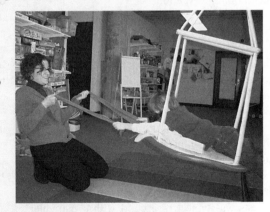

The goal in therapy was for Sam to be able to participate effectively in multiple opportunities for pleasurable and meaningful sensory experiences. Following the organizing sensory input, Rebecca had Sam participate in a fine or visual motor activity to improve his overall skill level. Sam would participate and utilize suspended equipment to "fly like a spaceship" on the platform swing. Here, Sam received organizing sensory input to help regulate his nervous system to make a meaningful and adaptive response while

Rebecca helps Sam fly like a spaceship.

interacting with his therapist. As he flew off to outer space, both Sam's internal motivation and excitement brought on an effective nervous system response. Sam's body was calm, attentive, and well-organized and he was able to maintain this level to then participate in a tabletop activity geared at improving his fine and visual motor abilities.

(box continues on page 216)

Box 13.2 (continued)

Throughout the course of sensory integration therapy, Sam became able to both tolerate and respond to sensory experiences within his school and home environments effectively and positively. Sam's attention and focus continued to lengthen and he was able to become an active participant in circle time. Textures, sounds, and daily transitions no longer caused Sam's nervous system to become disorganized and lose its regulation. Ultimately, Sam became a happier child as he was able to have more successful experiences both at home and in school.

Other guidelines reflect new ideas from the task-oriented approach (see Chapter 12), which emphasize attention to how the task and environment might contribute to observed difficulties in performance and include appropriate interventions directed at these issues. Overall, there is a shift in orientation from an exclusive focus on remediating the underlying problem in the client to focusing on how the problem interacts with external conditions that interfere with everyday performance and deciding on the most efficacious strategy of intervention.

A recent paper outlined what are considered core elements of sensory integration intervention (Parham et al., 2007). These are shown in Table 13.1. These guidelines were developed through expert review and nominal group process. Although the purpose of the guidelines was to assess treatment fidelity, they do represent a consensus of sensory integration leaders about what are the core elements of sensory integration intervention.

Research and Evidence Base

The sensory integration model has been the subject of a great deal of research. Ongoing research has contributed to the development of the SIPT (Bundy, 2002a) and, concurrently, to the validation of underlying sensory integration constructs. Pivotal studies in this area are the factor analytic studies, which identified meaningful clusters of test scores (Bundy 2002a). These studies demonstrated that poor performance in a specific cluster of tests was typical of a child with a particular kind of sensory integrative problem. Based on this research, it is thought that test score patterns can be indicative of whether and of what type of sensory integrative problem a person may have. Recent research has made use of electroencephalography to demonstrate that children diagnosed with

sensory processing disorders do exhibit differences in brain activity (Davies & Gavin, 2007).

A second area of research includes studies of the effectiveness of sensory integrative therapy. Examining studies completed between 1972 and 1981, Ottenbacher (1991) conducted a meta-analysis (a method of using data from several studies to determine whether there is evidence of a treatment effect) and concluded that there was evidence of treatment effectiveness. Hoehn and Baumeister (1994) criticized some of the studies Ottenbacher included as lacking sufficient rigor. Vargas and Camilli (1999) later used meta-analysis to examine studies reported between 1983 and 1993 and found very little evidence for treatment effectiveness, which is not surprising as many studies conducted in the last two decades failed to demonstrate positive outcomes of treatment on the specific variables measured.

Bundy et al. (2002) concluded that evidence concerning the effectiveness of sensory integration–based therapy was "mixed at best and downright negative at worst" (p. 22). They also noted that despite the lack of evidence for treatment effectiveness, parents and therapists were enthusiastic about their firsthand experience with sensory integration–based therapy. One possibility is that the therapy produces positive outcomes but not for the reasons specified by sensory integration theory and measured in studies (Kaplan, Polatajko, Wilson, & Faris, 1993). For example, it is hypothesized that the relationship between the therapist and child may account for outcomes or that sensory integration principles are used to reframe how problems are perceived by others in the child's environment, leading to positive outcomes. This was supported by Cohn and Cermak (1998), whose study focused on the parent perpective of changes with sensory integration therapy. Parents reported that

Table 13.1   **Core Elements of Sensory Integration Intervention Process**

Core Process Elements	Description of Therapist's Behavior and Attitude
Provide sensory opportunities	Presents the child with opportunities for various sensory experiences, which include tactile, vestibular, and/or proprioceptive experiences; intervention involves more than one sensory modality.
Provide just-right challenges	Tailors activities so as to present challenges to the child that are neither too difficult nor too easy, to evoke the child's adaptive responses to sensory and praxis challenges.
Collaborate on activity choice	Treats the child as an active collaborator in the therapy process, allowing the child to actively exert some control over activity choice; does not predetermine a schedule of activities independently of the child.
Guide self-organization	Supports and guides the child's self-organization of behavior to make choices and plan own behavior to the extent the child is capable; encourages the child to initiate and develop ideas and plans for activities.
Support optimal arousal	Ensures that the therapy situation is conducive to attaining or sustaining the child's optimal level of arousal by making changes to environment or activity to support the child's attention, engagement, and comfort.
Create play context	Creates a context of play by building on the child's intrinsic motivation and enjoyment of activities; facilitates or expands on social, motor, imaginative, or object play.
Maximize child's success	Presents or modifies activities so that the child can experience success in doing part or all of an activity that involves a response to a challenge.
Ensure physical safety	Ensure that the child is physically safe either through placement of protective and therapeutic equipment or through the therapist's physical proximity and actions.
Arrange room to engage child	Arranges the room and equipment in the room to motivate the child to choose and engage in an activity.
Foster therapeutic alliance	Respects the child's emotions, conveys positive regard toward the child, seems to connect with the child, and creates a climate of trust and emotional safety.

From Parham, L.D., Cohn, E.S., Spitzer, S., Koomar, J.A., Miller, L.J., Burke, J.P., et al. (2007). Fidelity in sensory integration intervention research. American Journal of Occupational Therapy, 61, 216-227 with permission.

one of the important outcome measures of intervention was developing the ability to understand and reframe their child's behavior as a way to support and advocate for the child.

Tickle-Degnen (1988) noted that studies have not yet examined mediating factors that might better explain when and how sensory integration–based therapy works and for what types of individuals. Recently more attention has been paid to the rigor of studies of the effectiveness of sensory integration intervention. For example, Parham et al. (2007) concluded that many sensory integration outcome studies have been threatened by weak fidelity to sensory integration treatment guidelines.

The variability in the treatments administered in sensory integration research studies may be in part due to the fact that sensory integration intervention is individualized and frequently adapted based on a child's changing needs. This lack of standardization makes the selection and use of sensitive outcome measures challenging. The population of children receiving sensory integration therapy (and the population that has been included in research) is heterogeneous, encompassing a vast number of diagnoses and problems in functioning. It may be the case that outcome measures that have been used in many sensory integration research studies are not ideal for capturing change in the participating children for the aforementioned reasons (Szklut & Philibert, 2006).

The fact that research on sensory integration has been so extensively discussed and critiqued reflects the fact that there is a substantial body of research upon which meaningful discussion and critique can be based. Increased emphasis on high-quality, randomized controlled studies should produce more rigorous assessments of the outcomes of sensory integration interventions in the future (Miller, Coll, & Schoen, 2007).

Discussion

The sensory integration model is an extensively researched and systematically developed model of practice. Nonetheless, the use of the model in practice has been subject to some criticism and controversy. Also, some professionals outside of occupational therapy have been skeptical about sensory integrative theory and interventions. This skepticism appears to be waning with increasing evidence (especially evidence that draws upon more basic science methods such as electroencephalogram to demonstrate the existence of sensory processing disorders). Moreover, sensory processing disorders are now included in interdisciplinary diagnostic frameworks (Miller, Anzalone, et al., 2007)

Therapists have applied this model to populations that others deemed inappropriate for sensory integration treatment. Others have borrowed ideas and techniques from the model incompletely, resulting in clinical practices not justified by the theory. Moreover, sensory integration is sometimes confused with other related approaches. For example, Bundy et al. (2002) noted that sensory integration treatment should be differentiated from sensorimotor approaches in that the latter emphasize specific motor responses, whereas the concern of the former is specifically with how the child processes sensation. They also differentiate sensory integration from sensory stimulation programs in that the latter apply sensation to the child, whereas in the sensory integrative approaches, the child seeks out the sensation.

This highly complex and well-developed model is both attractive to therapists and challenging to master. However, as noted, application of the model has not always been systematic. Clark et al. (1989) note that "entry level therapists should not expect to be able to provide sensory integrative procedures upon graduation" (p. 484). They point out that considerable skill is required for use of this practice model. Therapists who wish to administer the SIPT must become certified either through approved graduate or continuing education courses and an examination process. The model represents an area of specialty practice in occupational therapy that requires training and experience beyond that of the generically trained therapist.

Box 13.3

Sensory Integration Model Case Example: LAURA

Laura was born on May 31, 2001. She began life as a twin, but her sibling died at 14 weeks gestation. It is speculated that this may have influenced Laura's development. Her birth was uneventful and Laura was a quiet, easy baby from the start. She could smile and make eye contact. She preferred playing with sound toys and rocking, and at times she would do these things repetitively.

Laura's mom notes that she first became concerned when Laura was around six months old. She was sitting with Laura in her lap eating soup when she realized that Laura was "too good." At this age, Laura should have been squirming and trying to get the spoon and soup, but she could not easily move her hands and was not wiggling, reaching, or making messes. Also, she did not sit up independently or roll over yet. Laura's mother had an excellent pediatrician who encouraged her to see a neurologist. The initial neurologist, who saw Laura when she was a year old, did not feel he could provide a diagnosis so early. The pediatrician then referred Laura to the New England Medical Center where a developmental pediatrician connected Laura with a full team of professionals for evaluation. During this assessment process Laura first received the diagnosis of cerebral palsy at approximately 15 months and was diagnosed with PDD-NOS (Pervasive Developmental Disorder–Not Otherwise Specified) before she was two.

These diagnoses qualified her for extensive services through Early Intervention, and Laura received physical, occupational, and speech therapy, as well as an educator who came to the home. Laura's mother recalls that these providers helped her navigate through the maze of understanding her complex daughter with compassion and humor. She carefully listened to the advice they gave her and followed through on home programs. With this intervention Laura began to reach, roll over, and sit up.

When Laura turned three she became eligible for school-based services. Laura was enrolled into a summer pre-kindergarten program with limited support. On the first day of camp Laura's mother observed that the school staff had various expectations and demands that she considered to be above Laura's abilities. She remembers the day starting with a teacher putting Laura up on a stool at the sink and telling her to wash her hands. Laura's mother had to interject that Laura was unable to stand independently on a stool and could not yet wash her hands. After approximately 45 minutes in this chaotic program, Laura reacted as she never had before; she became completely vacant and "unreachable." This concerned Laura's mother so much that she took Laura home.

Laura appeared shut down and unreachable for the rest of the day. When put in her crib that night Laura began to bang her head, making the crib hit the wall. Over the next week Laura would not get off the bed or couch and began licking herself. This behavior frightened Laura's mother, who decided that Laura could not return to the school program. This decision was substantiated by Laura's neurologist who noted that her sensory processing issues were so great that Laura would need one-on-one services, with the long-term goal of transitioning to a regular education classroom.

Since Laura was unable to access the public school environment, she received her early education through home-based programming. Within two weeks, this home-based provider had Laura responding to her name and looking at others when they walked into the room. She appeared to unlock Laura's learning potential, and Laura flourished educationally with this structured, sequential approach to learning. In addition, Laura received occupational, physical, and speech therapy at the school. It was the school

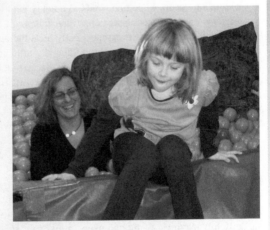

Laura works hard to get herself out of the ball pit.

(box continues on page 220)

Box 13.3 (continued)

occupational therapist who began to explain Laura's significant sensory issues to her mother and began to discuss strategies to help calm Laura. At that time, Laura would rock in a small rocking chair with such intensity that the chair moved across the room. Laura's mother felt that occupational therapy was the best service for Laura once the severity of Laura's sensory processing problems was explained to her. At this time Laura's mother sought out outside sensory integration sessions at South Shore Therapies.

When occupational therapist Stacey Szklut met Laura in November, 2004, Laura was three years old. Laura's mother described her to Stacey as a child who "gives 110% effort but is always hanging on by a string." Many typical daily events were extremely difficult for Laura to tolerate such as hair washing, hair combing, tooth brushing, and getting dressed. Laura and her family were not able to participate in social events outside the house such as going to McDonalds, a museum, a playground, or a birthday party. Both Laura and her mother appeared extremely fragile, due to the fact that Laura could so quickly and easily melt down in situations where sensory experiences or demands were too overwhelming. During the first interview, Stacey asked Laura's mother about her goals for Laura and she replied, "I would die happy if I could brush her hair or teeth."

Considering Laura's significant difficulties regulating sensory input from the world, Stacey selected sensory integration as her primary conceptual practice model. For Laura, her ability to understand the world around her was greatly hindered by defensiveness (overreactivity) to incoming sensations. Laura was overwhelmed by many typical daily sounds, sights, and touch experiences. Hair washing was so aversive that Laura might cry for 30 minutes during and after it. Trying to wear new shoes or a new coat was generally unsuccessful, involving bouts of kicking and screaming.

One of the first times Stacey met Laura, a hair from her head got wrapped around Laura's finger and Laura immediately began to panic and hyperventilate. Her mother, in turn, responded just as quickly to remove the aversive touch and catch Laura before she completely melted down. This observation helped Stacey to understand that part of Laura's defensive responses were also due to an inefficient ability to discriminate what was happening to her body and to plan an effective adaptive response. Rather than being able to quickly understand and label that there was a hair on her finger and use the other hand to attempt to remove it, Laura went into panic (fright) mode.

Laura was exhibiting many classic signs of overresponse in patterns of flight, fright, and fight. These are typical responses when one feels threatened, but for Laura these responses were occurring with simple daily events that should not have been perceived as aversive. The desire to flee a situation occurs when one wants to quickly get away from a noxious event, such as covering one's ears when someone scratches their fingernails down a chalkboard.

The fright stage occurs when one's body feels threatened; it is characterized by increased heart rate, shallow and rapid breathing, dilated pupils, increase in muscle tension, perspiration, and nausea. The emotional experience is similar to that following a near-accident such as almost getting hit by a car. Due to decreased motor mobility, Laura did not have the capability to remove herself from many overwhelming situations. Thus, she spent much of her time in a frightened and panicked mode.

The final protective stance is fight, reflected in outward or inward aggression (e.g., yelling, kicking, or biting others or self). Laura exhibited fight responses with new clothing, hair cutting, or at the end an overwhelming day. In these instances, she would bang her head.

Since these sensory-based reactions affected every aspect of Laura's and her mother's interactions, they were essential to address immediately. Moreover, Laura's limited mobility and poor motor planning confounded her ability to feel safe and empowered in the world. At age three, Laura was completely dependent on her family to help her feel safe and participate in basic daily life activities. Laura had many component areas to address to provide the foundation for more successful participation in daily occupations such as grooming, dressing, and social participation on the playground and in a school classroom. Those foundations included sensory

Box 13.3 (continued)

processing, postural control, respiratory support, motor planning, ideation and initiation, motor execution, bilateral coordination, eye-hand coordination, temporal-spatial adaptation, timing, and sequencing. They also included a sense of confidence and independence. Thus, while sensory integration was the central conceptual model for Laura's occupational therapy, Stacey also used concepts and approaches from motor control theories and the model of human occupation.

The first step in therapy was to develop Laura's:

- Ability to regulate and understand incoming sensations
- Capacity to act effectively on the world around her
- Feelings of effectiveness

These were addressed through play-based activities that involved organizing sensory input and exhibiting developmentally appropriate adaptive responses. Many of the first activities Laura could successfully participate in involved a simple level of adaptive response such as responding to passive stimuli or holding on and staying put. The first sensory-based activities always incorporated sensations that are known to be the most organizing (i.e., touch pressure, flexed positions, resistance to limb motion, rocking and bouncing, oral motor input, and rhythmical auditory simulation). It was essential to observe Laura carefully for signs of overload and to begin to identify for her mother what combinations and rhythms of sensation were organizing to Laura so that they could be incorporated into activities at home. Activities that involved touch pressure and movement could quickly engage Laura. She loved swinging and bouncing rhythmically in a spandex hammock with gentle singing. Her first adaptive response was to look at Stacey to indicate that she wanted more. Later, she could sign for more. Finally, she could vocalize for more. Since this activity was so motivating to Laura it also presented the opportunity to increase her motor planning and skilled motor responses. Stacey encouraged Laura to climb in on her own by positioning the hammock close to the floor.

As Laura's skill increased, Stacey assisted her in moving a sturdy platform to stand on while climbing into the hammock. Since oral input and memory activities were organizing for Laura, Stacey introduced whistles for Laura to indicate the type of motion she wanted. Laura's favorite motion was bouncing, and her hardest respiratory pattern was sustained blowing. Thus, for up and down motion, Laura had to blow one long blow. Her second favorite motion was side to side; for this she had to produce three short blows.

Over time this approach of using activities Laura liked and requesting new behaviors within her capacity was used to introduce increasingly difficult activities. An essential component to Laura's progress was an approach that enabled Laura to feel less threatened and more in control of sensory experiences and how she would respond. For instance, Stacey instructed Laura's mother that before she acted to wipe saliva from Laura's mouth or remove a hair stuck between her fingers, it was important to engage Laura in the process.

Stacey also used this approach in therapy. She labeled and showed Laura each thing that was happening to her. Stacey would present a mirror and show Laura the saliva on her face, give her a paper towel, and help her wipe it off. This yielded striking changes in Laura's confidence and independence.

Commenting on this process Stacey noted:

> I recall when Laura first found her body in the ball pit. I was sitting with her and we were searching for large stuffed animals I had hidden (a task that encourages touch discrimination, visual scanning, and rotational movement patterns). I "accidentally" found Laura's foot and exclaimed, "What could this be?" Rather than her earlier responses of panicking and overresponding to this unexpected touch she smiled, pulled her leg up, and stated, "Laura foot."

Over time Laura was able to use this improved sense of her body to plan more complex movement sequences in space. Through being involved as an active participant in the therapy process, Laura began to develop a sense of competency and success in her initiation and planning of actions.

(box continues on page 222)

Box 13.3 (continued)

Laura had a very strong reaction to moving visual input. For example, she would startle and cower when something or someone moved toward her. Laura was also fearful of stairs, walking on unsteady surfaces, climbing into her bed, or even sitting in a chair in which her feet did not touch the ground. To address these problems, therapy centered on the visual system and its ability to coordinate with vestibular and proprioceptive input.

In therapy sessions, Stacey began with a platform swing with a tire on it that gave Laura full postural support. Stacey followed the normal progression of visual-spatial development. Laura first worked on reaching for motivating objects (beanie babies), presented in varied visual planes, while she was still. Laura achieved this skill quickly and then she and Stacey moved to reaching while the swing was moving. They then moved to throwing these objects at a large target while the swing was still and, later, with the swing moving. To tap Laura's inner drive for these more challenging tasks and facilitate imaginative play, Stacey would set up the activity so that she was throwing the Beanie Babies into a pool for a swim or delivering Christmas presents.

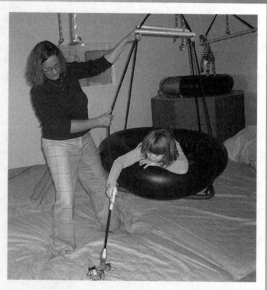
Laura "rescues" animals while in a moving swing.

As Laura became more competent, she developed more confidence in moving her body through a predictable environment. At this stage, Stacey added skills that required Laura to plan and move her body in new and changeable ways while looking for a still visual target, such as climbing up a ramp to pull a sticker off the wall, or finding eggs hidden on, under, behind, and on top of objects.

In addition, it was important to help Laura begin to deal with the unexpected things that might occur in the real-world environment. On a playground or in school, Laura would need to be able to move her body through a moving and changing environment. Stacey comments about this process:

> I call this "pushing the envelope" where I create an exciting, changeable activity to see if the child has developed the regulatory abilities and coping mechanisms to regroup when something challenges his or her system. If they cannot then I move back to more predictable, calming activities. If they can then I know they are on their way to success in the real world of play, school, and life.

The first time Stacey created an activity that was unpredictable and changeable, Laura's mother was in the room observing. Laura and her brother were riding a boat swing. Her brother was pulling rings so the motion of the swing was rhythmical and predictable. Stacey added the unpredictability in an imaginative play scheme by pretending to be a weather forecaster talking about an approaching storm. As the storm approached Stacey wiggled the swing and tossed some stuffed animal sea creatures into the boat.

As this level of excitement was readily accepted by Laura and her brother, Stacey added a stronger component, using large soft pillows and pretending that the waves were washing into the boat. This afforded Stacey the opportunity to apply touch pressure with the soft pillow to Laura's head and face, still her most sensitive areas. At first Laura was startled and unsure about the chaos of this activity.

Stacey knew that, at such times it is essential to "follow the child's lead" to ensure that the activity is being integrated effectively. Such situations require that a trusting relationship has

Box 13.3 (continued)

been set up over time so that the child feels safe and in control with the therapist. Laura looked at Stacey, her mother, and brother and saw them all laughing. At that point she laughed too and the storm continued, with breaks in the waves as needed. That was the first night that Laura's mother was able to wash Laura's hair without Laura crying.

Another example of using sensory-based play to encourage active participation occurred late in the fall with the first snowstorm. Laura was very agitated and did not want to go outside to come to therapy. Within the therapy session Laura and Stacey had a snowball fight with the large pillows. They rolled in the "snow" and bopped each other with soft pillows. They captured each other under larger pillows, pretending they were huge piles of snow. Following this session, Laura donned a hat and gloves and joined her brothers outside to play.

Laura is now six and is successfully integrated into a regular education first grade with a great deal of support. At school she has a full-time aide and receives intensive occupational and speech therapy, as well as supportive physical therapy. Laura continues to come to South Shore Therapies on an as-needed basis to develop new strategies for sensory regulation and focus on higher-level motor planning skills.

The stresses and demands of Laura's daily life can still be overwhelming, and when she gets sick many older behavior patterns emerge. On the other hand, Laura is a confident first grader who can participate in a wide variety of appropriate daily life tasks. She is working on her scissor and writing skills in occupational therapy, on pedaling a bike in physical therapy, and on clearer speech in speech therapy. She participates in gym class, art class, music class, assemblies, and on the playground. She is a friend to others and can participate in appropriate social activities such as birthday parties.

Table 13.2 **Terms of the Model**

Dyspraxia	An impairment in the ability to conceive of, plan, sequence, or execute novel actions.
Neural plasticity	The ability of the brain to change or be modified.
Postural disorder	A disorder characterized by difficulty stabilizing during rest or when moving.
Postural reactions	Changes in one's body position to maintain equilibrium.
Praxis	Planning of motor action; involves knowing how to do an action.
Proprioception	Perception of joint and body movement and of the position of the body and its segments in space.
Sensory discrimination disorder	Difficulty interpreting sensory information.
Sensory information	Sensations (e.g., from touch, movement).
Sensory intake	Taking in of sensations from the environment or internally from the body.
Sensory integration	The neurological process that organizes sensation from one's own body and the environment and allows for effective use of the body within the environment.

(table continues on page 224)

Table 13.2 **Terms of the Model** continued

Sensory modulation disorder	Disorder involving difficulty responding to sensory input with behavior appropriate to the degree, nature, or intensity of the sensory information.
Sensory overresponsivity	Responding with more speed, intensity, or duration than is typical to one or many types of sensory information.
Sensory seeking/craving	Having an insatiable desire for and seeking excessive amounts of sensory information or a specific type of sensory information.
Sensory underresponsivity	Disregarding or not responding to sensory information leading to apathy or lethargy.
Sensory-based motor disorder	A disorder that manifests as difficulties with postural or volitional movement.
Vestibular sensation	Sensory awareness of one's bodily position in relation to gravity.

SUMMARY: THE SENSORY INTEGRATION MODEL

Theory

Organization

+ Sensory integration is the neurological process that organizes sensation from one's own body and the environment and allows for effective use of the body within the environment

+ Sensory integration theory is based on five assumptions
  • The brain has neural plasticity, which is the ability to change or be modified as a result of ongoing experiences of sensory processing
  • There is a developmental sequence of sensory integrative capacities
  • The brain functions as an integrated hierarchical whole
  • Brain organization and adaptive behavior are adaptive
  • Persons have an inner drive to participate in sensory motor activities

+ Sensory integration is a process in which sensory intake, sensory integration and organization, and adaptive occupational behavior result in a spiral of development

+ Sensory integration is concerned with multimodal sensory processing (i.e., integrating at least two sources of sensory information) in which sensory data are organized and processed in the brain, converted to meaningful information, and used to plan and execute motor behavior

+ Vestibular and proprioceptive sensation consists of inputs derived from active body movements

+ Children have an inner drive to seek out organizing sensations

+ Mind and brain are interrelated; subjective experience is a necessary part of the adaptive spiral of sensory integration

Problems and Challenges

+ When individuals have deficits in processing and integrating sensory inputs, difficulties in planning and producing behavior occur that interfere with conceptual and motor learning

+ Recently, a new categorization has been proposed that identifies three main sensory processing disorders:

- Sensory modulation disorder
  - Sensory overresponsivity
  - Sensory underresponsivity
  - Sensory seeking/craving
- Sensory-based motor disorder
  - Postural disorders
  - Dyspraxia
- Sensory discrimination disorder

Therapeutic Intervention

✦ Aimed at remediation (change) of the sensory integrative problem

✦ Goal is to improve ability to integrate sensory information by changing organization of the brain

✦ Enhanced sensory intake, which occurs when a child plans and organizes adaptive behavior in a meaningful activity, improves ability of the CNS to process and integrate sensory inputs

Practice Resources

Assessment

✦ Assessment procedures traditionally included a formalized battery of tests (Sensory Integration and Praxis Tests), informal observation of performance, and data gathered from caretakers and other sources

✦ Data are used to arrive at an assessment of whether a person has a sensory integrative impairment and, if possible, to specify the nature of that impairment

✦ The Sensory Integration and Praxis Tests (SIPT) are a battery of tests designed to help

the therapist identify and understand sensory integrative impairments in children four through eight years of age

✦ Because the SIPT cannot be used with many clients who receive sensory integrative services and because of the training and time involved in learning and administering the SIPT, other assessment strategies are increasingly used

Treatment Approach

✦ Sensory integrative experiences selected to benefit a child are derived from identification of the child's problems and the theory concerning the underlying reasons for those problems (i.e., the particular difficulty processing sensory information)

✦ Play is a vehicle for therapy; in play the child is given control and enticement to choose appropriate sensory motor behaviors

✦ Three factors are critical for maintaining a playful approach to intervention
  - Perception of inner control
  - Intrinsic motivation
  - Freedom from the constraints of reality

✦ Overall, there is a shift in orientation from an exclusive focus on remediating the underlying problem in the client to focusing on how the problem interacts with the external conditions that interfere with everyday performance and deciding on the most efficacious strategy of intervention

REFERENCES

Arendt, R.E., MacLean, W.E., & Baumeister, A. (1988). Critique of sensory integration therapy and its application in mental retardation. *American Journal on Mental Retardation, 92,* 401–411.

Ayres, A.J. (1972). *Sensory integration and learning disorders.* Los Angeles: Western Psychological Services.

Ayres, A.J. (1979). *Sensory integration and the child.* Los Angeles: Western Psychological Services.

Ayres, A.J. (1989). *Sensory integration and praxis texts.* Los Angeles: Western Psychological Services.

Brown, C., Tolefson, N., Dunn, W., Cromwell, R., & Filion, D. (2001). The Adult Sensory Profile: Measuring patterns of sensory processing. *American Journal of Occupational Therapy, 55,* 75–82.

Bundy, A.C. (1991). The process of planning and implementing intervention. In A.G. Fisher, E.A. Murray, & A.C. Bundy (Eds.), *Sensory integration: Theory and practice* (pp. 333–353). Philadelphia: F.A. Davis.

Bundy, A.C. (2000). *Test of playfulness manual* (version 3). Ft. Collins, CO: Colorado State University.

Bundy, A.C. (2002a). Assessing sensory integrative dysfunction. In A.C. Bundy, S.J. Lane, & E.A. Murray (Eds.), *Sensory integration: Theory and practice* (2nd ed., pp. 169–198). Philadelphia: F.A. Davis.

Bundy, A.C. (2002b). Play theory and sensory integration. In A.C. Bundy, S.J. Lane, & E.A. Murray (Eds.), *Sensory integration: Theory and practice,* (2nd ed., pp. 227–240). Philadelphia: F.A. Davis.

Bundy, A.C., & Koomar, J.A. (2002). Orchestrating intervention: The art of practice. In A.C. Bundy, S.J. Lane, & E.A. Murray (Eds.), *Sensory integration: Theory and practice* (2nd ed., pp. 241–260). Philadelphia: F.A. Davis.

Bundy, A.C., Lane, S.J., & Murray, E.A. (Eds.) (2002). *Sensory integration: Theory and practice* (2nd ed.). Philadelphia: F.A. Davis.

Bundy, A.C., & Murray, E.A. (2002). Introduction to sensory integration theory. In A.C. Bundy, S.J. Lane, & E.A. Murray (Eds.), *Sensory integration: Theory and practice* (2nd ed., pp. 3–33). Philadelphia: F.A. Davis.

Clark, F., Mailloux, Z., Parham, D., & Bissell, J.C. (1989). Sensory integration and children with learning disabilities. In P.N. Clark & A.S. Allen (Eds.), *Occupational therapy for children* (2nd ed., pp. 457–509). St. Louis: C.V. Mosby.

Cohn, E.S., & Cermak, S.A. (1998). Including the family perspective in sensory integration outcomes research. *American Journal of Occupational Therapy, 52,* 540–546.

Davies, P.L., & Gavin, W.J. (2007). Validating the diagnosis of sensory processing disorders using EEG technology. *American Journal of Occupational Therapy, 61,* 176–189.

Dunn, W. (1999). *Sensory profile: User's manual.* San Antonio: Psychological Corporation.

Dunn, W. (2006). *Sensory profile school companion.* San Antonio, TX: Pearson Education.

Fisher, A.G. (1991). Vestibular-proprioceptive processing and bilateral integration and sequencing deficits. In A.C. Bundy, S.J. Lane, & E.A. Murray (Eds.), *Sensory integration: Theory and practice* (pp. 71–107). Philadelphia: F.A. Davis.

Fisher, A.G., & Murray, E.A. (1991). Introduction to sensory integration theory. In A.G. Fisher, E.A. Murray, & A.C. Bundy (Eds.), *Sensory integration: Theory and practice* (pp. 3–26). Philadelphia: F.A. Davis.

Fisher, A.G., Murray, E.A., & Bundy, A.C. (Eds.) (1991). *Sensory integration: Theory and practice.* Philadelphia: F.A. Davis.

Hoehn, T.P., & Baumeister, A. (1994). A critique of the application of sensory integration therapy to children with learning disabilities. *Journal of Learning Disabilities, 27,* 338–350.

Kaplan, B.J., Polatajko, H.J., Wilson, B.N., & Faris, P.D. (1993). Reexamination of sensory integration treatment: A combination of two efficacy studies. *Journal of Learning Disabilities, 26,* 342–347.

Kielhofner, G., & Fisher, A.G. (1991). Mind-brain-body relationships. In A.G. Fisher, E.A. Murray, & A.C. Bundy (Eds.), *Sensory integration: Theory and practice* (pp. 27–45). Philadelphia: F.A. Davis.

King, L.J. (1974). A sensory-integrative approach to schizophrenia. *American Journal of Occupational Therapy, 28,* 529–536.

Lane, S.J. (2002). Sensory modulation. In P.N. Pratt & A.S. Allen (Eds.), *Occupational therapy for children* (2nd ed., pp 101–122). St Louis: C.V. Mosby.

May-Benson, T.A. (2001) A theoretical model of ideation. In E. Blanche, R. Schaaf, & S. Smith Roley (Eds.), *Understanding the nature of sensory integration with diverse populations* (pp. 163–181). San Antonio, TX: Therapy Skill Builders.

May-Benson, T.A., & Cermak, S.A. (2007). Development of an assessment for ideational praxis. *American Journal of Occupational Therapy, 61,* 148–153.

May-Benson, T.A., & Koomar, J.A. (2007). Identifying gravitational insecurity in children: A pilot study. *American Journal of Occupational Therapy, 61,* 142–147.

Miller-Kuhaneck, H., Henry, D.A., Glennon, T.J., & Mu, K. (2007). Development of the Sensory Processing Measure—School: Initial studies of reliability and validity. *American Journal of Occupational Therapy, 61,* 170–175.

Miller, L.J., Anzalone, M.E., Lane, S.J., Cermak, S.A., & Osten, E.T. (2007). Concept evolution in sensory integration: A proposed nosology for diagnosis. *American Journal of Occupational Therapy, 61,* 135–140.

Miller, L.J., Coll, J.R., & Schoen, S.A. (2007). A randomized controlled pilot study of the effectiveness of occupational therapy for children with sensory modulation disorder. *American Journal of Occupational Therapy, 61,* 228–238.

Ottenbacher, K. (1991). Research in sensory integration: Empirical perceptions and progress. In A.G. Fisher, E.A. Murray, & A.C. Bundy (Eds.), *Sensory integration: Theory and practice* (pp. 388–389). Philadelphia: F.A. Davis.

Parham, L.D., Cohn, E.S., Spitzer, S., Koomar, J.A., Miller, L.J., Burke, J.P., et al. (2007). Fidelity in sensory integration intervention research. *American Journal of Occupational Therapy, 61,* 216–227.

Parham, L.D., & Mailloux, Z. (2001). Sensory integration. In J. Case-Smith, A.S. Allen, & P.N. Pratt (Eds.), *Occupational therapy for children* (4th ed., pp. 329–351). St. Louis: Mosby.

Pratt, P.N., Florey, L.A., & Clark, F. (1989). Developmental principles and theories. In P.N. Pratt & A.S. Allen (Eds.), *Occupational therapy for children* (2nd ed., pp. 19–47). St Louis: C.V. Mosby.

Szklut, S., & Philibert, D. (2006). Learning disabilities. In D. Umphred, G. Burton, & R. Lazaro (Eds.), *Neurological rehabilitation* (5th ed., pp. 418–461). St. Louis: Mosby Elsevier Health Services.

Tickle-Degnen, L. (1988). Perspectives on the status of sensory integration theory. *American Journal of Occupational Therapy, 42,* 427–433.

Vargas, S., & Camilli, G. (1999). A meta-analysis of research on sensory integration treatment. *American Journal of Occupational Therapy, 53,* 189–198.

Williamson, G.G., & Anzalone, M.E. (2001). *Sensory integration and self-regulation in infants and toddlers: Helping very young children interact with their environment.* Washington, DC: Zero to Three.

Related Knowledge

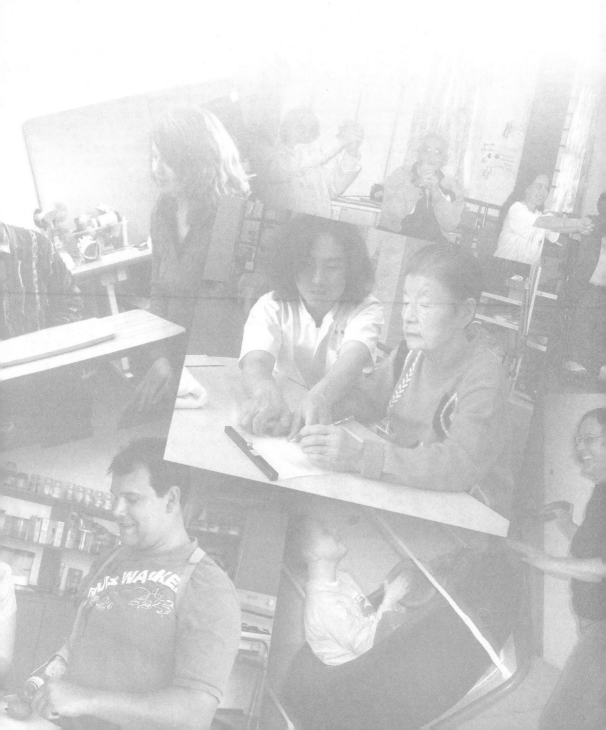

CHAPTER 14

The Nature and Use of Related Knowledge

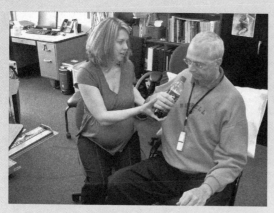

Heidi helps a client build strength in his affected arm following a stroke.

Heidi Fischer, Bacon Fung Leung Ng, and Karen Roberts all make use of appropriate conceptual practice models that were discussed in Section Two. These occupational therapy models, along with the field's paradigm, define and shape the nature of their occupational therapy services. Nonetheless, each of these therapists finds it necessary to make use of related knowledge that comes from other disciplines.

Heidi Fischer uses several occupational therapy models in her practice with persons with stroke. She also draws upon disability studies, an interdisciplinary field that emphasizes environmental barriers instead of simply impairments as factors that create disability. As a result, Heidi notes:

I see my clients as more than a list of impairments or a list of functional limitations. I see clients as persons who are adapting to a disability and trying to get back to their lives or create new lives in the face of an environment that is not always supportive or accessible to them.

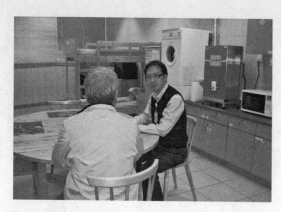

Bacon and a client discuss the progress of therapy.

Bacon Fung Leung Ng indicates that when he works with clients with depression, he supplements his use of occupational therapy models with cognitive behavioral theory and also with ideas that come from the field of positive psychology.

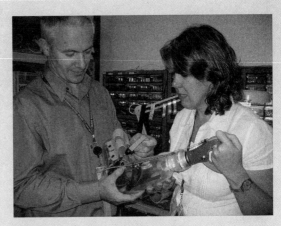

Karen consults with a prosthetist regarding a prosthetic arm for one of her clients.

Karen Roberts notes that, when working with amputees, it is important for her to have information from the medical model used by physicians; this includes:

Knowledge of edema management, wound healing, and scar maturation along with being aware of the inherent tensile strength in a scar and the time it takes to build this up, or the length of time it takes for a wound to heal. These all impact upon when someone can wear a prosthesis and also provide indications for OT intervention techniques such as massage and edema management.

As these examples illustrate, occupational therapists routinely use knowledge beyond that provided by the profession's paradigm and conceptual practice models. This related knowledge developed in other fields does not belong to occupational therapy but is related to the concerns and practice of the profession.

Types of Related Knowledge

Two types of related knowledge are often used to supplement conceptual practice models:

* Foundational knowledge related to the interdisciplinary base of the models
* Applied knowledge addressing issues not addressed by models

Foundational knowledge is generally knowledge linked to basic sciences or disciplines. For instance, the biomechanical model builds upon the knowledge of anatomy (particularly musculoskeletal anatomy) and physiology, and the sensory integration and cognitive-perceptual models build on knowledge from the neurosciences. Other models, such as the model of human occupation, build on knowledge from psychology and the social sciences. In fact, many readers will recognize that these bodies of knowledge often make up what are considered prerequisites to courses that teach occupational therapy conceptual practice models.

Applied knowledge is knowledge developed for application in other professions. One example is behaviorism, developed in psychology. This theory employs the concept of reinforcement (i.e., positive and negative consequences of behavior) to explain and manage the acquisition and relinquishing of behavior patterns. The feature box in this chapter provides an example of using this knowledge in combination with an occupational therapy model.

Three Exemplary Bodies of Related Knowledge

Potential related knowledge for occupational therapy includes a wide range of theories and models from many disciplines and professions.

> **Box 14.1 Using Related Knowledge in Combination with an Occupational Therapy Conceptual Practice Model**
>
> The following is an instance in which an occupational therapist might use related knowledge in combination with an occupational therapy model. Adolescent clients with behavioral problems may be engaged in occupations designed to allow them to explore, to pursue interests, and to develop a sense of efficacy, based on the model of human occupation. Those same adolescents may be informed that if they become verbally or physically aggressive, they may lose points in the token economy (i.e., a behavioral approach wherein clients may earn and lose points that can be cashed in for privileges and/or desired goods). In this instance, an occupational therapy model defines the major aspects of therapy, but knowledge and techniques drawn from behaviorism are used to manage behaviors interfering with participation in therapy.

To cover all of this knowledge is beyond the scope of this text. However, three applied bodies of knowledge that are frequently used in occupational therapy will be covered in this section. They are:

* The medical model
* Cognitive behavioral therapy
* Disability studies

The medical model is developed and used in medicine. It has always served as important related knowledge in occupational therapy. Techniques from cognitive behavioral therapy are often used to deal with specific emotional and behavioral reactions that clients have to the stress of illness and disability. The interdisciplinary field of disability studies emphasizes understanding disability from the perspective of persons who have disabilities (Albrecht, Fitzpatrick, & Scrimshaw, 2000; Longmore, 1995; Oliver, 1996; Scotch, 2001; Shapiro, 1993). Central to this perspective is the argument that many of the problems faced by persons with disabilities can be located more properly in the environment, in everything from physical barriers to stigmatizing attitudes to outright discrimination. Since the vast majority of occupational therapy clients have a disability, ideas from disability studies have many lessons to teach practitioners. This knowledge increasingly influences how and what kind of rehabilitation services are provided. Occupational therapists use related knowledge to supplement the conceptual practice models that define and guide the main elements of occupational therapy practice.

The three bodies of related knowledge that will be discussed in this section represent three distinct, sometimes opposing, and potentially complementary views of the condition of disability and how to go about changing it. The medical model locates the problem as a condition in the individual, which requires the ministrations of an authoritarian medical expert to remove or attenuate it. Cognitive behavioral therapy teaches clients to understand and manage their own emotional and behavioral reactions to stressful events and circumstances. Disability studies locate the

> **Occupational therapists use related knowledge to supplement the conceptual practice models that define and guide the main elements of occupational therapy practice.**

problem in social conditions that transform impairment into disability; it envisions social change and empowerment of disabled persons as groups. Each of these perspectives identifies a part of the complex situation faced by clients with chronic illness and disability.

Discussion

In most instances, an occupational therapist could not be an effective practitioner without recourse to related knowledge. Therefore, the use of related knowledge is a basic characteristic of good practice. It is important to remember, however, that related knowledge is not unique to occupational therapy. Thus, it cannot serve as a source of professional identity or as the defining component of an occupational therapist's competence. Rather, related knowledge serves as adjunctive and complementary to the field's paradigm and conceptual practice models.

REFERENCES

Albrecht, G.L., Fitzpatrick, R., & Scrimshaw, S.C. (Eds.). (2000). *Handbook of social studies in health and medicine.* London: Sage.

Longmore, P.K. (1995). The second phase: From disability rights to disability culture. *The Disability Rag and ReSource, 16,* 4–11.

Oliver, M. (1996). *Understanding disability: From theory to practice.* New York: St. Martin's Press.

Scotch, R.K. (2001). *From good will to civil rights: Transforming federal disability policy* (2nd ed.). Philadelphia: Temple University Press.

Shapiro, J.P. (1993). *No pity: People with disabilities forging a new civil rights movement.* New York: Random House.

CHAPTER 15

The Medical Model

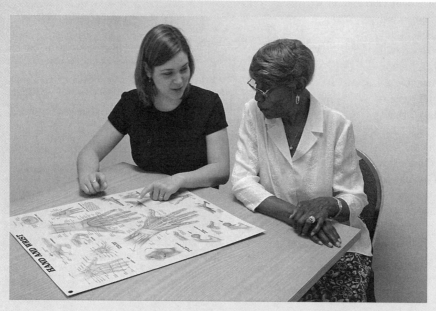

An occupational therapist works with a client following an upper extremity injury that required surgery. As part of her approach, the therapist explains to the client the post-surgical healing process and its implications for safely engaging in occupations. In a wide range of circumstances, therapists must have an understanding of their clients' disease processes and prognoses, the expected side effects of medication, or the pathway of recovery from trauma and/or surgical procedures. In these instances, occupational therapists are drawing on related knowledge from the medical model.

The medical model was developed in and for the practice of medicine, although aspects of it are used in many health disciplines, including occupational therapy. This model addresses disease and trauma that interrupt ordinary bodily function. The model has resulted in a steady growth of scientific knowledge concerning:

- Biochemical constituents of the human body and their cause-and-effect relationships
- The nature, causes, and management of disease and trauma (Dubos, 1959)

Practitioners using this model aim to eliminate or contain the effects of disease or trauma through manipulation or alteration of bodily structures and processes.

Theory

The medical model reflects beliefs about healing that have origins in the medical system of the ancient Greeks (Dubos, 1959). According to Grecian mythology, the god Asclepius was a healer who cured with medicinal plants and surgery. Asclepius wielded esoteric knowledge as part of his healing art. With absolute authority, he ministered to a passive and compliant recipient of the healing action. The idea of the physician as an authority and the client as a compliant recipient of care derives from this mythological divine healer (Siegler & Osmond, 1974).

In the 20th century, medicine increased its scientific base dramatically. Scientists made great strides in understanding the physical world through careful examination of the building blocks of nature and their interrelationships (Capra, 1982). Medicine emulated the intellectual models of early physical sciences (Capra, 1982; Riley, 1977), adopting a view in which:

- The body was considered a complex machine
- The task of medicine was conceived as repairing breakdowns in the machine (i.e., disease and trauma) (Capra, 1982)

Knowledge foundational to and incorporated into the medical model has been generated by many disciplines including basic sciences such as genetics, biochemistry, anatomy, and physiology, as well as applied sciences such as pharmacology, nutrition, and bioengineering (Bertalanffy, 1966; Capra, 1982).

Medicine has implicitly, if not always explicitly, employed the concept of health to define organization in the human body. In the medical model, health is generally defined by three themes:

- The absence of disease
- Homeostasis
- Normative states

Because of its focus on illness, the medical model approach to defining health has been primarily to proceed "inductively by enumeration of examples [of disease] and then health is the absence of all of those states" (Brody, 1973, p. 75). Although some efforts have been made to define health as more than the mere absence of disease (e.g., concepts of wellness) (Berliner & Salmon, 1980), these efforts are largely outside of the traditional medical model.

Homeostasis is the notion that living systems try to maintain certain predetermined states (Bertalanffy, 1966). Examples of homeostatic processes are the maintenance of blood pressure and body temperature. An extension of the idea of homeostasis is how the body seeks to restore order when it has been disturbed by disease or trauma. Thus, for example, understanding of immunological process by which the body fends off infections or the healing process following accidental or surgical trauma is important to medicine.

Finally, the study of anatomical and physiological dimensions of the body resulted in descriptions of what is normative. For example, the understanding of the organization of the musculoskeletal system has resulted in the idea of what constitutes the average body. Similarly, descriptions of physiological processes have resulted in descriptions of typical physiological

> **Although some efforts have been made to define health as more than the mere absence of disease (e.g., concepts of wellness), these efforts are largely outside of the traditional medical model.**

states. These norms have become accepted as standards for health, and deviation from them is the basis for identification of problems.

The medical model identifies problems in terms of:

• Disease and trauma
• Disturbances in homeostasis
• Deviations from body norms

Disease, homeostatic disturbance, and bodily abnormality are seen as negative states that need to be altered or eradicated. Disease is viewed as disrupting the homeostatic order of biological processes because it forces somatic functions beyond normative limits.

Critical to understanding disease are its:

• Syndromatic signs and symptoms
• Etiology
• Prognosis

Signs of disease refer to the cluster of physical indicators (e.g., swelling, fever, abnormal physiological values) that represent a deviation from bodily norms. **Symptoms** refer to individuals' experiences and complaints (e.g., pain, fatigue, and difficulties with bodily processes and functions). An important step in understanding any disease or trauma is identification of the attendant signs and symptoms.

Etiology refers to the underlying cause of the disease process. Careful description of the root source and unfolding of physical events that constitute each disease process is basic to the medical model. Typical causes of disease include:

• Infectious or noxious agents entering the body (e.g., viral infections, lead poisoning, exposure to asbestos)
• Genetic disorder (e.g., Down syndrome)
• Externally imposed physical trauma to the body (e.g., spinal cord injury) or breakdown of the body due to wear and tear (e.g., carpal tunnel syndrome or cerebrovascular accident)

Medical researchers originally sought to identify a single cause of a disease process; however, it is now recognized that many if not most diseases are a result of many contributing and interacting factors. Originally, the medical model was only interested in biological factors

that contributed to disease status (Blaney, 1975; Ludwig & Othmer, 1977; Siegler & Osmond, 1974). It is now known that biological factors need not be the sole cause of disease and that such factors as psychological stress contribute to some disease processes.

Prognosis refers to the natural course that a disease will take. Prognosis includes understanding both the underlying unfolding of the physiological processes and their consequences (e.g., impairment, pain, or death). Prognosis is important in making decisions about whether, when, and how to intervene. For example, the consequences of letting a disease take its natural course versus risking the side effects of medical procedures must sometimes be weighed. Also, identification of how far a disease has progressed along its natural course may also influence the type of medical intervention chosen.

Prognostic information is often important for occupational therapy because it provides an understanding of how impairments are likely to change. For example, some diseases are progressive and will result in functional decline over time. Other diseases are characterized by exacerbations (periods in which symptoms and impairments may increase) and remissions (periods in which symptoms and impairments may decline) over time. In other cases, the onset of a problem such as stroke will be followed by a period of recovery of function. By being able to project the future course of diseases and their functional implications, occupational therapists are better able to set goals and establish treatment priorities for clients.

Medicine has applied the basic approach of investigating the syndrome, etiology, and prognosis of disease to a vast number of disease and trauma states. Many of these are now well understood, and others are still partly or poorly understood. Because of the emergence of new disease processes (AIDS being one example), medicine is constantly investigating and generating understanding of new problems.

Rationale for Action

The aim of medicine is to identify the appropriate therapeutic agents that could be applied to eradicate or arrest the disease process (Brody,

1973). Control of disease is accomplished by attacking the causative agent or focusing treatment on that part of the body affected by disease (Dubos, 1959). Therapeutic agents include drugs and procedures (e.g., surgery, radiation) that attack the disease or remove or repair the diseased component (Ludwig & Othmer, 1977). This requires that the physician carefully collect data on the signs and symptoms manifested by the client in order to arrive at a correct diagnosis. When the client's disease is correctly identified, the physician, depending on the existing knowledge about the disease, will have some ability to predict and control the course of illness. The diagnosis is critical in the medical model, because it predicts the path of the disease and indicates the appropriate treatment or treatment options.

Nonetheless, only in a limited number of diseases does medicine have sufficient knowledge to proceed in this fashion (Brody, 1973). In fact, there is a continuum from those diseases for which there is rather certain knowledge of etiology, course, and treatment to those about which little is known. Consequently, physicians often operate with only partial knowledge about a disease and its treatment. Even when there is fairly good knowledge about the efficacy of medical interventions, there will be substantial variation in how individual clients react to the treatments. For example, optimal dosage of medication and the experience of side effects is a matter of great variation among clients for certain conditions and their treatment. Thus, medication sometimes involves a trial-and-error period during which both the desired results and side effects are monitored in order to achieve correct prescription.

Often, treatment cannot be directed at underlying causes (which may not be known) and instead focuses on managing symptoms without affecting the underlying problem (Ludwig & Othmer, 1977). This means that medical model treatment may be curative, compensatory, syndromatic, or symptomatic (Mechanic, 1978). In **curative treatment**, causative agents are attacked, and the condition is reversed. **Compensatory treatment** aims to minimize further problems and maintain function; **syndromatic treatment** manages major problems related to

the disease without cure. Finally, **symptomatic treatment** simply alleviates some problems without altering basic causes or effects of the disease. Only a very small percentage of medical treatment is curative (Ludwig & Othmer, 1977).

In many instances, medical treatment aims to limit or reduce impairment and occupational therapy interventions are complementary to medical efforts. So, for example, the physician may prescribe medication or perform surgery designed to reduce impairments. For such clients, occupational therapy often aims to maximize remaining capacities or to capitalize upon the potential for increased function that results from medical interventions. In such instances, occupational therapists must be aware of the nature of the medical intervention, its purpose, and its consequences. For example, when physicians prescribe medication, therapists must be aware of the intended positive outcomes of the medication as well as possible side effects. Moreover, when surgery is performed, therapists must understand the precautions following surgery, the process of recovery, and healing after surgery. In this way, occupational therapists routinely make use of knowledge from the medical model.

Research and Evidence Base

Medical research includes ongoing research into basic physiological processes of the body; investigation of the nature, causes, and course of diseases; and investigation to develop and test therapies for various diseases. Biomedical research has yielded one of the largest scientific bodies of knowledge available to modern societies. In the 20th century, great strides were made in understanding the human body, the most notable of which was unraveling the human genome. Vast amounts of money are directed to the study of various disease processes and how they can be cured or attenuated. As a consequence, medical model knowledge continues to grow substantially. Nonetheless, knowledge about diseases can range from those about which very little is still known or for which little can be done to those that are more completely understood and can be readily eradicated or managed. This circumstance reflects the fact that new problems are always emerging and indicates the vast number of medical problems that must be investigated on an ongoing basis.

Discussion

The medical model is clearly the most influential and successful force in modern health care. The knowledge of this model underlies the successful management of a large range of illnesses and traumatic conditions. Many of the accomplishments of applying this model represent truly remarkable achievements that result in significant life saving and reduction of pain and suffering. As a technical achievement, the medical model is remarkable.

The medical model has both ideological and knowledge components. The ideological component of the medical model includes a set of beliefs about the physician's role as a healer with authority over clients. The knowledge component is a biochemical body of information that explains disease as an interruption of normal physiological processes and yields procedures to eliminate disease through manipulation or alteration of somatic structures and processes.

The medical model can thus be defined as the beliefs and knowledge that define physicians as authoritative healers and that enable them to cure, ameliorate, or arrest disease through recognition and alteration of its manifestation in bodily states. Despite its important accomplishments, a number of limitations and weaknesses of the medical model have been identified.

The idea of the physician as an authoritative healer and the client as a passive and compliant recipient of medical care has been criticized. Authors have called for a more egalitarian and collaborative model in which the client shares in the process of managing the disease and recovery. This becomes especially true in cases in which medicine cannot provide a cure or reverse the medical problem, and the client must have an active role in ongoing management of the disease process.

Engel (1962, 1977) criticizes the medical model for its lack of concern for factors other than the biomedical. He argues that the medical model has led to undesirable treatment practices, such as overuse of surgery and drugs and inappropriate use of diagnostic procedures. The value of diagnostic procedures is directly related to the certainty of etiological and therapeutic implications of the diagnosis. This requires that much be known about the disease, its course, its alterability, and the agents that have power to control the disease processes. Where knowledge is less certain, the physician's ability to effectively apply the medical model is limited. For example, many persons have criticized the use of the medical model in psychiatry, where many diagnoses do not approach the degree of knowledge and certainty needed for effective delineation of etiology, course (prognosis), and treatment (Goffman, 1961; Leifer, 1970; Szasz, 1961).

Another criticism of the medical model is its stance that disease is a negative state. In cases in which disease can be identified and eradicated, this stance is largely unproblematic. However, this aspect of the medical model falters when a disease process is chronic, produces impairments, and cannot be eradicated by medical procedures. In such instances, the medical model stance on disease and impairment as negative can result in devaluation of the person (Gill, 2001; Leifer, 1970). Moreover, the negative identification of disease can be used to justify practices that amount to social control, as in the case of psychiatric illness (Leifer, 1970; Szasz, 1961).

Any discussion of the medical model must also recognize that in many instances occupational therapists work alongside physicians who derive their status and expertise from the medical model. Rogers (1982) points out that there are critical differences between occupational therapy's approach to identifying problems and

> **The medical model can thus be defined as the beliefs and knowledge that define physicians as authoritative healers and that enable them to cure, ameliorate, or arrest disease through recognition and alteration of its manifestation in bodily states.**

doing therapy and that of the medical model. Medicine is primarily concerned with eradicating disease. Siegler and Osmond (1974) go so far as to argue that the physician's role does not include addressing impairment. Occupational therapy seeks primarily to influence how people conduct their lives in the face of permanent impairments (Reilly, 1962). In that sense, the respective contributions of the medical model and occupational therapy can be complementary. Occupational therapists should be aware of both the strengths and limitations of the medical model. It is also important to recognize that while therapists use information from the medical model as related knowledge in practice, the overall approach and contributions of occupational therapy are different from those of the medical model.

Table 15.1 **Terms of the Model**

Compensatory treatment	Treatment that aims to minimize further problems and maintain function.
Curative treatment	Treatment in which causative agents are attacked and the condition is reversed.
Etiology	Underlying cause of the disease process.
Homeostasis	The notion that living systems try to maintain certain predetermined states.
Prognosis	The natural course that a disease will take.
Sign	One of a cluster of physical indicators that represents a deviation from bodily norms.
Symptom	An individual's experience or complaint.
Symptomatic treatment	Treatment in which some problems are alleviated but no basic causes or effects of the disease are altered.
Syndromatic treatment	Treatment that manages major problems related to the disease without cure.

SUMMARY

✦ The medical model is concerned with:
  • Biochemical constituents of the human body and their cause-and-effect relationships
  • The nature, causes, and management of disease and trauma
  • Eliminating or containing the effects of disease or trauma through manipulation or alteration of bodily structures and processes

Theory

✦ Beliefs about healing that define the physician as an authority and the client as a compliant recipient of care derive from the Greek mythological divine healer, Asclepius

✦ Intellectual models of early physical sciences resulted in:
  • The body being seen as a complex machine
  • The task of medicine being conceived as repairing breakdowns in the machine
  • Basic sciences, such as genetics, biochemistry, anatomy, and physiology
  • Applied sciences, such as pharmacology, nutrition, and bioengineering

+ Health is defined by three themes:
  • Absence of disease
  • Homeostasis (the notion that living systems try to maintain certain predetermined states)
  • Normative physiological states

Problems and Challenges

+ The medical model identifies problems in terms of:
  • Disease and trauma
  • Disturbances in homeostasis
  • Deviations from body norms

+ Disease is viewed as disrupting the homeostatic order of biological processes because it forces somatic functions beyond normative limits

+ Critical to understanding disease are its:
  • Syndromatic signs (physical indicators) and symptoms (individuals' experiences, complaints, and symptoms)

• Etiology (underlying cause of the disease process)
• Prognosis (natural course that a disease will take)

Rationale for Action

+ Action derived from the medical model is somatic and guided by the germ theory of disease (attacking the causative agent or focusing treatment on that part of the body affected by disease)

+ Diagnosis is critical in the medical model because it predicts the path of the disease and indicates the appropriate treatment or treatment options

REFERENCES

Berliner, H.S., & Salmon, J.W. (1980). The holistic alternative to scientific medicine: History and analysis. *International Journal of Health Services, 10,* 133–147.

Bertalanffy, L. von (1966). General systems theory and psychiatry. In S.R. Arieti (Ed.), *American handbook of psychiatry* (vol. 3). New York: Basic Books.

Blaney, P.H. (1975). Implications of the medical model and its alternatives. *American Journal of Psychiatry, 132,* 911–914.

Brody, H. (1973). The systems view of man: Implications for medicine, science, and ethics. *Perspectives in Biology and Medicine, 17,* 71–92.

Capra, F. (1982). *The turning point: Science, society, and the rising culture.* New York: Simon & Schuster.

Dubos, R. (1959). *The mirage of health.* New York: Harper & Row.

Engel, G.L. (1962). The nature of disease and the care of the patient: The challenge of humanism and science in medicine. *Rhode Island Medical Journal, 65,* 245–252.

Engel, G.L. (1977). The need for a new medical model: A challenge for bio-medicine. *Science, 196,* 129-135.

Gill, C.J. (2001). Divided understandings: The social experience of disability. In G. Albrecht, K. Seelman, & M. Bury (Eds.), *Handbook of*

disability studies (pp. 351–372). Thousand Oaks, CA: Sage.

Goffman, E. (1961). *Asylums.* New York: Doubleday.

Leifer, R. (1970). Medical model as ideology. *International Journal of Psychiatry, 9,* 13–34.

Ludwig, A.M., & Othmer, E. (1977). The medical basis of psychiatry. *American Journal of Psychiatry, 134,* 1087–1092.

Mechanic, D. (1978). The doctor's view of disease and the patient. In D. Mechanic (Ed.), *Medical sociology* (2nd ed.). New York: Free Press.

Reilly, M. (1962). Occupational therapy can be one of the great ideas of 20th century medicine. *American Journal of Occupational Therapy, 76,* 1–9.

Riley, J.N. (1977). Western medicine's attempt to become more scientific: Examples from the United States and Thailand. *Social Science and Medicine, 11,* 549–560.

Rogers, J. (1982). Order and disorder in medicine and occupational therapy. *American Journal of Occupational Therapy, 36,* 29–35.

Siegler, M., & Osmond, H. (1974). *Models of madness, models of medicine.* New York: Harper & Row.

Szasz, T. (1961). *The myth of mental illness: Foundations of a theory of personal conduct.* New York: Harper & Row.

CHAPTER 16

Cognitive Behavioral Therapy

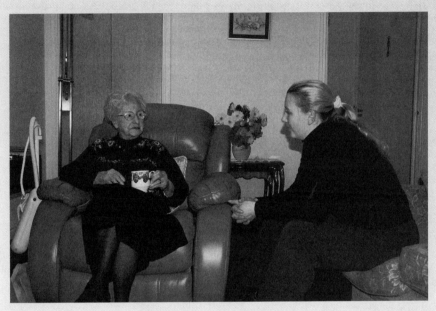

Alice Moody works in a pain management program as part of a multidisciplinary team that utilizes knowledge from cognitive behavioral therapy. Alice notes:

Many people who come through the memory clinic appear to isolate themselves for fear of social embarrassment due to word-finding difficulties or following a fall. My use of cognitive behavioral therapy enables them to consider their fears about particular occupations and perhaps utilize new strategies, aids, or anxiety management techniques.

Cognitive behavioral therapy (CBT) is an approach used by psychotherapists and other medical and rehabilitation professionals to address clients' cognitions along with related emotions and behavior. CBT is used to help clients reframe the way they think about themselves and their impairments and to change related behaviors. CBT can be applied to a wide range of clients. Like Alice, (previous page), occupational therapists often use CBT as a component of the services they offer to clients.

CBT was developed primarily by psychologists as a specific method of psychotherapy. However, CBT and concepts of CBT have been applied to a wide range of clients in many contexts. A useful resource for occupational therapists applying CBT to persons with disabilities is the text *Cognitive Behavioral Therapy for Chronic Illness and Disability* (Taylor, 2006). In addition to providing a comprehensive treatment of the theory, evidence, and methods of CBT, it also discusses how CBT can be integrated with occupational therapy and other relevant bodies of knowledge for persons with disabilities.

Theory

Cognitive behavioral therapy is guided by the cognitive model. This model proposes that dysfunctional thinking and unrealistic cognitive appraisals of life events can negatively influence feelings and behavior (Beck, 1995, 1999). The cognitive model (Beck, 1991, 1995, 1999) identifies three levels of cognition:

* Core beliefs
* Intermediate beliefs
* Automatic thoughts and images

According to cognitive theory, core beliefs drive intermediate beliefs that, in turn, influence automatic thoughts.

Core beliefs are the deepest level of beliefs; they organize how people interpret and deal with incoming information (Beck, 1996). Adaptive core beliefs allow one to interpret, appraise, and respond realistically to life events. Dysfunctional core beliefs distort reality and are characteristically global, rigid, and overgeneralized (Beck,

1995). According to Taylor (2006), there are four types of core beliefs that are of primary concern in working with individuals who have disabilities:

* Core beliefs about self
* Core beliefs about others
* Core beliefs about the health-care system
* Core beliefs about the impairment or disability

The following are examples of dysfunctional core beliefs corresponding to the four types of core beliefs previously noted:

* "I don't have the strength to face my impairment"
* "My family members find me to be a burden now that I have a disability"
* "Rehabilitation professions are only optimistic because they don't have disabilities themselves"
* "People with my type of disability are never able to find happiness"

Intermediate beliefs are unarticulated attitudes, rules, expectations, or assumptions reflected in a person's thinking. Examples of intermediate beliefs are:

* "I shouldn't complain about my pain"
* "I can tell that the employer who interviewed me today doesn't want to hire a person with a disability"
* "My children will think I am not a good parent if they know I have depression"

Intermediate beliefs influence a person's views (thoughts and feelings) of situations as well as how they will behave regarding those situations. When these beliefs are dysfunctional, they result in unnecessary emotional pain and may interfere with performance and with achieving enjoyment and satisfaction with performance.

Automatic thoughts occur at the most superficial level of cognition. They are the ideas or images that go through one's mind concerning immediate circumstances. Negative automatic thoughts are verbal self-statements and/or mental images that are characterized by:

* Distortion of reality
* Emotional distress
* Interference with the pursuit and attainment of life goals (Beck, 1995)

Some examples of negative automatic thoughts are:

- "Since I won't be able to do this task without a lot of help, I'm going to appear really incompetent"
- "If I don't keep going, my therapist will think I am not trying hard enough"
- "That pain means I am having an exacerbation"

Hot thoughts are recurring automatic thoughts characterized by intense emotional experience. They are considered the most important automatic thoughts to work with in psychotherapy since they cause the most distress and interference with functioning (Beck, 1995; Greenberger & Padesky, 1995).

Automatic thoughts typically occur in association with **situational triggers,** which are events or circumstances that evoke certain thoughts or emotions in a given client. Situational triggers could include, for instance, a difficult task, a comment or facial expression by another person, or a physical sensation such as fatigue or pain.

In summary, the cognitive model argues that there are three levels of cognition. The innermost core beliefs are formed through the course of development and tend to be the most fixed in a person's cognitive system. These core beliefs influence the kind of intermediate thoughts that persons have about situations or circumstances in life. Intermediate thoughts, in turn, influence how people react to various situational triggers and, thus, the kind of automatic thoughts that occur in response to those triggers. Each of these levels of cognition can be adaptive or maladaptive.

Maladaptive Cognitions

Maladaptive cognitions can be realistic or unrealistic. What determines their adaptive status is how the cognitions affect a person's emotion and behavior. CBT was originally developed to address individuals whose cognitions were the primary source of their difficulties. Thus, CBT was a method for addressing disordered thinking that was part and parcel of psychiatric problems.

Persons with significant impairments often experience loss of abilities coupled with difficulty

and failure in performance. Moreover, they may also experience rejection, alienation, exclusion, and discrimination from others. Consequently, such persons—even those without histories of dysfunctional cognitions—are at risk for developing dysfunctional thinking and beliefs. Individuals with pre-existing or predispositions toward maladaptive cognition are at even higher risk. Persons who develop maladaptive cognitions experience negative emotional, behavioral, and physiological consequences. They tend to misinterpret otherwise neutral events or to develop exaggerated concerns about health and functioning that can exacerbate the consequences of their illness or impairment. An important dimension of these negative consequences is the result of increased stress, worry, anxiety, and other negative emotional experiences on physiological processes. Taylor (2006) reviews a wide range of literature that documents how negative emotional experiences (such as those emanating from cognitive distortions or preoccupations) can result in changes in endocrine and immune system functioning.

> **Persons who develop maladaptive cognitions experience negative emotional, behavioral, and physiological consequences.**

There are two types of maladaptive cognitions:

- Errors in thinking
- Preoccupations

Errors in Thinking

Errors in thinking are cognitive distortions that reflect incorrect logic and/or that do not reflect reality. Automatic thoughts, intermediate beliefs, and core beliefs typically cluster together in patterns that reflect errors in thinking. So, for example, a client who has a core belief that he cannot take pressure may have an intermediate belief that he will break down and cry if his occupational therapist asks him to increase performance in the next session. Such a client might have the following automatic thought: "I'll never get through the next occupational therapy session." The resulting automatic thought may elicit feelings of anxiety and dread whenever any event, object, or circumstance triggers thinking about occupational therapy. In this instance, the automatic thought about occupational therapy emanates from an underlying distorted belief about self (i.e., the client's belief that he cannot take pressure). It results in the distorted anticipation that he will not be able to handle increased expectations for performance, which in turn yields a dread of his next therapy session.

Typically, the cognitive distortions of a client will manifest as distinctive clusters and patterns of thinking that go together. For example, if the client discussed earlier held another core belief that others saw him as a weakling, then he might have an intermediate thought that if he breaks down during the next occupational therapy session, his therapist will think even less of him. This in turn could result in the automatic thought that if he goes to his next therapy session, the outcome will be that his therapist is no longer going to want to work with him. This in turn may lead to avoiding his next occupational therapy session. As the example illustrates, cognitive distortions can result in patterns of thinking that create emotional distress for clients and that lead to negative behaviors. Clients tend to manifest the same kind of distortions over and over so that the emotional distress and negative behavioral consequences tend to pile up.

> According to CBT, the beliefs that clients hold about situations, rather than the situations themselves, are what determine negative emotional experience, behavioral reactions, and physiological response.

Preoccupations

Even if clients do not have illogical ways of thinking, they can become preoccupied by negative cognitions about their impairment and functioning. Although such cognitions are based on reality, the preoccupation with the thoughts becomes problematic. Preoccupations are usually accompanied by difficult emotions, problematic behaviors, or aversive physiological reactions. Hence preoccupations can reduce functioning or quality of life. The following are three examples of clients with dysfunctional preoccupations:

- Clients who cannot enjoy activities because they worry that the activities will cause pain
- Clients who are so concerned about others' judgments or reactions to their impairment that they avoid social interaction
- Elderly clients who are at risk for falling, but whose preoccupation with the possibility of falling leads them to unnecessarily curtail

activities in order to avoid falling. Such clients may actually increase their risk of falling by deconditioning themselves through activity restriction

As these examples illustrate, the preoccupations are problematic for clients because they interfere with occupational satisfaction and adaptive behavior.

Rationale for Intervention

According to CBT, the beliefs that clients hold about situations, rather than the situations themselves, are what determine negative emotional experience, behavioral reactions, and physiological response (Beck, 1995; Beck, Rush, Shaw, & Emery, 1979). CBT intervention generally includes three assumptions (Dobson & Dozois, 2001):

- Cognition affects behavior
- Cognition can be monitored and altered
- Behavior change is mediated by cognitive change

Thus, while the focus of CBT is on cognitions, it is recognized that behavior change is also an important component of this approach.

CBT teaches clients to replace distorted thinking with more realistic and adaptive cognitions. During therapy, these distortions are typically identified by listening to the client's automatic thoughts and attempting to identify the specific type of error that the client seems to be making (Taylor, 2006). Clients are often educated to identify and correct their errors in thinking independently. Clients with preoccupations are helped to manage these concerns through approaches that stress coping, managing the impairment, and problem-solving.

Practice Resources

Assessment

The main thrust of CBT assessment is to identify the client's maladaptive cognitions (Taylor, 2006). Cognitive distortions and preoccupations are typically identified by interviewing clients and listening to them during therapy sessions.

Careful attention to what a client says can help to identify the client's automatic thoughts. Through interviewing the client and using objective knowledge about the client's condition and situation, cognitive distortions can be differentiated from preoccupations. When the client presents with a cognitive distortion, the therapist attempts to identify the specific type of error that the client seems to be making (Beck, 1995).

It is important in assessment to distinguish between distorted thinking (inaccurate thoughts) and accurate thoughts that constitute preoccupations. Each of these different thought patterns has different implications for the type of cognitive behavioral techniques for addressing them (Taylor, 2006). Distorted thinking is best addressed through cognitive techniques that seek to correct the thinking pattern, whereas realistic preoccupations are often best addressed through coping skills, symptom and impairment management training, and problem-solving.

It is not appropriate to challenge or try to correct the beliefs of clients who report negative thoughts that are valid based on their experiences and are well-grounded in reality (White, 2001). When working with clients who have chronic impairments it is especially important to be aware of when clients' thoughts are realistically negative versus when thoughts reflect errors in thinking.

It is also important to identify whether a client tends to have predominantly one or both thinking patterns (i.e., distortion and/or preoccupation). In the circumstance when clients have both types of maladaptive cognitions, it is typically useful to engage the client in a process of distinguishing thoughts into realistic and unrealistic categories.

Intervention

As noted previously, CBT intervention generally focuses on either helping clients with distorted thinking to correct their thinking patterns or assisting clients with realistic maladaptive cognitions to cope more effectively. Correcting thinking patterns or cognitive restructuring requires a careful and systematic approach to helping clients reexamine and reconstruct how they think. Coping techniques focus on changing how clients think about these problems or situations because

the clients' cognitions exacerbate the consequences of these negative circumstances. Both of these approaches to intervention are discussed here.

Cognitive Restructuring

Cognitive restructuring techniques that correct distorted thinking require a comprehensive and multi-level approach to cognitive change. Maladaptive automatic thoughts are addressed by identifying them and teaching the client how to respond to them (typically through the use of thought records). Intermediate and core beliefs are addressed by identifying them and teaching the client to modify them. Both techniques are discussed.

Use of Thought Records

CBT teaches clients how to identify their own automatic thoughts so that they can actively explore and respond to them. The primary means by which this is accomplished is through having clients complete a **thought record,** a form that allows the client to identify and respond to automatic thoughts. The thought record includes multiple targeted questions that allow clients to reflect upon and develop alternatives to their maladaptive thoughts. There are many types of existing thought records; the feature box in this chapter illustrates a thought record useful for clients with disabilities. Ordinarily the therapist works with the client to complete one or more thought records until the client feels comfortable using the tool independently. Then, the thought record is assigned as a homework assignment to be done outside the therapy time. Therapists will check in with clients during subsequent sessions to ascertain how effectively the client is using the thought record to manage automatic thoughts.

Identifying and Modifying Intermediate and Core Beliefs

The process of changing intermediate thoughts and core beliefs is complex and requires thorough knowledge of the theory and methods of CBT. Intermediate and core beliefs can be brought to consciousness through a very specific sequence of questioning that allows the client to probe progressively deeper levels of consciousness (Burns, 1980).

Box 16.1   A Thought Record for Persons with Disabilities

Taylor (2006) developed a "response record," which is a type of thought record for use with individuals with disabilities who have distorted cognitions. This response record, shown below, is designed to help clients record and respond to negative automatic thoughts.

Response Record			
Date:	Health event trigger (or other triggering event):		
What am I feeling right now? (Circle all that apply.)	panicked	numb	sad	angry
	hopeless	worried	other:	
What thoughts or pictures are passing through my mind?			
Which of these thoughts or pictures makes me feel the worst? (circle one above)			
What are the emotional, behavioral, and physical consequences of thinking this way?			
Emotional:	Behavioral:	Physical:	

- What do I already know that supports this belief?
- What do I already know that does not support this belief?
- What might someone else think about this situation?
- What advice would I give to a friend if he or she was in this situation?
- What is the best possible outcome of this situation?
- What is the worst possible outcome of this situation?
- If (the worst outcome) were to happen, what could I do to minimize its impact?
- Given what I know so far, how likely is (the worst outcome) to happen?
- How do I benefit from keeping this belief?
- What negative consequences go along with keeping this belief?
- Is there anything else that could explain this situation?

Response Record. *From: Taylor, R.R. (2006). Cognitive behavioral therapy for chronic illness and disability. New York: Springer Science & Business Media with permission.*

Once a hot thought is identified, the therapist temporarily assumes it is true and queries the client as to its meaning using questions that identify intermediate beliefs (e.g., what a given thought, situation, or action means about their worldview, value system, or about the way the world works). This line of questioning coupled with the therapist's restating of the client's thoughts are used to identify the client's intermediate belief and then to probe for the core belief.

Once an intermediate or core belief is identified, a number of methods can be utilized to assist a client in modifying or restructuring that belief. Socratic questioning (a strategy of questioning that allows clients to see the illogic in their own thoughts) may allow some clients to talk themselves into a more adaptive belief. In other cases, different techniques are required; they include:

- Reframing the past, which involves guiding clients backward in time to think of personal examples that disconfirm the negative core belief
- Helping clients find more moderate ways of viewing their situation
- Imagining the extreme in order to recognize that one's circumstances are not as extreme as originally thought
- Finding positive examples that contradict negative thoughts

Each of these procedures involves specific strategies on the part of the therapist (Taylor, 2006). They are often undertaken in therapy and assigned as homework for clients to do outside the therapy time.

Behavioral Approaches in CBT

In addition to the cognitively oriented approaches to addressing maladaptive cognitions, there are some techniques that are more behavioral in nature. These include such techniques as systematic desensitization, meditation and relaxation techniques, and approaches that focus on activity modification. One of the more complex behavioral approaches is the behavioral experiment.

Behavioral experiments are activities that allow clients to test the validity of their beliefs directly (Taylor, 2006). They are most appropriate for use by individuals with unrealistic cognitions (e.g., systematic errors in thinking or excessive fears). Care must be taken in recommending behavioral experiments because they are the "ultimate test" of the validity of a client's thoughts (i.e., the therapist should be nearly 100% certain that the outcome of the experiment will be positive and disprove the client's faulty belief). Nonetheless, therapists should always inform their clients about the possibility that their engagement in an experiment might lead to a confirmation of their fears or concerns. Behavioral experiments are most appropriate for the client when other cognitive approaches are not working and when the client is open to the procedure. They are used with clients who tend to be avoidant or have difficulty coping with a situation (White, 2001).

The following is an example of a behavioral experiment. A client has avoided following through on a recommendation to increase walking time from 5 to 10 minutes twice daily. Her refusal is based on her belief that increasing her walking time would limit her energy to do other things she enjoys. The therapist recommends that she conduct an experiment by walking 10 minutes twice a day as recommended and keeping a log of her energy levels and participation in other activities during the rest of the day. In this instance, the therapist should be highly confident that the increased walking will not decrease the client's energy levels.

The Sequence of Cognitive Behavioral Therapy

CBT typically follows a very specific sequence (Taylor, 2006). First, clients are taught the relationships between situational triggers, automatic thoughts, and emotional, behavioral, and physiological reactions to their cognitions. The next stages of therapy involve creating homework assignments, behavioral experiments, and learning experiences according to the client's needs and abilities to participate in these activities. These activities teach clients to identify, monitor, and evaluate the validity of their automatic thoughts and they typically provide clients some relief from difficult emotions.

The later stages of therapy generally involve identifying and modifying the intermediate and core beliefs that underlie the automatic thoughts and predispose clients to engage in dysfunctional thinking across a variety of situations. The final stages of therapy generally focus on relapse prevention and on empowering clients to monitor and manage their own cognitions and behavior.

A number of cognitive behavioral techniques can be useful for maladaptive cognitions that do not involve cognitive distortion (i.e., preoccupations). Taylor (2006) developed a "reversal record," which is a thought record that emphasizes how to manage a painful or interfering cognition. Instead of focusing on challenging the cognition, the reversal record emphasizes recognition of its consequence and choosing a **reversal activity** (i.e., an activity that aims to reverse the mood, behavioral, or physiological consequence of the maladaptive thought). The reversal activity can consist of any one of the following categories of activities (Taylor, 2006):

- Coping mechanisms
- Self-care activities
- Pleasurable or gratifying activities
- Distraction exercises
- Motivating activities
- Goal-oriented activities

Since completion of the record is usually assigned as homework, it is part of the therapy session structure to check the homework and identify any difficulties the client has in following through on reversal activities.

Other approaches include (Taylor, 2006):

- Benefit-finding (i.e., finding examples of how a life event, such as an impairment, has been associated with positive changes or positive outcomes in one's life)
- Fast-forwarding (i.e., guiding a client to think about or picture him/herself at a future point in time that is fundamentally different from the present time)
- Positive imagery (i.e., brief or more involved meditation exercises such as imagining a difficult event and then imagining oneself coping effectively with that event)
- The responsibility jigsaw, which helps clients with anger, guilt, or shame to see that they are not responsible for all the consequences that emanate from their impairments
- Planning for the future, in which clients anticipate expected changes in their condition and plan for how to deal with those changes
- Treatment decision-making, in which clients facing difficult treatment decisions are helped to work though the decision-making process

- Problem-solving that focuses on dealing with practical issues that result from the disability
- Self-advocacy training that involves teaching and empowering clients to act in their own best interests when interacting with healthcare professionals, employers, friends, family, partners, and others
- Thought stopping that involves teaching a client to actively clear his or her mind of verbal messages or visual images that are negative or painful
- Distraction and meditation techniques for dealing with thoughts yielding painful emotions
- Coaching clients to observe and make lists of situations, people, and environments that are stress-reducing and stress-promoting and increasing or decreasing their interactions with those situations, people, or environments in the future
- Involving partners and family members in therapy

Research and Evidence Base

CBT is a widely researched approach. A growing number of research studies point to positive outcomes of cognitive behavioral approaches that involve reductions in symptom severity and improvements in self-efficacy, physical functioning, and quality of life (Antoni et al., 2001; Haddock et al, 2003; Lorig, Manzonson, & Holman, 1993).

Discussion

CBT is increasingly used in occupational therapy because errors in thinking and preoccupations are commonly experienced by clients facing impairments. These maladaptive cognitions often interfere with the therapy process and/or with the client's occupational adaptation. It should also be noted that cognitive distortions are often a part of a client's volition (a key concept of the model of human occupation discussed in Chapter 11). For instance, clients' personal causations may reflect inaccurate beliefs about their own capacities or may reflect realistic preoccupations with limitations of capacity. Further, clients' value systems may reflect distorted ideas about how it

is necessary to perform. Thus, CBT can be an important adjunctive tool when addressing problems of volition in clients that reflect maladaptive cognitions.

However, like all approaches, cognitive behavioral approaches in general do have limitations (Beck, 1996). These limitations may be more pronounced when considering chronic impairments that often involve complex circumstances. For example, many conditions that result in disability are inherently unstable. That is, they may be characterized by exacerbations and remissions, progressive decline, or recovery. In these instances, clients may have difficulty getting an accurate picture of their own abilities and limitations that do not reflect true cognitive distortions but are simply linked to their changing circumstances. In other instances, clients are facing newly acquired impairments and have not yet had adequate experiences to form an accurate picture. Thus, it is important not to label such clients' cognitions as maladaptive, but to carefully track the evolution of their thinking and coping over time and to support it through providing experiences that allow clients to discover their own circumstances.

Another caveat in using CBT is that the methods are inherently complex and require extensive training. Thus, before occupational therapists undertake CBT they should make sure that they are adequately educated in its concepts and methods. Further, not all clients will benefit from CBT. Clients who are good candidates for CBT are those with sufficient cognitive and emotional capacity to participate in the process (i.e., to reflect upon and evaluate their own thinking about their impairment). Thus, the occupational therapist should evaluate whether a client is a good candidate for CBT before undertaking it with the client.

Table 16.1 **Terms of the Model**

Automatic thought	An idea or image that goes through one's mind concerning immediate circumstances.
Behavioral experiment	An activity that allows a client to test the validity of his/her beliefs directly.
Core belief	The deepest level of beliefs; it organizes how people interpret and deal with incoming information.
Hot thought	A recurring automatic thought characterized by intense emotional experience.
Intermediate belief	An unarticulated attitude, rule, expectation, or assumption reflected in a person's thinking.
Reversal activity	An activity that aims to reverse the mood, behavioral, or physiological consequence of the maladaptive thought.
Situational trigger	An event or circumstance that evokes certain thoughts or emotions in a given client.
Thought record	A form that allows the client to identify and respond to automatic thoughts.

SUMMARY

✦ CBT is used to help clients reframe the way they think about themselves and their impairments and to change related behaviors

Theory

✦ Cognitive behavioral therapy is guided by the cognitive model, which proposes that dysfunctional thinking and unrealistic cognitive appraisals of life events can negatively influence feelings and behavior

✦ The cognitive model identifies three levels of cognition:
  • Core beliefs, which are the deepest level of beliefs; they organize how people interpret and deal with incoming information
  • Intermediate beliefs, which are unarticulated attitudes, rules, expectations, or assumptions reflected in a person's thinking
  • Automatic thoughts and images are the ideas or images that go through one's mind concerning immediate circumstances

▪ Hot thoughts are recurring automatic thoughts characterized by intense emotional experience and are considered the most important automatic thoughts to work with in psychotherapy

▪ Automatic thoughts typically occur in association with situational triggers, which are events or circumstances that evoke certain thoughts or emotions in a given client

✦ Maladaptive cognitions can be realistic or unrealistic

✦ What determines their adaptive status is how the cognitions affect a person's emotion and behavior

✦ There are two types of maladaptive cognitions:
  • Errors in thinking, which are cognitive distortions that reflect incorrect logic and/or that do not reflect reality

- Preoccupations, which are usually accompanied by difficult emotions, problematic behaviors, or aversive physiological reactions

Rationale for Intervention

+ CBT intervention generally includes three assumptions:
  - Cognition affects behavior
  - Cognition can be monitored and altered
  - Behavior change is mediated by cognitive change

+ CBT teaches clients to replace distorted thinking with more realistic and adaptive cognitions

+ During therapy, these distortions are typically identified by listening to the client's automatic thoughts and attempting to identify the specific type of error that that client seems to be making

Practice Resources

Assessment

+ Cognitive distortions and preoccupations are typically identified by interviewing clients and listening to them during therapy sessions

+ Careful attention to what clients say can help to identify the clients' automatic thoughts

+ Through interviewing the client and using objective knowledge about the client's condition and situation, cognitive distortions can be differentiated from preoccupations

+ It is important in assessment to distinguish between distorted thinking (inaccurate thoughts) and accurate thoughts that constitute preoccupations

+ Distorted thinking is best addressed through cognitive techniques that seek to correct the thinking pattern, whereas realistic preoccupations are often best addressed through coping skills, symptom and impairment management training, and problem-solving

+ It is also important to identify whether a client tends to have predominantly one or both thinking patterns (i.e., distortion and/or preoccupation)

Intervention

+ Cognitive restructuring techniques that correct distorted thinking require a comprehensive and multi-level approach to cognitive change

+ Maladaptive automatic thoughts are addressed by identifying them and teaching the client how to respond to them (typically through the use of thought records)

+ Intermediate and core beliefs are addressed by identifying them and teaching the client to modify them

+ A thought record is a form that allows the client to identify and respond to automatic thoughts

+ The thought record includes multiple targeted questions that allow clients to reflect upon and develop alternatives to their maladaptive thoughts

+ The process of changing intermediate thoughts and core beliefs is complex and requires thorough knowledge of the theory and methods of CBT

+ Intermediate and core beliefs can be brought to consciousness through a very specific sequence of questioning that allows the client to probe progressively deeper levels of consciousness

+ In addition to the cognitively oriented approaches to addressing maladaptive cognitions, there are some techniques that are more behavioral in nature

+ Behavioral techniques include systematic desensitization, meditation and relaxation techniques, approaches that focus on activity modification, and behavioral experiments

+ Behavioral experiments are activities that allow clients to test the validity of their beliefs

+ CBT typically follows a very specific sequence
  - First, clients are taught the relationships between situational triggers, automatic thoughts, and emotional, behavioral, and physiological reactions to their cognitions

- The next stages of therapy involve creating homework assignments, behavioral experiments, and learning experiences according to the client's needs and abilities to participate in these activities
- The later stages of therapy generally involve identifying and modifying the intermediate and core beliefs that underlie the automatic thoughts and predispose clients to engage in dysfunctional thinking across a variety of situations
- The final stages of therapy generally focus on relapse prevention and on empowering clients to monitor and manage their own cognitions and behavior

✦ A number of cognitive behavioral techniques can be useful for maladaptive cognitions that do not involve cognitive distortion (i.e., preoccupations)

✦ One example is a "reversal record," which is a thought record that emphasizes how to manage a painful or interfering cognition

REFERENCES

Antoni, M.H., Lehman, J.M., Kilbourn, K.M., Boyers, A.E., Culver, J.L., Alferi, S.M., et al. (2001). Cognitive-behavioral stress management intervention decreases the prevalence of depression and enhances benefit finding among women under treatment for early-stage breast cancer. *Health Psychology, 20*(1), 20–32.

Beck, A.T. (1991). Cognitive therapy as the integrative therapy. *Journal of Psychotherapy Integration, 1*(3), 191–198.

Beck, A.T. (1996). Beyond belief: A theory of modes, personality, and psychopathology. In P. Salkovskis (Ed.), *Frontiers of cognitive therapy* (pp. 1–25). New York: Guilford Press.

Beck, A.T. (1999). *Prisoners of hate: The cognitive basis of anger, hostility, and violence.* New York: HarperCollins.

Beck, A.T., Rush, A.J., Shaw, B.F., & Emery, G. (1979). *Cognitive therapy of depression.* New York: Guilford Press.

Beck, J. (1995). *Cognitive therapy: Basics and beyond.* New York: Guilford Press.

Burns, D.D. (1980). *Feeling good: The new mood therapy.* New York: Signet.

Dobson, K.S., & Dozois, D.J.A. (2001). Historical and philosophical bases of the cognitive-behavioral therapies. In K.S. Dobson (Ed.), *Handbook of cognitive-behavioral therapies* (2nd ed., pp. 3–39). New York: Guilford Press.

Greenberger, D., & Padesky, C. (1995). *Mind over mood: A cognitive therapy treatment manual for clients.* New York: Guilford Press.

Haddock, G., Barrowclough, C., Tarrier, N., Moring, J., O'Brien, R., Schofield, N., et al. (2003). Cognitive-behavioural therapy and motivational intervention for schizophrenia and substance misuse: 18-month outcomes of a randomised controlled trial. *British Journal of Psychiatry, 183*, 418–426.

Lorig, K., Mazonson, P.D., & Holman, H.R. (1993). Evidence suggesting that health education for self-management in patients with chronic arthritis has sustained health benefits while reducing health care costs. *Arthritis and Rheumatism, 36*, 439–446.

Taylor, R.R. (2006). *Cognitive behavioral therapy for chronic illness and disability.* New York: Springer Science & Business Media.

White, C.A. (2001). *Cognitive behavior therapy for chronic medical problems: A guide to assessment and treatment in practice.* Chichester, England: John Wiley & Sons.

CHAPTER 17

Disability Studies

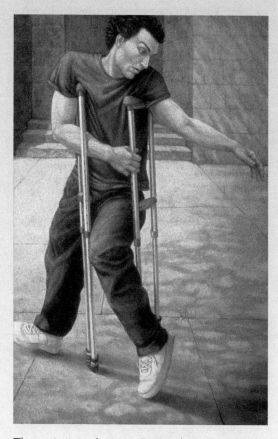

The painting above is Riva Lehrer's portrait of William Shannon, alias "Crutchmaster," an accomplished dancer, choreographer, and video artist. Shannon's choreography is based on his body and its movements, as affected by severe osteoarthritis and Legg-Perthes disease. Visual and performing artists like Lehrer and Shannon strive to challenge non-disabled notions of beauty and contest stereotypical notions of disability. Their work is part of disability studies, a diverse body of scholarly, reflective work that seeks to reframe our understanding of disability and how to respond to it.

Disability studies addresses the issue of disability from a unique perspective. The field emerged in the 1970s and 1980s as a counterpoint to the then-dominant view of disability (Scotch, 2001). The prevailing view of disability, which disability studies contravenes, can be summarized in three broad, interrelated themes.

First, disability was conceptualized by the medical model and related health professions as an abnormality or deficit requiring professional management (Linton, 1998; Nagi, 1991; Scotch, 2001; Zola, 1972). This framework considered disability synonymous with personal impairment, and its solution was to fix the disabled person* (Nagi, 1991; Rioux, 1997). The second viewpoint defining disability was an economic model. Disability was conceptualized in terms of disabled persons' inability to be self-sufficient and productive, thereby requiring economic and social support (Hahn, 1985; Oliver, 1990; Rioux, 1997). The third concept, a societal perspective, cast impairment as inherently negative, rendering disabled persons in a variety of images, from the malevolent deviant to the victim of a personal tragedy (Asch & Fine, 1988; Gill, 2001; Snyder, Brueggeman, & Garland-Thompson, 2002; Zola, 1972).

> As disability studies has evolved, it has also retold the story of disability, challenging the standing assumptions not only about the causes but also about the very nature of disability.

The medical and economic perspectives reflected and reinforced dominant cultural views that cast disability in negative terms. Furthermore, these professional and societal conceptualizations of disability have translated into public policies that have defined and shaped disabled persons' lives (Hahn, 1997; Scotch, 2001).

Disability studies has sought to challenge and correct these views of disability. Perhaps the most critical goal has been to identify the causes of disability as environmental barriers rather than

impairments and to relocate disability from residing in the individual to inhering in societal attitudes and actions. As disability studies has evolved, it has also retold the story of disability, challenging the standing assumptions not only about the causes but also about the very nature of disability. Finally, disability studies has sought to transform disability from an "individual or medical problem into a civil rights issue" (Paterson & Hughes, 2000, p. 30).

Theory

Disability studies has attracted scholars from a range of disciplines. Many of the themes represented in the field were first articulated in the social sciences. Disability studies draws on political and economic concepts as well as gender and race studies in its articulation of how disabled persons are oppressed. It builds on concepts from the humanities in the examination of various ways disability is represented in popular culture, literature, and art. Especially important to disability studies is **social constructivism,** the argument that both everyday and specialized (e.g., scientific) ways of knowing are not absolute and, instead, reflect historical, ideological, and cultural forces and biases (Jeffreys, 2002). This postmodern perspective has been used as a platform from which to critique and deconstruct predominant cultural and professional conceptions of disability.

Deconstructing and Reconstructing Conceptions of Disability

Disability studies is fundamentally different from the other typical bodies of knowledge occupational therapists encounter. Because its aim has been to critique and deconstruct the extant notion of disability, it has:

- Illuminated biases and fallacies in standing societal and professional conceptions and approaches to addressing disability

---

*The matter of language is an important theme in disability studies. In considering how best to refer to persons who have impairments that result in disability this chapter was guided by the many scholars today who prefer the term "disabled person."

• Offered alternative conceptions and action implications of disability

Thus, it has sought to achieve a number of fundamental shifts in thinking about and taking action with reference to disability.

The following sections describe in detail the three traditional, dominant conceptions of disability. Moreover, this chapter examines how disability studies scholars have critiqued these perspectives and presented alternative conceptualizations of disability.

Disability as a Medical Problem Rooted in Impairment

The medical model perspective developed by rehabilitation professionals generated the view that disability was rooted in the disabled person's physical, emotional, sensory, or cognitive impairments that, in turn, were the consequence of some disease process or trauma (Longmore, 1995a; Longmore, 1995b; Wendell, 1996; Zola, 1993a). This approach firmly located disability in the person (Linton, 1998; Nagi, 1991; Rioux, 1997; Scotch, 2001). This perspective was reinforced by efforts to describe and measure the disabled person's impairments and document their relationship to limitations in activities of daily living and work (Rioux, 1997; Zola, 1993a).

Because of its grounding in the medical model, rehabilitation's impairment approach to disability views the impairment and its underlying causes as problems (i.e., negative states to be removed or reduced). Rehabilitation emerged as an effort to prevent, minimize, and, to the extent possible, reduce the consequences of impairment (Zola, 1993a). The unquestioned assumption of rehabilitation has been that disability (defined as deviation from normative physical and psychological structures and processes) is undesirable to both the disabled person and to society at large. This perspective rationalized efforts to prevent and reduce impairment (and, if not the impairment itself, then its public appearance) (Linton, 1998; Nagi, 1991; Scotch, 2001; Zola, 1972). The emphasis of rehabilitation has been to transform the disabled person toward a state that most approximates "normal" function and appearance.

The Impairment Model as a Tool of Social Control

The positive impact of many rehabilitation services notwithstanding, disability scholars have pointed out that rehabilitation also has important downsides for disabled people. These include three interrelated elements. First, rehabilitation practices reinforce the idea that the disability is the disabled person's problem (to the relative omission of considerations of how environmental factors, especially the social environment, contribute to disability*) (Linton, 1998; Nagi, 1991; Scotch, 2001; Zola, 1972). Consequently, they "cannot account for, let alone combat … bias and discrimination" (Longmore, 1995b, p. 6).

Second, the rehabilitation professional is seen as the expert on the disabled person's condition, the implication being that the essence or meaning of disability is to be located in professional classifications and explanations of disability. Moreover, the disabled person is expected to be the compliant recipient of care (Zola, 1972). Together these elements tend to take away the "voice" of the disabled person.

Third, rehabilitation efforts enforce a version of normalcy that pressures disabled persons to fit in by appearing and functioning as much like non-disabled persons as possible (Jeffreys, 2002; Scott, 1969; Zola, 1972). A consequence of these three elements is that the rehabilitation becomes a form of **social control.** That is, rehabilitation aims to eliminate client characteristics that threaten the legitimacy of mainstream norms.

In a classic study, Scott (1969) documented how the rehabilitation of blind persons, contrary to aims of enabling them to be more functional, systematically socialized them into becoming compliant and dependent. The first stage in this process involves an invalidation of the disabled persons' understanding of their own disability.

---

*Most current concepts of disability in rehabilitation include consideration of how the environment contributes, along with impairment, to creating disability. To the extent that the current paradigm of rehabilitation does admit of the environmental dimension of disability, it has been influenced by disability scholars. Another feature that differentiates the current incorporation of environmental factors in the understanding of disability is the much stronger (if not exclusive) emphasis that disability studies puts on environmental factors (especially social, political, and economic aspects of the environment).

For instance, Scott (1969) notes that the blind person is

> *rewarded for showing insight and subtly reprimanded for continuing to adhere to earlier notions about his problems. He is led to think that he 'really' understands past and present experiences when he couches them in terms acceptable to his therapist. (p. 79)*

In this way, the disabled person's understanding of his own disability is invalidated and replaced with an official, professional definition. The blind person is persuaded to learn ways of behaving that follow the professional conception of the problem of blindness, however much the conceptions may contradict personal experience.

Another example of how rehabilitation efforts can impose definitions and solutions to problems to the detriment of the disabled persons' self-sufficiency is illustrated in Jeffreys' (2002) description of his brother, Jim, who did not have legs because of a congenital condition. He recalls Jim "swaying precariously in his custom-fitted bucket atop his latest pair of DuPont artificial legs, all their straps and plastics cloaked in slacks, the idea being to make him look as standardized as possible, even though the contraption imprisoned him" (p. 36).

Contrast Jim's fate with McBryde Johnson's (2003) description of what happened when her muscle-wasting disease left her too weak to hold up her spine: "At 15, I threw away the back brace and let my spine reshape itself into a deep twisty s-curve. . . . Since my backbone found its own natural shape, I've been entirely comfortable in my own skin" (p. 51). The irony is that while her strategy resulted in a more comfortable physical existence, it clearly violated what would be considered medical good sense, as surgery and braces would have given her a more "normal" appearance and function.

McBryde Johnson's rejection of such medical advice and Jim's subsequent discarding of his prosthetic limbs not only violate what is considered appropriate medical counsel but also evoke negative social reactions. The dilemma they face is faced by many disabled people. They must either choose an uncomfortable mode of embodiment not suited to their actual physical selves or face the discomfort of others who cannot abide their disruption of physical

norms (as defined medically and socially). To the extent that rehabilitation efforts shepherd disabled people toward conformity with social norms, they reinforce the dilemma (Jeffreys, 2002; Linton, 1998; Zola, 1972).

Disability as an Economic Problem

The perceived economic consequences of disability (i.e., the required resources for persons who could not care for themselves or work) (Albrecht & Verbrugge, 2000) have always been a matter of public and political concern. Although nations have addressed disability differently, depending on their social philosophies (Albrecht & Bury, 2001), the development of welfare policies globally has underscored the perception that disabled persons are essentially a negative factor in the economic marketplace (Longmore & Goldberger, 2000).

The development of rehabilitation services designed to reduce dependence on services and enhance entry into the workforce has been shaped by concern to reduce the perceived burden of disabled persons on a modern society (Albrecht, 1992; Albrecht & Bury, 2001; Albrecht & Verbrugge, 2000). The rehabilitation idea of independence carries a subtext that dependence is an undesirable human state that both reduces the dignity of the individual and, importantly, creates a burden for others. Concern with the economic costs of disability is highlighted in the creation of disability as an administrative category (Stone, 1984). Indeed, a complex bureaucracy exists in most countries to determine who is properly classified as disabled and therefore deserving of disability services and public support.

Rehabilitation efforts to document functional limitations and their relationship to self-care and work reinforce the image of the disabled person as productively incapable. Finally, rehabilitation oppresses disabled people when the problem is identified as being located in the client rather than in the environment. For example, Abberley (1995) documented that occupational therapists consistently attributed failures in therapy to client problems such as a lack of motivation rather than to economic problems such as lack of resources or opportunities. Conversely, they attributed successes to their expertise rather than to client efforts.

Disability studies scholars have sought to turn the prevailing economic perspective on its head. They argue that, instead of disabled persons being a drain on public resources, they have been the victims of **social oppression**. This oppression, rather then personal impairments or traits, has made them unnecessarily dependent and barred them from access to the marketplace and other forms of civil participation.

Reformulating Disability as Oppression

One of the most powerful assertions to come from disability studies is that "people with disabilities are oppressed" (Charlton, 1998, p. 5). By this it is meant that disabled people are treated by society in ways that diminish their social, personal, physical, and financial well-being and are cast as members of a socially disadvantaged minority group (Charlton, 1998). Supporting the argument that disabled people represent an oppressed minority group are data illustrating that these people fare much worse than non-disabled persons in housing, education, transportation, and

> **Disabled people are treated by society in ways that diminish their social, personal, physical, and financial well-being and are cast as members of a socially disadvantaged minority group.**

National activists participate in the Garrett Rally, held in October 2000, to demonstrate support to uphold the American with Disabilities Act (ADA) in the Supreme Court case Garrett vs. University of Alabama. Frustrating to disability rights advocates, the court ruled that Congress did not have the authority when it passed this act to allow individuals to sue states for employment discrimination. To the detriment of the disability community, the decision grants states immunity from damages as a result of lawsuits brought by their employees against states under the ADA. *Photo courtesy of Sharon Snyder and Suburban Access Squad.*

employment (Louis Harris & Associates, 1998; McNeil, 1997). Disabled people consistently report that discrimination and attitudinal barriers negatively affect their self-sufficiency and participation in society (Charlton, 1998; Hahn, 1985; Oliver, 1996).

Using a Marxist analysis, Finkelstein (1980) and Oliver (1990) argue that disability was identified as a problem for medical management because of the demand of capitalist economies for unimpaired labor. Finkelstein's historical analysis proposes that disability emerged with the transformation from a feudal to a capitalist society. Prior to this transition, persons with impairments worked at the lower end of the socioeconomic spectrum. With the advent of modern industrial economies, they were deemed unfit for the marketplace, barred from employment, and relegated to being problems for medical management, which often meant segregation in institutions. Oliver's analysis compares societies, arguing that the view of disability as an individual medical problem is not universal. Rather, it is a feature of societies that emphasize individualism and capitalist production.

Longmore and Goldberger (2000) argue that by casting disability as a matter of pathology, the medical perspective "individualized and privatized disability" (p. 2). This paved the way for what Albrecht and Bury (2001) refer to as the commoditization of disability goods and services. This is not without consequence. For example, economic incentives can lead rehabilitation providers to socialize clients toward some amount of ongoing dependence on their services (Scott, 1969).

Charitable organizations for persons with disabilities have also been the object of critique from disability scholars. Two points are made. First, a large number of able-bodied people work within such charities that operate as big business and inevitably generate motives of personal gain. As such, these organizations can be seen as exploiting the disabled population. Second, and more important, charitable organizations reinforce the idea that support for disabled persons is "not a social responsibility to be fulfilled by governments, but an act of kindness" (Wendell, 1996, p. 53). Public disability policies that, in effect, restrict persons from attaining self-sufficiency (e.g., encourage nursing home placement over community living and discourage entry into the labor market) have also been the target of criticism (Longmore, 1995b; Oliver, 1990; Shapiro, 1993).

In sum, disability studies scholars contradict the longstanding view that disabled persons are merely an economic drain on society because of their limitations in self-sufficiency. Rather, they argue, society economically disadvantages disabled persons. This occurs when disabled persons are barred from the marketplace, are transformed into targets of a disability industry that profits from products and services that are largely imposed, and are prevented by policies from living more self-sufficient lives.

Social Constructions of Disability

According to Longmore and Goldberger (2000), disabled persons historically have been cast as:

> Victims and villains in popular culture, dependent sentimentalized children in charity fund raising, mendicants who should be allowed to beg, "unsightly disgusting objects" who should be banned from public places, potentially dependent or dangerous denizens of society, worthy subjects of poor relief but unworthy citizens of the nation. (p. 5)

The misunderstanding and misconstruction of disability by society have led scholars to examine how popular cultural conceptions of disability are generated and perpetuated in art, literature, and film. For instance, Mitchell (2002) points out that although story lines freely employ the anomaly of disability as literary devices that embody and underscore other personal aberrations and social ills, they rarely address disability as either a source of personal knowledge or as a social or political injustice. Poignant recent examples are the use of physical disfigurement and mobility limitation as a metaphor for malevolence in the books and subsequent films, *Hannibal* (Lustig & Scott, 2001) and *The Red Dragon* (Davis & Ratner, 2002). The image of disability as negative and undesirable is reinforced by the pairing of the disability trait with personal or social ills.

The humanities approach to disability points out that disability is a multifaceted experience that has always been a part of the human condition. It seeks to counter the assumption that eliminating or reducing disability is necessary or even desirable. Rather, it argues for recognition of disability as a phenomenon integral to the fact that humans have bodies. Bodies are inherently vulnerable; they age and almost invariably experience some kind of impairment. Thus, rather then being an aberration, disability is part of the human condition.

Goffman's (1963) concept of **stigma** is the foundation for many elements of current arguments about societal reactions to disability. His basic argument, derived primarily from the study of persons with mental illness, is that disabled persons, by virtue of their physical or behavioral aberrations, breach cultural norms. As a result, they are assigned a spoiled identity (as bad, undesirable, dangerous, or weak) and subjected to pressure and/or efforts of others (often in the guise of medical or rehabilitation services) to minimize their deviation from norms. These social reactions serve not only to coerce disabled persons toward fitting in but also to highlight and reaffirm the very social norms that have been breached. As Davis (2000) argues, disabled persons are singled out as part of a process in which individuals without impairments can be reassured they fit within a norm.

As a consequence of the stigmatizing process, Gill (2001) argues that disabled people grapple with mistaken identity, repeatedly encountering and struggling to overcome others' misconceptions of what it means to be disabled. She concludes, "A core element of the experience of disability is being seen as something you are not, joined with the realization that what you are remains invisible" (Gill, 2001, p. 365). Exemplifying this argument, French (1993) notes:

> Disbelief remains a common response of able-bodied people when we attempt to convey the reality of our disabilities...when I try to convey the feelings of isolation associated with not recognizing people or not knowing what is going on around me, the usual response is "you will in time" or "it took me ages too." This type of response renders disabled people "just like everyone else"...knowing how different we really are is problematic and it is easy to become confused

and to have our confidence undermined when others insist we are just the same. (p. 74)

Not surprisingly, then, negative stereotypes about disability are often internalized by the disabled individual (Fine & Asch, 1988; Gill, 1997). According to disability studies scholar Harlan Hahn (1985), one of the most pressing problems facing the political struggle of people with disabilities is developing a positive identity. An important distinction that disability scholars make is that this identity development is not an individual, but rather a social, cultural, and political process (Longmore, 1995a; Longmore, 1995b). That is, the fundamental change that needs to take place is a transformation in societal values that devalue and stigmatize disabled people in the first place. As Zola (1993a) notes, disabled persons must free themselves "from the negative loading of the concept of disability" (p. 27).

Summary

The various ways in which disability studies scholars have critiqued the traditional social and

professional perspectives on disability can be summarized in the idea that disability is socially constructed. Wendell (1996) explains that the social construction of disability includes a range of social conditions from those "that straightforwardly create illnesses, injuries, and poor physical functioning to subtle cultural factors that determine standards of normality and exclude those who do not meet them from full participation in their societies" (p. 36). Taken together, the various arguments of disability studies have transformed the understanding of disability from being the inevitable and tragic consequence of impairment to being a neutral human difference. Disability is transformed into a negative condition by social definitions, attitudes, practices, and policies that devalue, exclude, and disenfranchise persons with disabilities.

Action Implications

As noted earlier, disability studies comprises a unique body of knowledge unlike others encountered in medicine and rehabilitation. One of the

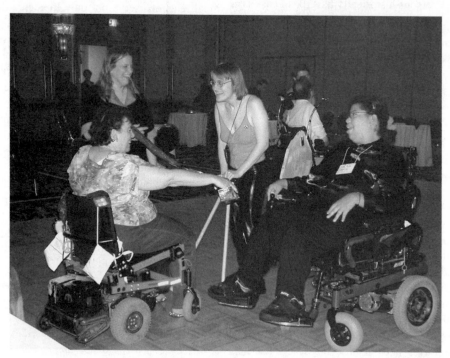

Attendees of the 2003, 16th Annual Meeting of the Society for Disability Studies, share in fellowship at the annual SDS dance. The theme "Disability and Dissent: Public Cultures, Public Spaces" explored the role of disability, dissent, and the creation of new public spaces (e.g., architectural, attitudinal, representational, and empirical) in the 21st century. *Photo courtesy of Sharon Snyder, 2003 SDS program co-director.*

features that distinguishes these studies is the emphasis on actions that are directed not at fixing the disabled person, but rather on:

- Empowering persons with disabilities to engage in self-advocacy and combat discrimination
- Transforming social conditions that create barriers and oppression (including cultural beliefs and attitudes and public policies) (Charlton, 1998; Scotch, 2001)

Longmore (1995b) characterizes these as two phases:

> The first phase sought to move disabled people from the margins of society to the mainstream by demanding that discrimination be outlawed and that access and accommodations be mandated....the second phase has asserted the necessity for self-definition...[and] repudiated nondisabled majority norms. (p. 8)

Empowerment and Civil Rights Advocacy

Charlton (1998) adopted the phrase "Nothing about us without us" as a way of urging "people with disabilities to recognize their need to control and take responsibility for their own lives and urging political-economic and cultural systems to incorporate people with disabilities into the decision-making process" (p. 17). Political activism aimed at achieving social justice and civil rights is naturally associated with the argument that disabled persons are socially oppressed (Baylies, 2002; Charlton, 1998). Activism takes on many forms, such as the kind of political advocacy in the United States that resulted in the Americans with Disabilities Act of 1990, which established civil rights for disabled persons. On the other end of the spectrum are efforts to combat movements such as eugenics and euthanasia that imply disabled persons are a negative to be avoided and that disabled persons' lives are not worth saving or maintaining. One example is Not Dead Yet, a national organization that "opposes legalized assisted suicide along with

disability-based killing" (McBryde Johnson, 2003, p. 53).

Disability Identity, Culture, and Pride

Disability studies identifies the development of a positive identity among persons with disabilities as a key step in reversing the social construction of disability (Gill, 1997; Hahn, 1985; Zola, 1993a; Zola, 1993b). The conceptual shift in understanding disability has naturally led to changes in how disabled persons see themselves (e.g., as persons who are different but not less valuable than non-disabled persons and as members of a minority group that faces oppression). It is resulting in changes in values. For instance, Longmore (1995b) identifies the following transformation in values: "not self-sufficiency but self-determination, not independence but interdependence, not functional separateness but personal connection, not physical autonomy but human community" (p. 9). Disabled persons are increasingly identifying themselves as members of a minority group and identifying with a disability community (Longmore, 1995a; Longmore, 1995b; Phillips, 1990). One example of how disability is being redefined is the identification of deafness and consequent use of sign not as a handicap but as a language and culture (Shapiro, 1993).

> **Disabled persons are increasingly identifying themselves as members of a minority group and identifying with a disability community.**

Transforming Social Perceptions

Disability studies also seeks to achieve transformations in intellectual and population conceptions of disability. Efforts to transform perceptions of the causes and nature of disability are wide-ranging in nature. By illuminating the hidden assumptions, biases, and practices that constitute disability, scholars are aiming to change attitudes among scholars, disciplines, professions, systems, and society at large.

A major contribution of disability studies comprises phenomenological accounts of disability experience. As Jeffreys (2002) notes, such accounts give voice to disability as an "authentic experience through the privileging of first-person narratives" (p. 33). Moreover, as Davis (2002) argues, such accounts underscore the variety of human experience rather than enforcing ideals of normality.

Many of these works are autobiographical texts in which disabled persons documented their own experiences. Examples are Zola's (1982) chronicle of coming to accept his disability during a sojourn in a Dutch community for disabled persons, Williams' (1992) description of how her experiences as a child with autism placed her in a extraordinary world, Jamison's (1995) portrayal of her roller-coaster existence with manic-depressive illness, and Price's (1994) conclusion that his illness and paralysis resulted in a new and better life.

Disabled writers have asserted that living with a disability is consistent with living a fulfilling and joyful life. As Vash (1981) notes, disability can be "a positive contributor to life in its totality—a catalyst to psychological growth" (p. 124). However, as Deegan (1991) notes, it has little to do with living a life that is normative or dictated by one particular set of values.

Research and Evidence Base

Because disability studies has incorporated concepts and methods from the humanities, different forms of scholarship (e.g., literary and art criticism) make up part of the process of inquiry and critical analysis of data. Thus, scholarship has included historical analyses such as those by Finkelstein (1980) and Longmore (1995b); philosophical works such as the one by Toombs (1992); phenomenological inquiry; and critical analysis such as the Mitchell (2002) and Snyder et al. (2002) discussions of literature, art, and film.

Disability studies also includes the traditional empirical traditions of the social sciences. Qualitative research in the field focuses on the "lived experience" of disability, and quantitative research is used to point toward the condition of disability. The former includes studies that range from the various ethnographic studies of disabled persons' experiences to autobiographical works. Quantitative studies are much less visible, but they do document the conditions and perceptions of disabled people and are part of the lexicon of the literature.

Participatory action research, which involves disabled persons as co-investigators, is an important and growing area of research (Balcazar, Keys, Kaplan, & Suarez-Balcazar, 1998). This approach has been fueled by the argument that disabled persons' voices are absent from much research; thus the research does not represent and, in fact, actively ignores disabled persons' experiences, perspectives, and knowledge (Kitchin, 2000; Oliver, 1992). Participatory action research seeks to respond to Oliver's call for research that is both emancipatory (i.e., seeking to change social structures) and empowering (i.e., allowing individuals to be transformed through participating in the research process).

Discussion

Because it is a new discipline, disability studies is still being defined. Disability studies today consists of a collection of scholarly approaches that participate in examining how disability comes into existence, what forces create it, how it affects people, and what it reveals about the human condition. Disability studies consists of a rapidly growing body of scholarship that has reformulated our understanding of disability.

The field is not without its own controversies. For example, Crow (1996) criticizes disability studies for having focused too exclusively on the environmental causes of disability. She differentiates the situation of disability from that of other oppressed groups based on gender, sexual orientation, or race. The latter groups are based on neutral differences, whereas impairment does produce suffering and difficulty. Crow notes that many disabled persons struggle with impairment even when disabling barriers are eradicated. She recommends reinstating impairment into the study of disability and considering it at three levels:

* The objective restriction or limitation of function
* The personal experience and interpretation of the limitation
* The societal context, which can misrepresent, exclude, and discriminate

Others, such as Wendell (1996) and Jeffreys (2002), have also argued for the importance of inserting the nature and experience of impairment into disability studies discourse. Hence, whereas impairment was understandably de-emphasized both as a counterpoint to medicine and rehabilitation's focus on impairment and society's tendency to translate impairment into tragedy, there is now a growing movement to rethink the place of impairment as a topic and concept in disability studies.

Another criticism of disability studies is that it does not represent the experience and perspectives of many disabled persons. Devlieger and Albrecht (2000) note that disability scholars are largely middle-class, white, well-educated, and empowered. They argue that the ways in which these persons construe disability may well be at variance with the disability experience and perspectives of persons who do not share these demographics. Indeed, one of the important realities is that many persons with disabilities (especially in the early states of an acquired disability) may hold attitudes much more aligned with the medical model or rehabilitation conceptions (i.e., they want their impairment minimized as much as possible).

These and other controversies and criticisms notwithstanding, disability studies represents a vibrant, emerging area of scholarship that will continue to transform thinking and action. Occupational therapists will need to consider seriously the critiques of rehabilitation in general, and of occupational therapy in particular, that are found in this literature.

For example, personal chronicles of disability experience sometimes include negative encounters with occupational therapy. For example, Callahan (1990), in discussing his rehabilitation experience following a spinal cord injury, recalls occupational therapy, noting: "I remember having my hands harnessed for long periods of time to a rolling-pin–like apparatus that sanded a piece of wood" (p. 74). He then notes, with appropriate sarcasm: "A bright future as a finish sander stretched before me if I played my cards right" (p. 74).

The anthropologist Murphy (1990) recalls about his experience of occupational therapy:

> I thought some of the exercises ridiculous. Nonetheless, visitors to our house still scrape their feet on the doormat that I made in O.T. [My wife] is the only person who knows its origins, a sign of the care I have taken to keep secret the indignities visited upon me…(pp. 54–55)

In contrast, Robert McCrum (1998), in his account of rehabilitation and recovery from a cerebrovascular accident, recalls:

> The part of convalescence that I found most profoundly humiliating and depressing was occupational therapy… I was reduced to playing with brightly colored plastic letters of the alphabet, like a three-year-old, and passing absurdly simple recognition tests. Sitting in my wheelchair with my day-glo letter-blocks I could not escape reflecting on the irony of the situation. (p. 139)

These and other descriptions in the literature reinforce the earlier argument that disabled persons' voices and knowledge are routinely ignored in rehabilitation.

There certainly have been efforts in occupational therapy to correct many of the failures of rehabilitation noted earlier in this chapter. For example, occupational therapists have attempted to recognize and address barriers in the environment that affect persons with disabilities. However, the focus tends to be on physical barriers or social factors in the immediate environment (e.g., family, school, workplace). Therapists have not generally been involved in helping to remove broader social barriers (i.e., political and economic). These issues play out in practice and could be addressed through occupational therapists engaging in advocacy and empowerment of clients.

Disability studies systematically criticizes and seeks to replace the dominant paradigm of disability. As such, this body of knowledge has laid down important challenges to occupational therapy practice. It calls for occupational therapists to go beyond incremental changes in practice and, instead, to radically alter perceptions of, and practices with, disabled persons.

Table 17.1 **Terms of the Model**	
Social constructivism	The argument that both everyday and specialized (e.g., scientific) ways of knowing are not absolute and, instead, reflect historical, ideological, and cultural forces and biases.
Social control	Efforts to eliminate individual characteristics that threaten the legitimacy of mainstream norms.
Social oppression	The treatment of disabled people by society in ways that diminish their social, personal, physical, and financial well-being and that casts them as members of a socially disadvantaged minority group.
Stigma	The assignment of a spoiled identity (e.g., bad, undesirable, dangerous, or weak) on the basis of a physical or mental deviation from what is considered normal.

SUMMARY

+ Disability studies has sought to challenge and correct dominant views of disability

+ It challenges standing assumptions about the causes and the very nature of disability

Interdisciplinary Base

+ Disability studies draws on concepts from a range of disciplines:
  • Social sciences
  • Politics and economics
  • Gender and race studies
  • Humanities

Deconstructing and Reconstructing Conceptions of Disability

+ Disability studies has:
  • Illuminated biases and fallacies in societal and professional conceptions and approaches to addressing disability
  • Offered alternative conceptions and action implications of disability

Disability as a Medical Problem Rooted in Impairment

+ The medical model perspective developed by rehabilitation professionals generated a concept of disability as rooted in the disabled person's physical, emotional, sensory, or cognitive impairments

+ Disability scholars have pointed out that rehabilitation perspectives:
  • Reinforce the idea that disability is the disabled person's problem
  • Cast the professional as expert on the disabled person's condition
  • Enforce a version of normalcy that pressures disabled persons to fit in by appearing and functioning as much like non-disabled persons as possible

The Impairment Model as a Tool of Social Control

+ The positive impact of many rehabilitation services notwithstanding, rehabilitation also has important downsides for disabled people

+ First, rehabilitation practices reinforce the idea that the disability is the disabled person's problem

+ Second, the rehabilitation professional is seen as the expert on the disabled person's condition, the implication being that the essence or meaning of disability is to be located in professional classifications and explanations of disability

+ Third, rehabilitation efforts enforce a version of normalcy that pressures disabled persons to fit in by appearing and functioning as much like non-disabled persons as possible

+ A consequence of these three elements is that the rehabilitation becomes a form of social control

Disability as an Economic Problem

+ The development of welfare policies globally has underscored the perception that disabled persons are essentially a negative factor in the economic marketplace

+ The development of rehabilitation services designed to reduce dependence on services and enhance entry into the workforce has been shaped by concern to reduce the perceived burden of disabled persons in a modern society

Reformulating Disability as Oppression

+ Disability studies scholars contradict the longstanding view that disabled persons are merely an economic drain on society because of their limitations in self-sufficiency

+ Disabled persons are barred from the marketplace, transformed into targets of a disability industry that profits on products and services that are largely imposed on them, and prevented by policies from living more self-sufficient lives

Social Constructions of Disability

+ Disabled persons historically have been misunderstood and misconstrued

+ The humanities approach to disability:
  • Points out that disability is a multifaceted human experience that has always been a part of the human condition
  • Counters the assumption that amelioration of disability is necessary or even desirable
  • Recognizes disability as a phenomenon integral to the fact that humans have bodies that are vulnerable and that age and almost invariably experience some kind of impairment

+ As a consequence of stigma:
  • Disabled people grapple with mistaken identity, repeatedly encountering and struggling to overcome others' misconceptions of what it means to be disabled
  • Negative stereotypes about disability are often internalized by the disabled individual

Action Implications

+ Disability studies emphasizes:
  • Empowering persons with disabilities to engage in self-advocacy and combat discrimination
  • Transforming social conditions that create barriers and oppression (including cultural beliefs and attitudes and public policies)

REFERENCES

Abberley, P. (1995). Disabling ideology in health and welfare: The case of occupational therapy. *Disability and Society, 10,* 221–232.

Albrecht, G.L. (1992). *The disability business: Rehabilitation in America.* Newbury Park, CA: Sage.

Albrecht, G.L., & Bury, M. (2001). The political economy of the disability marketplace. In G.L. Albrecht, K. Seelman, & M. Bury (Eds.), *Handbook of disability studies* (pp. 585–609). Thousand Oaks, CA: Sage.

Albrecht, G.L., & Verbrugge, L.M. (2000). The global emergence of disability. In G.L. Albrecht, R. Fitzpatrick, & S.C. Scrimshaw (Eds.), *Handbook of social studies in health and medicine* (pp. 293–307). London: Sage.

Americans with Disabilities Act of 1990. Pub. L. No. 101–336, 1991.

Asch, A., & Fine, M. (1988). Disability beyond stigma: Social interaction, discrimination and activism. *Journal of Social Issues, 44*(1), 3–22.

Balcazar, F.E., Keys, C.B., Kaplan, D.L., & Suarez-Balcazar, Y. (1998). Participatory action research and people with disabilities: Principles and challenges. *Canadian Journal of Rehabilitation, 12*(2), 105–112.

Baylies, C. (2002). Disability and the notion of human development: Questions of rights and capabilities. *Disability and Society, 17*(7) 725–739.

Callahan, J. (1990). *Don't worry, he won't get far on foot.* New York: Vintage Books.

Charlton, J. (1998). *Nothing about us without us.* Berkeley, CA: University of California Press.

Crow, L. (1996). Renewing the social model of disability. In C. Barnes & G. Mercer (Eds.), *Exploring the divide: Illness and disability* (pp. 55–72). Leeds, UK: The Disability Press.

Davis, A. (Executive Producer), & Ratner, B. (Director). (2002). *The red dragon* [Motion picture]. United States: Universal.

Davis, L. (2002). Bodies of difference. In S.L. Snyder, B.J. Brueggemann, & R. Garland-Thompson (Eds.), *Disability studies: Enabling the humanities* (pp. 100–106). New York: The Modern Language Association of America.

Deegan, P.E. (1991). Recovery: The lived experience of rehabilitation. In R.P. Marinelli & A.E. Dell Orto (Eds.), *The psychological and social impact of disability* (3rd ed.). New York: Springer-Verlag.

Devlieger, P.J., & Albrecht, G.L. (2000). Your experience is not my experience: The concept and experience of disability on Chicago's near west side. *Journal of Disability Policy Studies, 11*(1), 51–60.

Fine, M., & Asch, M. (1988). Disability beyond stigma: Social interaction, discrimination and activism. *Journal of Social Issues, 44*(1), 3–19.

Finkelstein, V. (1980). *Attitudes and disabled people: Issues for discussion.* New York: World Rehabilitation Fund.

French, S. (1993). Can you see the rainbow? The roots of denial. In J. Swain, V. Finkelstein, S. French, & M. Oliver (Eds.), *Disabling barriers, enabling environments* (pp. 69–77). Thousand Oaks, CA: Sage .

Gill, C. (1997). Four types of integration in disability identity development. *Journal of Vocational Rehabilitation, 9,* 36–46.

Gill, C.J. (2001). Divided understandings: The social experience of disability. In G.L. Albrecht, K. Seelman, & M. Bury (Eds.), *Handbook of disability studies* (pp. 351–372). Thousand Oaks, CA: Sage.

Goffman, E. (1963). *Stigma: Notes on the management of spoiled identity.* New York: Simon & Schuster.

Hahn, H. (1985). Disability policy and the problem of discrimination. *American Behavioral Scientist, 28*(3), 293–318.

Hahn, H. (1997). An agenda for citizens with disabilities: Pursuing identity and empowerment. *Journal of Vocational Rehabilitation, 9,* 31–37.

Jamison, K.R. (1995). *An unquiet mind: A memoir of moods and madness.* New York: Vintage Books.

Jeffreys, M. (2002). The visible cripple: Scars and other disfiguring displays included. In S.L. Snyder, B.J. Brueggemann, & R. Garland-Thompson (Eds.), *Disability studies: Enabling the humanities* (pp. 31–39). New York: The Modern Language Association of America.

Kitchin, R. (2000). The researched opinions on research: Disabled people and disability research. *Disability and Society, 15*(1), 25–47.

Linton, S. (1998). Disability studies/not disability studies. In S. Linton, *Claiming disability: Knowledge and identity* (pp. 132–156). New York: New York University Press.

Longmore, P.K. (1995a). Medical decision making and people with disabilities: A clash of cultures. *Journal of Law, Medicine & Ethics, 23,* 82–87.

Longmore, P.K. (1995b). The second phase: From disability rights to disability culture. *The Disability Rag and ReSource, 16,* 4–11.

Longmore, P.K., & Goldberger, D. (2000). The league of the physically handicapped and the Great Depression: A case study in the new disability history [Electronic version]. *The Journal of American History, 87,* 888–922.

Louis Harris & Associates. (1998). *Highlights of the N.O.D./Harris 1998 survey of Americans with disabilities.* Washington DC: National Organization on Disability.

Lustig, B. (Executive Producer), & Scott, R. (Director). (2001). *Hannibal* [Motion picture]. United States: MGM/Universal.

McBryde Johnson, H. (2003, February 16). Unspeakable conversations or how I spent one day as a token cripple at Princeton University. *The New York Times Magazine, 152,* 50–79.

McCrum, R. (1998). *My year off: Recovering life after a stroke.* New York: W.W. Norton.

McNeil, J.M. (1997). Americans with disabilities: 1994–1995. In *U.S. Bureau of the Census current population reports* (pp. 70–61). Washington, DC: U.S. Government Printing Office.

Mitchell, D. (2002). Narrative prosthesis and the materiality of metaphor. In S.L. Snyder, B.J. Brueggemann, & R. Garland-Thompson (Eds.), *Disability studies: Enabling the humanities* (pp. 15–30). New York: The Modern Language Association of America.

Murphy, R.F. (1990). *The body silent: An anthropologist embarks on the most challenging journey of his life: Into the world of the disabled.* New York: W.W. Norton.

Nagi, S.Z. (1991). Disability concepts revisited: Implications for prevention. In A. Pope & A. Tarlou (Eds.), *Disability in America: Toward a national agenda for prevention* (pp. 309–327). Washington, DC: National Academy Press.

Oliver, M. (1990). *The politics of disablement.* London: Macmillan.

Oliver, M. (1992). Changing the social relations of research production. *Disability, Handicap and Society, 7*(2), 101–114.

Oliver, M. (1996). *Understanding disability: From theory to practice.* New York: St. Martin's Press.

Paterson, K., & Hughes, B. (2000). Disabled bodies. In P. Hancock, B. Hughes, E. Jagger, K. Paterson, R. Russell, E. Tulle-Winton, & M. Tyler, *The body, culture and society: An introduction* (pp. 29–44). Buckingham: Open University Press.

Phillips, M.J. (1990). Damaged goods: Oral narratives of the experience of disability in American culture. *Social Science and Medicine, 30,* 849–857.

Price, R. (1994). *A whole new life.* New York: Atheneum Macmillan Press.

Rioux, M.H. (1997). Disability: The place of judgment in a world of fact. *Journal of Intellectual Disability Research, 41,* 102–111.

Scotch, R.K. (2001). *From good will to civil rights: Transforming federal disability policy* (2nd ed.). Philadelphia: Temple University Press.

Scott, R. (1969). *The making of blind men.* New York: Russell Sage.

Shapiro, J.P. (1993). *No pity: People with disabilities forging a new civil rights movement.* New York: Random House.

Snyder, S.L., Brueggemann, B.J., & Garland-Thomson, R. (Eds). (2002). *Disability studies: Enabling the humanities.* New York: The Modern Language Association of America.

Stone, D. (1984). *The disabled state.* Philadelphia: Temple University Press.

Toombs, K. (1992). *The meaning of illness: A phenomenological account of the different perspectives of physician and patient.* Dordrecht, Netherlands: Kluwer Academic.

Vash, C.L. (1981). *The psychology of disability.* New York: Springer.

Wendell, S. (1996). *The rejected body: Feminist philosophical reflections on disability.* New York: Routledge.

Williams, D. (1992). *Nobody nowhere.* New York: Times Books.

Zola, I.K. (1972). Medicine as an institution of social control. *Sociological Review, 20,* 487–503.

Zola, I.K. (1982). *Missing pieces: A chronicle of living with a disability.* Philadelphia: Temple University Press.

Zola, I.K. (1993a). Disability statistics: What we count and what it tells us: A personal and political analysis. *Journal of Disability Policy Studies, 4*(2), 9–39.

Zola, I.K. (1993b). Self, identity, and the naming question: Reflections on the language of disability. *Social Science and Medicine, 36*(2), 167–173.

Using the Conceptual Foundations in Practice

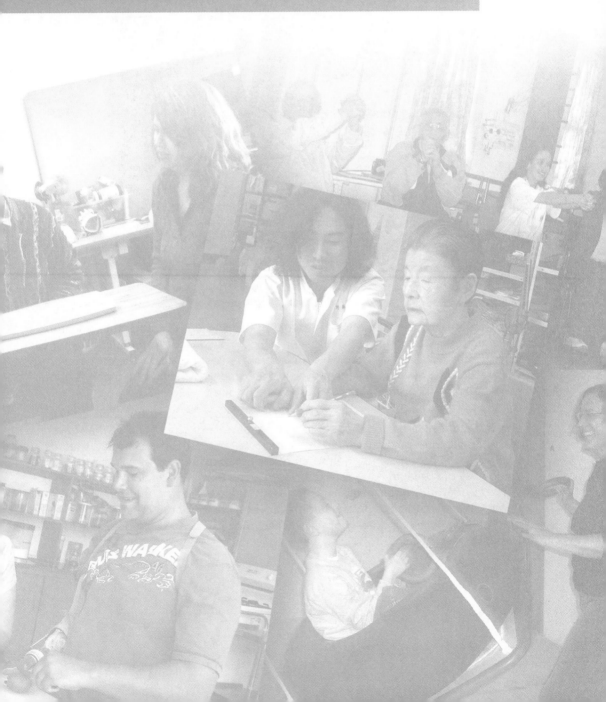

CHAPTER 18

Conceptual Foundations in Practice: Creating a Personal Conceptual Portfolio

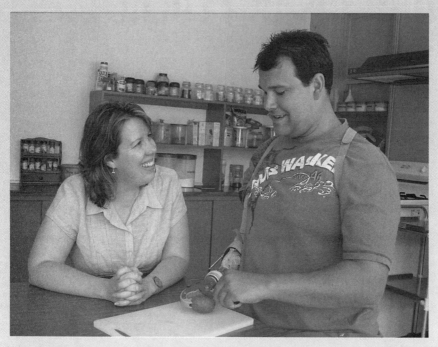

The occupational therapists featured throughout the previous chapters were selected because they make active use of occupational therapy's conceptual foundations in their practice. Each was asked to respond to a number of questions about the concepts they use in practice and how they use that knowledge. Among many insightful points about this topic was the following reflection from Karen Roberts:

> I think one of the challenges for new OTs (and possibly more experienced OTs too) is that they learn a lot about theory when they are in school and so they have a mass of concepts "buzzing around in their heads" and it's hard to sort out what fits where. That's not surprising given some of the complexity of concepts and the complexity of clients that they are faced with when they are actually working as OTs. When I work with students and new graduates within a clinical setting they often say to me, "We learned all of this stuff at the university but it doesn't really apply in practice." Of course, it does apply in practice; they just need some guidance to work out where it fits.

This chapter aims to provide some guidance as to how occupational therapists can integrate the field's conceptual foundations into their practice.

This text has demonstrated that the conceptual foundations of occupational therapy include the field's paradigm and conceptual practice models along with relevant related knowledge. This chapter considers how therapists select and use these three types of knowledge to inform their professional identity and competence. It will culminate with discussion and illustration of the personal conceptual portfolio, an individualized collection of values, beliefs, concepts, and expertise.

Solidifying One's Identity as an Occupational Therapist

Professional identity is grounded in the field's paradigm. We saw earlier in this text that occupational therapy's identity has changed with transformations in its paradigm. The profession was founded on a paradigm that recognized occupation as a domain of human life and as a therapeutic tool. During this era, the identity of the profession was organized around a mission of supporting the occupational well-being of clients through engaging them in occupations that enabled adaptation to the challenges posed by disability.

During its subsequent, mechanistic, paradigm, the field adopted a view of occupational therapy as the use of activities to remediate underlying impairments. This shift resulted in confusion about the definition and nature of occupational therapy. Individual therapists experienced this identity confusion as discomfort and frustration in not being able to describe what occupational therapy was.

During this period, occupational therapists sometimes borrowed identity from other professions (O'Shea, 1977) or defined themselves by their work setting or specialty (Barris, 1984). Some therapists became generic workers without unique occupational therapy perspectives or skills (Harrison, 2003).

Such problems of professional identity led occupational therapy to return to a focus on occupation. Occupational therapists are fortunate in that the field's contemporary paradigm provides a rich formula for what it means to be an occupational therapist. In short, the current paradigm defines occupational therapy practice as:

- Focused on supporting occupational well-being of clients
- Concerned with occupational problems (i.e., difficulty participating in work, leisure/play, and activities of daily living)
- Based on a holistic viewpoint that integrates concern for the person, occupation/task, and environment
- Addressing client problems of performing and participating in occupations
- Using occupational engagement as the central mechanism of therapy
- Client-centered and based on a positive therapeutic relationship

> **Occupational therapists are fortunate in that the field's contemporary paradigm provides a rich formula for what it means to be an occupational therapist.**

Occupational therapists should be aware of the field's collective paradigm. Moreover, it is a professional responsibility to decide how that paradigm will be reflected in:

- One's own definition of occupational therapy
- How one views one's services and what they accomplish for one's clients
- The values that guide one's practice

Later in this chapter we will see examples of occupational therapists who have articulated these elements for themselves and their practice.

The Complexity of Practice and the Need for Knowledge

Karen Roberts' reference to the complexity of occupational therapy practice is worth considering. This complexity is reflected in the following features that characterize occupational therapy practice:

- Occupational therapists practice with a wide variety of clients whose impairments may be physical, emotional, and/or cognitive in nature. Occupational therapists must understand those diverse impairments and how to address them
- Occupational therapy practice is based on the belief that practice should be holistic. Thus, practitioners must attend to multiple aspects of the clients' abilities, roles, routines, lifestyle, motives, emotions, and aspirations, as well as the client's physical and social context
- Occupational therapy practice primarily involves supporting clients to engage in occupations. Thus, clients' motives, perspectives, and cooperation are all critical to achieving positive occupational therapy outcomes
- Occupational therapy practice involves a relationship between the client and the therapist. That relationship is critical to therapy outcomes
- Occupational therapists not only see clients individually but often deal with clients in groups

> **Therapists must carefully select from the field's models those that are most suited for seeing and explaining the challenges faced by their clients and that address what to do in therapy.**

Each of these features of occupational therapy makes the field's practice complex. Moreover, each of these features of practice demands expertise. A good part of this expertise requires the kind of knowledge that is represented in conceptual practice models and related knowledge. Consequently, being a good practitioner means selecting the knowledge from these conceptual foundations that best supports one's practice.

Choosing Conceptual Practice Models

Given the complexity of practice noted previously, occupational therapists find it necessary to draw upon more than a single conceptual practice model. Therapists must carefully select from the field's models those that are most suited for seeing and explaining the challenges faced by their clients and that address what to do in therapy. Table 18.1 lists each of the models discussed in the previous section, summarizing which aspects of the client each model addresses and the aspect of therapy about which each model provides guidance. This table can serve as a kind of shorthand for thinking about which models one may wish to include as part of one's expertise.

The process of choosing models can be exemplified by considering a client with a recent spinal cord injury who is currently in rehabilitation and presents as unmotivated and emotionally volatile (see Fig. 18.1). The biomechanical model would serve as a way of understanding the specific effects of the spinal lesion on muscle enervation and the consequent loss of active and passive range of motion, strength, and endurance. This model also provides a way to consider how these impairments will impact the movement capacity of the individual in occupational tasks. It is important to note that the biomechanical model is silent on the emotional or motivational dimension of the client's situation. Hence, there is a need for more than one model if one wishes to address other problems experienced by the client.

For instance, the model of human occupation could be used to address the client's motivational status. This model would be concerned with how the spinal cord injury has affected the client's personal causation (sense of competence), interests, and values. This model orients the therapist to construct a picture of the client's intense feelings of loss of capacity and control, his fears about the future, the disruption of his ability to participate in and enjoy old interests, and the disintegration of long-term life goals. These factors, viewed together, provide a way to name the client's unmotivated status as a disruption of volition.

Moreover, the intentional relationship model could provide information critical to understanding situational characteristics of a client who is facing a major life-changing disability

Table 18.1 **Aspects of Clients and Explanations of Practice Offered by Conceptual Practice Models**

Model	Biomechanical Model	Cognitive Model	Functional Group Model	Intentional Relationship Model	Model of Human Occupation	Motor Control Model	Sensory Integration Model
Aspect of the client addressed by the model	Motion based on joint integrity, strength, and endurance	Cognitive capacities underlying performance	Group process influencing individual performance	Client interpersonal characteristics	Choices, organization, and performance of occupations in environment	Organization of skilled motor action based on CNS organization	Organization of sensory information in brain for adaptive movement
What the model explains about practice	How to enhance or compensate for limitations in range of motion, strength, and endurance	How to remediate or compensate for cognitive impairments	How to use functional groups to enhance client engagement in occupations	How to interact effectively with clients in order to support occupational engagement during therapy	How to enhance motivation, roles, habits, and skills	How to enhance the control of movement during occupational performance	How to enhance sensory processing and help clients cope with their unique sensory processing difficulties

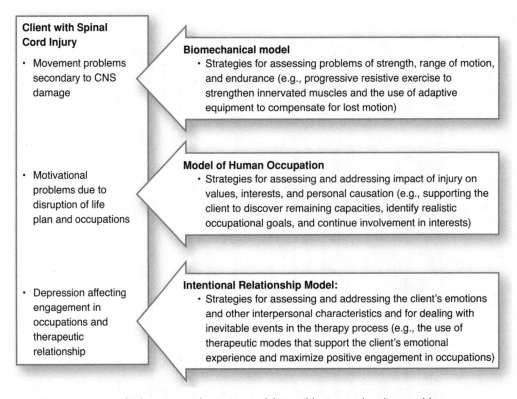

FIGURE 18.1 Using multiple conceptual practice models to address complex client problems.

and the loss of multiple capacities. This model would provide guidance for how the therapist could effectively interact with a client who is emotionally distraught and how to deal with tasks of therapy that are likely to be emotionally charged because they underscore for the client capacities that he or she has lost.

The three models, together, provide ways of conceptualizing the impact of spinal cord injury on the client more holistically, and they allow the therapist to see in more depth the nature of very different aspects of the client's circumstances. The biomechanical, human occupation, and intentional relationship models provide ways to understand the client's musculoskeletal, motivational, and emotional problems and to frame their meaning for function (e.g., limited movement affecting functional tasks and disrupted volition affecting motivation). They also provide a rationale for what can be done for the client in therapy, as shown in Figure 18.1.

Other circumstances may call for different models. The sensory integration model may be used to make sense of the clumsiness of a schoolchild. The cognitive model may shed light on the memory and problem-solving difficulties of someone with a head injury. Sensory integration or cognitive services might be offered to clients in a group format in which case the functional group model would serve as a helpful framework for planning and implementing those groups.

The Use of Conceptual Practice Models in Practice

The biomechanical, cognitive, motor control, and sensory integration models are designed to address movement, cognitive, motor, and sensory impairments. For this reason, these models will be selected when clients present with these types of impairments and when the aim of the therapy is to improve movement, cognitive, motor, and sensory capacities. The type of client group or purpose of the intervention will determine whether or not these models are used.

Because occupational therapists work with clients who are likely to have problems associated with one or more of these models, they are frequently used in occupational therapy (National Board for Certification in Occupational Therapy, 2004).

The model of human occupation addresses the occupational consequences of impairments (i.e., how interests, values, sense of capacity, roles, habits, and skills are influenced by impairments). Since these factors are likely to be influenced by any type of impairment, most clients seen by occupational therapists will have one or more issues that can be addressed by this model. Not surprisingly, 80% of occupational therapists in a recent national survey indicated that they use this model (Lee, Taylor, Kielhofner, 2009; Lee, Taylor, Kielhofner, & Fisher, 2008).

The intentional relationship model addresses the interaction between the occupational therapist and the client that is always a part of the occupational therapy process. Moreover, according to the opinions of practicing therapists (Taylor, Lee, Kielhofner, & Ketkar, in press), the therapeutic use of self by the occupational therapist is the single most important determinant of occupational therapy outcomes. Arguably, since this model addresses therapeutic interactions and the therapeutic use of self, this model should always be a part of occupational therapy practice.

The functional group model is designed to guide occupational therapy services when they are provided in groups. Since the use of groups is widespread in occupational therapy, this model should be relevant frequently.

Being a Multi-Model Therapist

As the previous discussion illustrated, decisions about using conceptual practice models inevitably lead occupational therapists to choose a combination of models to guide practice. Rather than adhering to or emphasizing a single model, the best therapists will be multi-model therapists who can draw upon a wealth of concepts and practical strategies that are afforded by

several models that are relevant to one's circumstances.

The effectiveness of strategies suggested by one model can also be enhanced through insights provided by another model. If we consider the earlier example of combining the biomechanical model, the model of human occupation, and the intentional relationship model, we see that intervention goals derived from all three models may be met together. For example, if a person with spinal cord injury participates in a therapeutic occupation that has meaning because of a connection to a life role, biomechanical goals may be enhanced (since a client may feel less fatigue and exert more effort in a meaningful activity). Volitional goals may be realized simultaneously (a sense of possibilities for competence and a regeneration of interest and meaning may emerge from the activity). Careful attention to the client's interpersonal characteristics and the intentional use of therapeutic modes will also support a productive relationship with the client and enhance the client's participation in therapy. By combining conceptual practice models, therapists can achieve a more holistic and efficacious approach to their work.

> By combining conceptual practice models, therapists can achieve a more holistic and efficacious approach to their work.

Selecting and Using Related Knowledge

While the paradigm and models of occupational therapy provide the most basic knowledge used in practice, there are always situations in which practitioners must draw on knowledge from outside the field. In these instances, therapists employ related knowledge. For example, consider the type of client discussed earlier.

In providing services to a client with spinal cord injury, a therapist may employ a range of information from outside the field. Consider the field of disability studies discussed in Chapter 17. The person who acquires a spinal cord injury enters a new experience and social status as a disabled person. The occupational therapist working with this client should be aware of concepts from disability studies and use these concepts at appropriate points. Similarly, if the therapist recognizes that the client is struggling with emotional coping, cognitive behavioral therapy may provide useful concepts and strategies.

When employing related knowledge it is important that therapists:

- Select appropriate and relevant related knowledge to complement their conceptual practice models
- Derive their identities and the main elements of their practice from the paradigm and practice models, and not from the related knowledge

In this way, related knowledge ensures that therapists have the full range of knowledge necessary for practice while functioning within the parameters of their professional role.

Developing a Conceptual Portfolio

Because the conceptual foundations are so important for being an excellent occupational therapist, it is worth taking time to reflect upon and develop one's conceptual portfolio. A conceptual portfolio should contain the following elements:

- A personal definition of occupational therapy
- A clear sense of the nature of one's clients and of the services one offers to them
- A personal set of values to guide practice
- Identification and clear understanding of the conceptual practice models one uses to address client needs
- Identification of concepts from related knowledge that inform one's practice

In the following section, two of the occupational therapists introduced earlier in this text present their conceptual portfolios.

Andrea Girardi

Andrea works in a community center serving adolescents and adults with a wide range of challenges related to mental illness, dementia, aging-related loss of function, and head injuries. She notes of her work:

I feel very proud to be an occupational therapist and I do believe in the power of occupation as a change agent. I have started

several programs, always basing my work in the principles of our professional paradigm and conceptual practice models. I have been able to demonstrate that occupational therapy is unique and effective.

Andrea's *definition of occupational therapy* is as follows:

OT is the art of helping people to rebuild their occupational lives by giving them the precise support they require. At the same time, it is a science that aims to know the client as an occupational being and understand the processes that influence, empower, or limit the client's participation in occupations.

Andrea's *views of her services and how they meet her clients' needs* are as follows:

I help clients recover occupational life. My clients are all facing a major disruption in their lives. Their challenges stem from emotional, physical, and cognitive impairments along with social and cultural barriers (i.e., prejudices, lack of acceptance, and stigma) that interfere with participation in daily occupations.

I work, hand in hand, with my clients using occupational engagement to rebuild their lives. I search to find the occupations that will be meaningful for each client, given who each person is and wants to be. My assessment is designed to understand what my clients want and what they need to do, given their life circumstances. As an occupational therapist, I work with clients in their ordinary occupational environments (e.g., school, work, home, and community meeting places). I also use environmental strategies to empower my clients and remove external barriers. It is important to my clients that I work with them in the real circumstances of their lives.

Andrea is guided by the following *values*:

- Respect for each client
- Recognition of the uniqueness of each client
- Careful attention to and recognition of the importance of occupation in the client's life
- Centering therapy on the specific client, his/her circumstances, and his/her environment
- Recognition of and belief in the strengths of each client

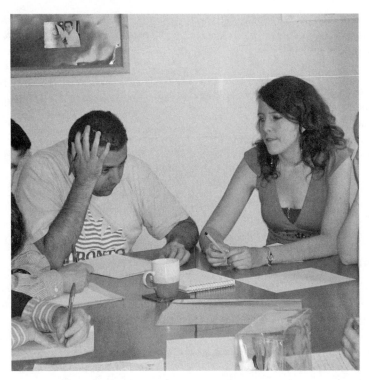

Andrea encourages a client who has become frustrated during a writing group.

- Belief in the power of occupation to produce change

    Andrea uses the following *conceptual practice models* in her practice.

- The model of human occupation (MOHO) is Andrea's leading model

According to Andrea:

    MOHO allows for the understanding of the multiple and complex aspects involved in human occupation. It allows me to understand and analyze the dynamics of occupational participation. The coherence among its theoretical base, practical tools, and research evidence gives me the confidence I need to work as an OT.

- Andrea specialized in this model through attending a series of three post-graduate courses and by working for a year and a half in a center specializing in MOHO where she received supervision from an expert. She has learned to administer a range of the MOHO-based assessments, which she uses routinely in her practice
- Andrea uses the intentional relationship model, which guides her in being able to relate to her clients in the most therapeutic manner. Andrea emphasizes the empathizing and collaborating modes in her work with clients and is able to draw upon other modes when clients need them. For example, with a client who has dementia and needs clear guidance, she uses the instructing mode and with a client who needs to figure out how to deal with a specific challenge, she uses the problem-solving mode
- Andrea uses the cognitive model to understand and address cognitive problems when working with clients who have dementia, severe mental illness, or cognitive sequellae to brain injury

Andrea draws on a wide range of *related knowledge* in her practice. She acquired much of this related knowledge through post-graduate course-work in community psychology. The related knowledge she employs includes:

- Concepts related to empowerment, social net-working, and social support (Fawcett, White, Balcazar, & Suarez-Balcazar, 1994)
- Clubhouse principles and concepts of supported and independent employment (Fountain House, n.d.)
- Concepts from Maslow's Theory of Needs (Maslow, 1970)
- Cognitive behavioral therapy (see Chapter 16)
- Concepts related to life meaning from the logotherapy work of Victor Frankl (1959)

Maya Tuchner

Maya works in the rehabilitation department in the Hadassah-Mount Scopus Hospital in Jerusalem. About a third of her clients have experienced cerebrovascular accidents; other clients have neurological conditions such as traumatic brain injuries or brain damage secondary to excision of tumors. She also sees clients with multiple sclerosis and spinal cord injury. Still other clients she sees have orthopedic problems or chronic pain.

Maya notes of her work:

> The uniqueness of occupational therapy comes from engagement in meaningful occupations being the essence of the treatment. I believe in a client-centered approach and consider our clients active partners in the treatment process, whenever this is possible. The challenge in my practice is to give every patient the best treatment according to his background, culture, habits, and way of living and to establish good therapeutic relationships with different clients.

Maya's *definition of occupational therapy* is as follows: "Occupational therapy is a rehabilitation service that helps clients return to their previous occupations or find new meaningful occupations that improve quality of life and support well-being."

Maya's *views of her services and how they meet her clients' needs* are as follows:

> As an occupational therapist I address not only impairments but also how they affect

my clients' performance and participation. I also address my clients' habits, daily routine, roles, and level of satisfaction and enjoyment in different areas of occupation. I also take into consideration the possible environmental barriers faced by my clients. Addressing and understanding all of these components together is unique to our profession.

Maya identified three *values* that guide her practice:

- To establish a good therapeutic relationship with all of her clients. According to Maya, "this is the most important value that guides my therapy and it includes the ability to feel empathy and to 'discover' who the client is and what the client's needs are"
- To respect every client independent of the client's background and religion. This means that Maya uses a client-centered approach, taking into consideration the client's specific needs
- To show professional responsibility for her clients by always being aware of best practice. This means that she must read in order to keep up with new knowledge in the profession and expand her knowledge by taking courses and doing continuing education

Because Maya sees clients with a range of problems she uses the following *conceptual practice models*:

- Maya uses the motor control model to address motor problems that follow brain damage due to stroke or traumatic brain injury. This includes principles that reflect neurodevelopmental treatment (NDT), Brunnstrom's movement therapy, and the contemporary task-oriented motor control approach, all of which were discussed in Chapter 12. Within the motor control model, Maya also uses constraint-induced therapy for clients who can benefit from this technique. This model is central to her work with most clients. Maya has received specific training and is certified in NDT
- Maya uses the biomechanical model when her clients present with orthopedic problems of muscle weakness, limited range of motion, or lack of endurance

- Maya uses the model of human occupation to address client motivation, habits, and roles
- Maya uses the cognitive model to guide her treatment of cognitive problems following brain damage. She emphasizes the dynamic interactional approach of this model along with functional and remedial cognitive training techniques. Maya has learned to administer a range of cognitive-perceptual assessments. Being versed in a number of cognitive assessments allows her to do comprehensive and in-depth assessment when a client presents with cognitive problems
- Maya recently learned about the intentional relationship model, which resonates with her view that the therapeutic relationship is the most important aspect of her therapy. She notes, "The most critical aspect of my therapy that makes a difference for my clients is my ability to show empathy and understanding, to create a unique and different treatment for every client, to explain what I am doing in the therapy and why." She is currently integrating this model into her practice

Maya uses the following *related knowledge* in her practice:

- Neuropsychological concepts that help her better understand the cognitive profile of her clients. She routinely reads articles from this field
- The medical model to better understand the consequences of the different kinds of brain damage she encounters in her clients

Conclusion

Andrea's and Maya's conceptual portfolios demonstrate how occupational therapists can achieve a thoughtful and theory-based approach to their practice. By making reflective use of the field's conceptual foundations, therapists can have a better sense of their own professional identity, a clear vision of the values that guide their work, and a thorough understanding of the concepts that underlie their approach to understanding and meeting client needs. Readers are encouraged to complete their own conceptual portfolios and to reflect upon them periodically.

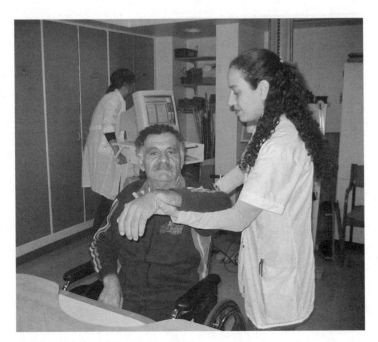

Maya works with a client on his passive range of motion.

REFERENCES

Barris, R. (1984). Toward an image of one's own: Sources of variation in the role of occupational therapists in psychosocial practice. *Occupational Therapy Journal of Research, 4*(1), 3–23.

Fawcett, S.R., White, G.W., Balcazar, F.E., & Suarez-Balcazar, Y. (1994). A contextual-behavioral model of empowerment: Case studies involving people with physical disabilities. *American Journal of Community Psychology, 22,* 471–496.

Fountain House. (n.d.). *Fountain house.* Retrieved April 25, 2008, from http://www.fountainhouse.org/

Frankl, V. (1959). *Man's search for meaning.* London: Hodder & Stoughton.

Harrison, D. (2003). The case for generic working in mental health occupational therapy. *British Journal of Occupational Therapy, 66,* 110–112.

Lee, S.W., Taylor, R.R., Kielhofner, G. (2009). Choice, knowledge, and utilization of a practice theory: A national study of occupational therapists who use the model of human occupation. *Occupational Therapy in Health Care, 23*(1), 60–71.

Lee, S.W., Taylor, R.R., Kielhofner, G., & Fisher, G. (2008). Theory use in practice: A national survey of therapists who use the model of human occupation. *American Journal of Occupational Therapy, 62,* 106–117.

Maslow, A.H. (1970). *Motivation and personality* (2nd ed.). New York: Harper & Row.

National Board for Certification in Occupational Therapy. (2004). A practice analysis study of entry-level occupational therapist registered and certified occupational therapy assistant practice. *Occupational Therapy Journal of Research: Occupation, Participation and Health, 24,* S1–S31.

O'Shea, B.J. (1977). Pawn or protagonist: Interactional perspective of professional identity. *Canadian Journal of Occupational Therapy, 44,* 101–108.

Taylor, R., Lee, S.W., Kielhofner, G., & Ketkar, M. (in press). The therapeutic relationship: A nationwide survey of practitioners' attitudes and experiences. *American Journal of Occupational Therapy.*

CHAPTER 19

Therapeutic Reasoning: Using Occupational Therapy's Conceptual Foundations in Everyday Practice

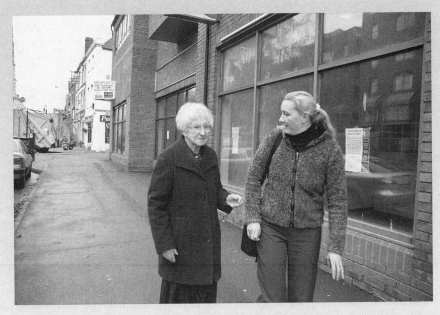

It is really important to carry out a full occupational screening in order to better understand clients' lives rather than jumping on the first "deficit" that is highlighted. When therapy does work, it is because it is not only tailored to the person's routine, values, and performance skills, but also because the therapy is a partnership between the client and myself. We are working toward whatever is important or essential for that person. I would like to think that over the years, I have taken the role of "doing" a lot more seriously from individual to individual based on their values, not mine. I feel it is important with all therapy to be flexible and to problem-solve throughout the therapy process. Needs change, along with priorities and often health, so I feel that it is important not to be too rigid along the way.

Alice Moody

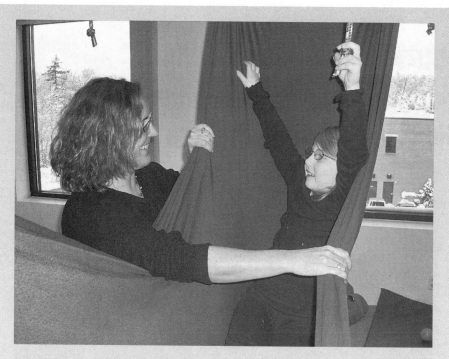

My goal is to help the child be more successful, to create "results that make a difference." I do this by working with each child as an individual, gearing the therapy program towards that child's unique needs and strengths. I can effect the greatest changes when I address three levels of intervention. I understand that the brain has plasticity and can make meaningful changes with carefully guided intervention. Through working with children in a safe and nurturing environment, I can provide the intensity of sensory input they need to help them become regulated and to "find their bodies." By creating a continually increasing challenge level that is appropriate to each child's development, I can effect change in that child's integration and developmental skills. Through working with families, I can help them learn how to support their child in the varied environments they need to function in outside of the therapeutic clinic setting. Last, by working with children at a level they can understand, I help them become advocates for themselves through understanding what they need to do to sustain better participation and success.

Stacey Szklut

As these therapists' descriptions of their work illustrate, occupational therapy is a complex process. In their everyday work, practitioners must:

- Understand their clients as occupational beings and as people with unique interpersonal characteristics
- Identify their clients' occupational problems and underlying impairments, along with environmental supports and barriers
- Identify reasonable goals and objectives that reflect their clients' desires, occupational lives, and potential for performance
- Engage clients in carefully selected occupations designed to promote attainment of treatment objectives
- Provide optimal interpersonal support and collaboration for occupational engagement and for change
- Monitor the therapy process and make necessary modifications when circumstances change or when the process is not going as intended
- Determine client progress and outcomes

> **Learning to think with theory means that the theory becomes a way of seeing clients, their impairments, their occupational circumstances, and their interpersonal characteristics.**

These tasks all require careful and reflective reasoning that is supported and guided by the field's conceptual foundations. Therapeutic reasoning is a process of using the concepts and practical resources of conceptual practice models and related knowledge to understand a client and choose an ongoing course of action to achieve positive outcomes for the client.

This chapter discusses and illustrates the process of therapeutic reasoning. Thus, it describes how theory is put into practice. It illustrates how the therapists featured in this text go about their own therapeutic reasoning processes. It will share their thoughts about therapeutic reasoning and illustrate the process through two case examples.

Therapeutic Reasoning: Thinking With Theory

Using a conceptual practice model or related knowledge requires understanding and use of the underlying theory. Learning to think with theory means that the theory becomes a way of seeing clients, their impairments, their occupational circumstances, and their interpersonal characteristics.

Just studying a theory (e.g., learning the concepts) does not ensure that one will actively use the theory in therapeutic reasoning. Rather, one must consciously go back and forth between theoretical concepts and the clients one sees in practice. For instance, one may use the concept of range of motion while watching a client move his arm or think about the concept of praxis while examining how a client goes about planning and executing a task.

Reflecting on the meaning of the concept and comparing it to what one sees helps to integrate the conceptual with the practice. Over time and with practice, the two will blend together and one will find oneself observing such things as "personal causation," "executive function," and "expression of emotion" in clients. When this process becomes second nature, one is truly thinking with theory. The concepts become the way that one sees and understands clients and the therapeutic process.

Client-Centeredness in Therapeutic Reasoning

Therapeutic reasoning emphasizes that the occupational therapist is exercising competence or expertise by using concepts to better understand a client's situation and how to address it. Sometimes, the idea of professional expertise has been seen as interfering or incompatible with the notion of client-centered practice and the kind of respect, empathy, and partnership that client-centered practice implies. However, this need not be the case. Rather, a therapist who is actively using theory can be much more client-centered than one who is not.

For instance, Bacon Fung Leung Ng notes that as he gained expertise and experience he became increasingly client-centered:

> *I switched my focus to emphasize the importance of coaching my clients for self-discovery to find and live a meaningful life of their choice. I try to empower my clients to obtain their valued life roles by making the best use of their functional capabilities.*

Similarly, Karen Roberts, who is an expert in the medical and biomechanical aspects of dealing with amputees, notes of practice:

> *If we truly spend time getting to know our clients, listening to their wants, needs, values, hopes, and dreams, and if we reflect these back to our clients, they feel valued, heard, and respected. I believe that therapy cannot really work well unless both the therapist and the client are committed to the process and are engaged in the process together. So I think making plans for therapy together, identifying goals of therapy together, and evaluating outcomes of therapy together help the process of therapy work.*

While these therapists emphasize the importance of collaborating with and empowering clients, not all clients are capable of this level of involvement. Clients who have limited ability to indicate their needs and assert their wants require different client-centered strategies. Clients who are newly disabled and/or who are feeling particularly vulnerable may require more directive or supportive, but nevertheless client-centered, strategies of therapy.

For those clients who are unable to verbalize and/or be active in collaboration, the therapist must work to understand the client's view of the world, what matters to the client, what the client enjoys, and how the client feels about his or her abilities. Only then can the therapist be truly client-centered. When the client has limited ability to verbalize his or her perspectives or participate in therapy, the therapist can also collaborate with family members or others who care about and can serve as advocates for the client.

In the end, being client-centered in one's therapeutic reasoning means:

- Working carefully to understand what the client is experiencing and what the client wants (independent of the client's ability to express these things)
- Being an advocate for the client's welfare and desires
- Recognizing what the client is capable of bringing into the therapy process and capitalizing on it for the client's benefit

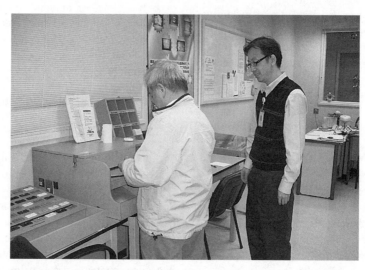

Bacon and a client work toward mutually agreed upon treatment goals established by discussing the client's future roles and current challenges in daily functioning.

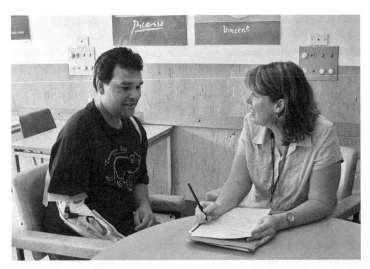

Karen and a client with an amputation plan the course of therapy together.

Being client-centered may involve empowering the client and collaborating with the client. It may mean simply taking the time and having the expertise to be able to appreciate and respect a client's experience in the therapy process. It may mean being an advocate for clients with limited ability to advocate for themselves.

Holism in Therapeutic Reasoning

Chapter 18 emphasized the importance of selecting more than a single conceptual practice model or body of related knowledge in order to achieve a comprehensive understanding of a client from multiple perspectives. The therapists featured in this book all emphasized this aspect of practice, which they typically referred to as having a holistic perspective.

Achieving a holistic view is more than simply using different concepts and focusing on different aspects of a client's life. It also involves being able to consider all of these factors as a whole and make judgments. For instance, Alice Moody describes the following:

> I worked with a lady with moderate dementia who chose to ride a bicycle regularly despite being physically frail and having little insight as to her memory impairment. There were very obvious risks to this activity. However, taking into account the environment and her rigid routine and difficulty in adapting to changes, I felt that the risks were well

worth enduring at the time. Moreover, I considered the client's minimal insight and poor tolerance to change. With all of these factors considered, I reasoned that, if we were to stop her from riding her bicycle, her agitation levels would probably hit an all-time high and her quality of life would be severely affected. Finally, her family would bear the brunt of this.

In this instance, Alice was able to consolidate several factors that included an understanding of the client's cognition (memory and awareness), volition, habituation, and interpersonal characteristics (i.e., need for control and emotional expression), along with consideration of the family context into her therapeutic reasoning and to arrive at a client-centered decision to support the client's bicycle riding. Holism enables therapists to make such complex judgments based on the simultaneous consideration of many aspects of the clients and their contexts. Good therapeutic reasoning always implies such a holistic approach. Hiroyuki Notoh explains how he aims to be holistic in his therapeutic reasoning:

> When I assess a client's ability to move part of his body, I only get part of the picture. I want to know what having difficulty or an inability to move means to my client. My clients are older and they have experienced many things in their lives that are far from my

own experiences (e.g., world wars or mar-
riages arranged by their parents). I always
try to keep in my mind that my intervention
must be based in my client's life. I try to listen
intently and carefully to their life events and
what is important for them. Only after careful
listening will I suggest my intervention plans.

The Six Steps of Therapeutic Reasoning

As illustrated in Figure 19.1, therapeutic reasoning involves six steps:

- Generating questions about the client
- Collecting information on, from, and with the client to answer the questions one has generated
- Using the information gathered to create an explanation of the client's situation
- Generating goals and strategies for therapy
- Implementing and monitoring therapy
- Determining outcomes of therapy

Importantly, these steps are not strictly sequential. Therapists generally move back and forth between the first five steps over the course of therapy. One must always be willing and ready to generate new questions, rethink one's understanding of a client, and arrive at new goals and intervention strategies.

Step One: Generating Questions to Guide Information Gathering

Client-centered therapeutic reasoning requires that therapists come to know their clients thoroughly. Getting to know clients is facilitated when one is systematically guided by questions about the client. In order to generate a holistic understanding of clients, therapists must ask a range of questions that reflect their underlying conceptual practice models and related knowledge.

Figure 19.1 illustrates the most general questions that are raised by the conceptual practice models discussed in this book. Each model, of course, will guide the therapist in asking much more detailed questions. For instance, the motor control model will guide the therapist to look for the multiple personal and environment factors that affect a client's difficulties with movement (e.g., muscle tone, the objects used,

the task being performed). The cognitive model will alert the therapist to ask about the status of executive functions, awareness, and specific cognitive processes in a client with cognitive problems. The model of human occupation will guide the therapist to ask about the client's personal causation, interests, values, roles, and habits. The intentional relationship model will provide questions about the client's interpersonal characteristics such as the need for control, affect, communication style, orientation toward relating, and capacity to receive feedback.

The concepts of each model help therapists to generate questions about the client's status. These questions create a mindset about the client that allows the therapist to be vigilant in coming to know the client. These questions also guide the therapist in collecting information necessary to know the client thoroughly.

Step Two: Gathering Information On, From, and With the Client

In order to answer the questions generated in the first step, therapists must gather information. This may mean reviewing existing documentation about a client, observing a client, talking with a client, and talking with others (family members, caretakers, and other professionals) who know the client. Therapists will generally go about gathering this information using both structured and unstructured approaches.

Structured assessments follow a set protocol whereas unstructured approaches take advantage of naturally occurring opportunities to gather information. Each of the conceptual practice models offers a range of assessments that can be used to generate information about the client and about the therapy process once it begins to unfold. Knowing the concepts of these models also guides therapists in using unstructured approaches that occur more naturally in interacting with or observing a client as the opportunity presents.

Step Three: Creating an Understanding of the Client

The information gathered to answer questions about a client should be used to create an understanding of that client that is informed by one's conceptual practice models and related

---

Step One: Generate questions to guide information gathering
What do I need to know about this client?
- What areas of occupational participation are problematic/at risk for this client?
- What is the status of this person's performance capacities and how do they affect occupational participation?
    - Motion (strength, range of motion, endurance)?
    - Control of movement?
    - Cognition?
    - Sensory processing?
- What is the status of this person's motivation for occupation, ability/opportunity to fulfill occupational roles, sustain functional habits, and perform necessary skills for occupational participation?
- What physical and social environmental factors are contributing to the client's situation (positively and negatively)?
- What interpersonal characteristics does this person bring to the therapy process and what interpersonal needs must be addressed?
- How might this person benefit from being involved in groups?

Step Two: Gather information on, from, and with the client
- Select and implement appropriate informal means (observation, talking, reviewing available information) and formal assessments in order to answer questions

---

Step Three: Create an understanding of the client
- What characteristics and circumstances contribute to the client's difficulties in occupational performance?
- Who is the client as an occupational being, including the client's desires and lifestyle?
- Given this client's characteristics, how is he/she likely to approach and participate in the therapy process and what interpersonal needs should be addressed?

Step Four: Identify goals and plans for therapy
- What are the goals for therapy?
- What occupational engagement will the client do and will these activities be done individually or in groups? (Occupation-based activity analysis guides this step.)
- What strategies will the therapist use to support occupational engagement and sustain a good working therapeutic relationship?

Step Five: Implement and monitor therapy
- Prepare for and support the client's occupational engagement individually and/or in groups (Requires ongoing occupation-based activity analysis).
- Maintain a good working therapeutic relationship.

Step Six: Determine outcomes of therapy
- Terminate therapeutic relationship.

FIGURE 19.1 The Process of Therapeutic Reasoning.

knowledge. This conceptualization of the client's situation represents a synthesis of the general concepts of the theory with the particular information about the client. The aim of this step is to create an understanding of:

- What characteristics and circumstances contribute to the client's difficulties in occupational performance
- Who the client is as an occupational being, including the client's desires and lifestyle
- Given the client's characteristics, how he or she is likely to approach and participate in the therapy process and what interpersonal needs should be addressed

In arriving at an understanding of one's client, it is important to get it right (i.e., to accurately understand the client's situation). For this reason, therapists should involve clients (and their surrogates if necessary) to the extent possible. By collaborating, the therapist and client can often generate insights into a client's situation that neither had at the outset. Clients know their own experiences. However, clients do not always have a clear picture of all the factors that contribute to that experience. The aim of this step, then, is to generate new insights that will form the basis for formulating a course of action to achieve desired change.

Step Four: Identifying Goals and Plans for Therapy

The next step is to plan the therapy process. This involves:

- Creating therapy goals for, or preferably with, the client
- Deciding what kinds of occupational engagement will enable the client to change
- Determining what kinds of therapeutic and interpersonal strategies will be needed to support the client to achieve the goals

This step requires a great deal of reflective thought. Karen Roberts notes, "I have to continually ask the question of myself: 'What do I want the outcome of this intervention to achieve?' I also have to plan well, be prepared, and think through my choices of therapeutic media carefully."

Similarly, Bacon Fung Leung Ng notes: "Each client requires different remedial techniques as the key to unlock their situation. Some require skills acquisition, some require habit formation, and some require motivation."

Successful therapy also depends on a client's willingness to accept the goals and strategies of therapy at some level. Therefore, the therapist must communicate and collaborate with the client to identify the therapy plan. How this is done will depend on the client and must be built around the client's perceptions and desires.

Step Five: Implementing and Monitoring Therapy

Once goals and general strategies of intervention are identified the therapist must prepare for and implement the therapy process. This requires the therapist to prepare for and support the client's occupational engagement individually and/or in groups.

An important element of this step is activity analysis, which involves selecting and, if necessary, adapting the occupations in which the client will engage as part of the therapy process. Activity analysis is discussed in detail in Chapter 20.

This step requires constant vigilance and reflection in order to make necessary adjustments in the occupation or context to facilitate optimal occupational engagement. Implementing therapy also involves building a positive therapeutic relationship as the therapy process unfolds. It requires the therapist to be aware of the client's experiences in therapy, to anticipate and note inevitable interpersonal events, and to make decisions about the use of self that support the client's occupational engagement and maintain a strong therapeutic alliance with the client. Additionally, if therapy is provided in groups, the therapist must plan for and monitor the group and manage dynamics so that the client is positively impacted.

Step Six: Determining Outcomes of Therapy

The final step involves noting the progress of the client, deciding when and how to terminate therapy, and documenting the outcomes of the therapy process. Ideally the occupational therapist and client mutually decide when to terminate therapy; however, termination is often determined by other factors such as insurance, team decisions to discharge, the end of the school year, and so on. When the therapist is aware of such external, structured ends to therapy, it is important to plan for them and to collect sufficient information to note and document outcomes.

The Dynamic Nature of the Therapeutic Reasoning Process

The steps of clinical reasoning discussed here can be cyclical in nature. That is, a therapist may begin with questions about the client and proceed to assessment, creating a conceptualization of the client and then planning the goals and the process of therapy. However, once therapy is implemented, the therapist may have new questions and gather further information to better understand the client. Or, once the client has made progress, new goals and a new therapy plan may be required. Thus, the steps in clinical reasoning may not be entirely sequential. They are presented and illustrated in the two following cases as sequential only to simplify the presentation.

Two Case Examples

In order to illustrate the process of therapeutic reasoning, two cases follow. The first is a case provided by Alice Moody from her practice in the area of chronic pain in England. The second is a case from Hiroyuki Notoh from his rehabilitation practice in Japan. Each of these cases illustrates how the therapists made thoughtful use of the conceptual foundations to conduct high-quality therapy for their clients.

Case One: Susan

Susan is a 41-year-old woman who lives in a quiet suburb in England with her husband. Nearly two decades ago she developed chronic fatigue syndrome following encephalitis. She fell during 2006, resulting in an injury to her lower back. Spinal injections and acupuncture provided only short-term relief to her chronic pain. Susan received physical therapy as an outpatient with some slight improvement. However, the pain persisted along with her chronic

fatigue; both significantly influenced her daily life and occupations. Susan was referred to a pain management program where Alice Moody served as her occupational therapist.

Questions Derived from the Conceptual Practice Models

Alice used three conceptual practice models as well as related knowledge to address Susan's situation. She used the model of human occupation as a guide to understanding how the pain and fatigue were influencing Susan's occupational life and the biomechanical model to understand the specific impact of the pain and fatigue on performance. Because pain management often requires Alice to deal with difficult emotions and interpersonal challenges, she also used the intentional relationship model and drew upon related knowledge from cognitive behavioral therapy. Here are the initial questions that Alice generated to guide her assessment of Susan.

Model of Human Occupation:
- How have Susan's pain and fatigue influenced her sense of personal causation?
- What is Susan's sense of efficacy in dealing with her symptoms and being able to go on with her occupational life despite them?
- How have her symptoms affected her interests and values?
- How do Susan's values influence how she reacts to the pain and fatigue?
- How have Susan's roles and habits been influenced by the pain and fatigue?
- What is the status of her motor, process, and communication/interaction skills?
- How does her environment influence her performance and coping with her illness?

Biomechanical Model
- How is Susan's ability to perform the movements necessary for everyday occupations affected by pain and fatigue?
- What is the extent of her pain and fatigue and when does it most affect her?

Intentional Relationship Model
- What are Susan's interpersonal characteristics and how are they affected by the stress she is experiencing from the pain and fatigue?

- How is she likely to respond to the therapy process given that it will not be able to influence her pain and fatigue but will instead focus on cognitive, emotional, and behavior changes that she must make to cope better?

Cognitive Behavioral Therapy

- What worries and anxieties does Susan express and do they interfere with her coping?

Gathering Information On, From, and With Susan

Following receipt of a referral letter from Susan's physician, Alice reviewed Susan's medical notes in order to gain an initial overview of her pain history and previous treatments she had undergone. As part of intake to the pain management program, Susan completed general questionnaires that asked about how her symptoms affected her everyday life in terms of self-efficacy, mood, and disability. Alice also informally interviewed Susan to gather supplementary information about the impact of the pain and fatigue on her occupational life and to provide Alice with an opportunity to know Susan interpersonally.

Alice did not use traditional biomechanical assessments (e.g., observing range of motion or strength) with Susan because her limitations were only related to fatigue and pain. Thus, Alice obtained information on the extent of pain and fatigue and their impact on daily functioning from Susan.

Alice used the information gleaned from these sources to complete the Model of Human Occupation Screening Tool (MOHOST) (Parkinson, Forsyth, & Kielhofner, 2006). The MOHOST provided a comprehensive overview of Susan's personal and environmental characteristics and how they influenced her occupational participation, as shown in Figure 19.2. The MOHOST was also used to structure the explanation of Susan's occupational status that is discussed here.

Alice's Explanation of Susan's Occupational Situation

Alice's assessment process allowed her to learn a great deal about Susan. She created the following explanation of Susan's situation, which guided her approach to therapy.

Volition (Personal Causation, Interests, and Values)

Susan's occupational functioning was dependent on her levels of pain and fatigue. Because her pain and fatigue were variable over time, Susan had difficulty identifying her own strengths and limitations on a daily basis. Hence, she would sometimes overdo things and experience a significant increase in her fatigue and/or pain, requiring her to rest for several days in order to recover. When asked to engage in upcoming social or family activities, Susan would feel uncertain as to whether or not she would be able to participate when the time came. This uncertainty limited her

Motivation for Occupation				Pattern of Occupation				Communication & Interaction skills				Process skills				Motor skills				Environment: Home			
Appraisal of ability	Expectation of success	Interest	Choices	Routine	Adaptability	Roles	Responsibility	Non-verbal skills	Conversation	Vocal expression	Relationships	Knowledge	Timing	Organization	Problem-solving	Posture & Mobility	Coordination	Strength & Effort	Energy	Physical space	Physical resources	Social groups	Occupational demands
F	**F**	F	**F**	**F**	F	F	F	**F**	F	F	**F**	F	F	**F**	**F**	F	F	F	F	**F**	**F**	F	**F**
A	A	**A**	A	A	**A**	**A**	**A**	A	**A**	**A**	A	**A**	**A**	A	A	**A**	**A**	**A**	A	A	A	A	A
I	I	I	I	I	I	I	I	I	I	I	I	I	I	I	I	I	I	I	**I**	I	I	**I**	I
R	R	R	R	R	R	R	R	R	R	R	R	R	R	R	R	R	R	R	R	R	R	R	R

FIGURE 19.2 Susan's MOHOST ratings.

sense of efficacy for overcoming obstacles and left her feeling that she could not control her occupational life.

Susan identified a number of interests including potting bulbs and plants and engaging in craft activities. While these leisure occupations were important to her, Susan was unable to engage in them consistently. While she valued being independent and being able to socialize and participate in family events, she felt that she was not consistent in being able to do what she valued. Although able to make choices about occupations, Susan would often avoid activities outside of her self-care routine if she was having a bad day or fearful that her symptoms might increase if she did the activity.

Susan had strong values about maintaining social appearances. When meeting with friends or family, Susan felt that she had to "put on a front." So she routinely smiled and presented herself as functioning normally, despite being tired or in pain. She felt that showing her difficulties would be a sign of weakness.

Habituation

Susan's pain and fatigue were variable, which made it hard for her to maintain a constant routine. She often had difficulty getting a good night's sleep, resulting in even lower energy levels. This, in turn, required her to rest frequently during the daytime, further disrupting her daily routine. In sum, Susan was constantly adapting her routine according to her pain and/or fatigue.

Susan also showed signs of being stuck in a pattern of activity cycling (i.e., doing more when the pain allowed and then experiencing increased pain levels that required rest or activity restriction for several days or weeks until the pain settled). During long periods of rest, Susan would become less physically fit, often experiencing stiff joints and low mood. When faced with a good day, she was tempted to make the most of it, despite the "payback" of increased pain later. In the long term, this pattern of activity cycling had led to frustration, deconditioning, and the worry that she was getting worse.

Her roles of wife, friend, family member, and hobbyist therefore were significantly limited by her pain and fatigue and its variability and unpredictable nature. Susan's responsibilities within the home had been changed to accommodate her pain and fatigue. Heavy tasks such as housework had been taken over by her husband. She placed importance on being able to attend to her own personal care, prepare a fresh fruit salad for herself each day, carry out paperwork tasks for the home, and engage in craft and gardening activities when she was able. Her friendship role was similarly dependent on her pain and fatigue levels.

Communication and Interaction Skills

Susan was able to communicate effectively and assert her needs. Her vocal expression was appropriate in tone, volume, and pace, but she often tired during interaction, having increased difficulty mentally processing information and talking more and more quietly. Susan enjoyed social contact and her manner was warm, polite, and friendly.

Process Skills

When feeling more alert, her ability to seek and retain information, plan, sequence, and problem-solve was unaffected. However, when fatigued all of these process skills were negatively affected. She had difficulty reading and conversing when fatigued. When engaging in hobbies, Susan would arrange the environment carefully for her needs ahead of time, organizing necessary tools and problem-solving in advance. Despite these efforts, she would often end up in increased pain.

Motor Skills

Susan could get around independently, but she moved slowly and carefully due to fatigue and pain. Walking, standing, and sitting for more than a few minutes at a time all caused increased pain and Susan changed her position constantly. At home, she would pursue her daily occupations in chunks (according to her fatigue levels) until the pain prevented her from continuing. Any activity outside of her routine (e.g., meeting a friend for coffee) would cause her to have to rest both before and after.

Environment

Susan's home was well maintained and comfortable, offering her opportunities for gardening and craft projects. While she still often received social invitations, she was frequently unable to attend.

Interpersonal Characteristics

Susan clearly wanted help and instruction in order to manage her occupations more effectively. She was placing a great deal of hope on the idea that the pain management program would be able to help her. It was clear that Alice needed to limit use of the encouraging mode to avoid instilling unrealistic hopes that might be detrimental for Susan. Rather, it was important for Alice to use the instructing mode to establish realistic expectations and to proceed in therapy at a modest pace.

Alice also recognized that Susan could be vulnerable to becoming overly compliant on instruction given by pain management services. This possibility highlighted the need to use the collaborating mode in therapy, providing choices for Susan and ensuring that Alice did not take on the more powerful role.

Alice also anticipated that Susan might be disappointed if occupational therapy did not quickly lead to results. Anticipating the possibility of such an empathic break, Alice felt it would be important to clarify that therapy was not a "magic formula" and that there were likely to be some things they would attempt that might not work but that could still serve as learning experiences.

Cognitions and Emotions

Alice anticipated that Susan's current method of carrying out her daily activities would need to be challenged in therapy in order for her to develop better strategies with which to manage her activities.

Susan's need to present a competent image to the outside world and to avoid others seeing her difficulties as a sign of weakness made her vulnerable to certain maladaptive thoughts. Thoughts such as, "If I admit that I can't keep up, they will think I am lazy" appeared to be driving Susan to overdo certain things, resulting in increased fatigue and pain. Alice realized she would need to gently challenge the basis of such maladaptive thoughts if Susan were to be able to pace her activities, especially within the public arena.

Therapy Goals and Plans

It was clear that Susan would not have the physical capacity to attend the typical 12-session pain management program due to her fatigue. Thus, the pain management team suggested that Susan meet with Alice individually to begin to explore the link between her activity levels and increased pain. Susan seemed pleased with this recommendation, as she was keen to be able to get some control back over her daily functioning. An appointment at a suitable time of day for her was arranged.

In their first meeting, Alice discussed possible goals for therapy with Susan. They agreed on the following goals:

- Be able to make a daily fruit salad on a consistent basis without increasing pain
- Feel more in control of gardening and craft activities through planning and pacing
- Be able to make social plans and stick to them (without extensive rest before and after)
- Better manage social activities through honest communication with others with regards to own physical needs
- Understand how unrealistic thinking patterns currently "drive" occupational functioning and come up with more helpful ways of thinking

They also agreed that the therapy process would involve Susan meeting with Alice at approximately six-week intervals for the next several months. Because her fatigue was an ongoing limitation, Susan did not feel able to make changes and think things through quickly and wanted a slower pace of therapy. The long time gap between sessions was also designed to give Susan the opportunity to fully digest reading materials that Alice planned to give her, to consider the discussions she had had with Alice, and to make small changes within her daily routine. In these ways, Susan could test out strategies that Alice would teach her and then return to therapy with questions of her own.

Implementing and Monitoring Therapy

During the initial session, Susan and Alice talked about pacing and activity cycling. Because Susan was breaking up her activities according to pain severity, she was unsure as to how long she could

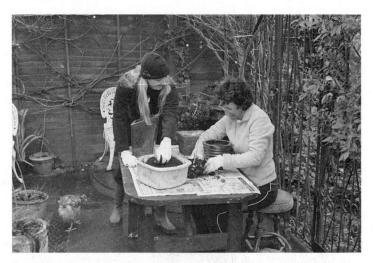

Susan practices using a stool while planting bulbs with Alice during therapy.

sit, stand, and walk before her pain began to increase. Alice and Susan agreed that it was not natural to take a break from an enjoyable activity when the pain level was manageable.

Alice recommended that Susan aim to achieve a more consistent pattern of engagement in occupations she enjoyed. To achieve this, Alice further recommended that Susan try changing positions to keep her pain at a more manageable level in order to complete a modest activity. This would, in theory, reduce the number of "bad days" she experienced. Alice also cautioned Susan about overdoing activity on days when she felt better. By evening out her level of effort, Alice explained, Susan might achieve more consistency to her activity levels and be more in control of her pain.

In order to achieve this consistency of effort, Alice and Susan engaged in problem-solving. For instance, Susan felt that she could stand for only five-minute intervals on a bad day while making her fresh fruit salad. Alice introduced the idea of using a stool. She recommended that Susan stand for five minutes, then sit on the stool for five minutes while continuing to work on the salad. In this way she could change her positioning rather than interrupting her activity to rest. By beginning to pace activities according to time limits determined by bad days, in theory, Susan would be able to maintain a consistent activity level whatever the day (good or bad).

Susan returned after the first six-week interval stating that she had been surprised to find that her standing tolerance on a bad day had in fact been only about three minutes. She had found it frustrating to have to pace her positioning and still need to take breaks to preserve her energy level. On the other hand, her sitting tolerance while doing activities had turned out to be about 10 minutes. So, despite her frustration about her standing tolerance, she remained determined to succeed and agreed that she would continue to use the stool.

In this session, Susan also talked about the ongoing conflict between her desire to be seen as useful and to fulfill social commitments and her fear of "pain and fatigue crashes" that often followed social engagement. Alice was aware that Susan's strong values were reflected in such thoughts as, "If I don't complete this today, everyone will think that I am lazy," or "If I can't do it this way, I might as well not bother." Alice decided to use a cognitive behavioral approach (CBT) to address these deeply ingrained thought patterns.

For instance, Susan was horrified at the idea of setting her own boundaries by explaining to friends that sitting in a restaurant for two hours would exhaust her and make her pain worse, resulting in several days of rest in order to recover. She worried that in showing "signs of weakness," friends would judge her poorly and think that she was making excuses. These fears reinforced her "boom and bust" or avoidance approaches to social activities, causing ongoing frustration and worry. She also found it a challenge to walk away from an incomplete craft project when pacing, as she was very talented and liked to complete projects perfectly.

Therefore Alice, utilizing elements of the CBT approach, asked Susan more about her thoughts, frustrations, and fears related to making changes in her occupational life. Susan was able to identify a number of thoughts upon which she judged herself. For example, Susan thought: "If I only attend a short lunch and then go home rather than follow lunch with a shopping trip, my friends will think I'm making excuses not to see them. They will think that I don't care." Another thought of Susan's was: "If I have to sit down at intervals, I'll never get my bulbs planted."

Alice gently challenged the authenticity of some of Susan's thoughts. For example, Alice asked Susan whether she would think any less of a friend who was experiencing a health problem and had physical limitations. Susan agreed that of course she would not judge the friend harshly, but she made the point that with pain being an invisible condition, it would probably be more difficult for others to understand. She did, however, with gentle guidance, begin to consider the idea that her thoughts might not be accurate, and that her friends had never actually accused her of being lazy or thoughtless when she had to go home early from an outing due to pain or fatigue. By the end of the session, she could tolerate the idea that it might be possible, if she were to explain her needs, that her friends might actually understand.

Alice discussed communication and assertiveness techniques with Susan and helped her begin to think about how she could communicate her needs. They also brainstormed ways that Susan could negotiate when planning a social engagement with a friend or relative. Finally, they talked about how Susan could recognize and challenge her own fears about the reactions of others. Alice coached Susan on how to entertain alternative and more helpful thoughts relating to her social life, such as, "If I don't explain my needs to

people, how can I expect them to understand and support me?"

Alice also addressed the issue of Susan's values and how they affected her occupational life. Susan was able to recognize that her need for perfection increased her frustration levels when attempting to pace herself during activities. She showed great strength and insight into her thinking patterns, recognizing how her pre-pain values ("I need to get as much done as I can while I have the chance") were acting as a mental "push" for her to overdo things, resulting in increased pain. At the end of the session, Susan planned not only to monitor her thoughts related to activity and social engagements, but also to actively challenge these in order to pursue both her pacing goals and her approach to social activities.

As Alice anticipated, Susan was a serious client who tended to just want Alice to tell her what to do for the best outcome. So, Alice was careful to collaborate with rather than direct Susan. For instance, Alice initially asked Susan to talk about a typical day and week in her life so they could together identify her strengths and needs. This allowed them to mutually formulate specific goals that were important to Susan. Alice also empathized with how challenging it was for Susan to make changes. She sought to avoid an emphatic break (i.e., making Susan feel judged) by emphasizing that it was challenging for anyone to make changes in thought and activity patterns. Alice also examined the advantages of Susan's current activity patterns along with their disadvantages to avoid Susan feeling judged about the way she had gone about her everyday life before beginning occupational therapy.

Therapy Outcomes

Following several additional sessions in which Alice and Susan reviewed her activity pacing and thinking patterns, they decided to evaluate Susan's progress. The following was their mutual assessment of her progress.

Pacing
Susan had experienced a big breakthrough with pacing techniques. After several months of perseverance, she found it almost second nature to divide her daily tasks into timed chunks of

sitting, perching, standing, and walking. She had become an expert in changing positions before her pain increased. This meant that, though still having to take regular breaks due to fatigue, she was able to more consistently engage in craft and gardening projects. She was able to accomplish more and experience fewer periods of increased pain. She continued to pace her fruit salad preparation. She was also able to accompany her husband to the supermarket to choose her own fruit for 5 to 10 minutes. Afterwards, she would sit in the car and stretch while he finished shopping. As a result, she felt more control over activities of importance to her.

She also managed to rethink her orientation to activities she enjoyed. Rather than experiencing pacing as frustrating when she had to stop an incomplete craft or gardening activity, she came to view it as "spreading out the enjoyment" over time. She had managed to plant all of her winter bulbs by permanently having her pots set out on a raised surface with all necessary tools, carrying out several minutes of potting at a time, and using her stool for breaks from standing. She felt satisfied that she was able to successfully plan and succeed at her chosen occupations on a consistent basis.

Planning and Communicating

Susan's planning skills also extended to her goal of being able to participate in more social activities. She began to talk to friends about her limitations and how she needed to accommodate them. For example, instead of a lunch and shopping with friends that previously had exhausted her, she planned to have the meal followed by visiting one shop and then taking a taxi home. When a friend asked Susan to tour a local stately home and grounds, Susan was able to explain her need to plan regular periods of sitting to break up her walking.

Despite her initial fears, Susan found that her friendships improved and strengthened. They were now based on more honest interactions. She was amazed when one of her friends said, "I'm so glad to know you are human just like the rest of us!" As a result, Susan had begun to feel more confident in explaining her needs clearly and calmly when planning to attend bigger social events such as weddings and weekends away. She found that generally people were not annoyed when she chose only to attend certain parts of planned group activities in order to better manage her pain and energy levels.

Limitations and Ongoing Goals

At this point, Susan identified that she felt much more in control of her chosen occupations and social interactions. She felt much more in charge of her pain. She was aware that things would not always go according to plan and that she still had to manage a tendency to overdo things. She also identified that it would be an impossible goal to try to please everyone in her life. She was able to recognize that she was not a failure because of her physical limitations. The reactions of others had reinforced her new positive belief in herself.

She had set for herself future pacing goals and hoped to join a craft class either at a local college or school. She felt that she had the courage to explain that she would not be able to sit, or even stay, for a whole session without fear of rejection. One of Susan's final comments was, "I may not be able to change other people, but I can change myself." Susan does not now feel the need to meet with Alice on such a regular basis, so she and Alice decided that her next review would take place in four months time.

Case Two: Kinu

Kinu was in her late eighties and had lived an active life. She had managed a family business while raising her son and daughter. For the past decade, despite high blood pressure and diabetes mellitus, she had been a caretaker for her husband who was disabled following a cerebrovascular accident (CVA). Since her husband's death, Kinu had lived with her son's family. She was proud that each child and grandchild was well-educated and successful. Over the past few years, Kinu had begun to take haiku lessons at the elders club in her community. She had wanted to pursue more education in her youth but her father had refused, as he had believed that education was not necessary for women. Participating in the elders club and writing haiku fulfilled her lifelong desire to study.

While shopping with some members of the club, Kinu was suddenly unable to walk or speak.

She was rushed to the hospital where she was diagnosed with left hemiplegia caused by a cerebral infarction. Five days later, she began to receive rehabilitation services. From the beginning of her rehabilitation program, Kinu was eager to exercise, but she often tired quickly. She had severe pain caused by left shoulder dislocation and shoulder-hand syndrome, a disorder resulting in pain and limited range of motion in the shoulder and hand. Kinu needed assistance in all self-care occupations except eating and always used a wheelchair.

Three weeks into her rehabilitation, Kinu fractured the left distal edge of her ulna as a result of a nursing staff error. The fracture produced severe pain in her wrist. Shortly thereafter, Kinu moved to a long-term rehabilitation setting, where Hiroyuki Notoh was assigned as her occupational therapist.

Questions Derived from the Conceptual Practice Models

Hiroyuki chose four models to guide his therapeutic reasoning with Kinu. Because of the pain, sensory, and motor impairments documented in her medical record, Hiroyuki chose to use the biomechanical and motor control models. Because Kinu's impairments were likely to have an impact on her motivation and occupational roles and habits, Hiroyuki chose the model of human occupation. Finally, due to the emotionally charged changes Kinu had been facing and the challenging nature of her rehabilitation, Hiroyuki chose the intentional relationship model. The questions he derived from these models are listed here.

Biomechanical Model
- What is the exact nature of Kinu's pain, sensory loss, muscle weakness, and limited range of motion?
- How do these impairments affect her self-care and other valued occupations?
- How will these impairments likely influence reconstruction of her occupational routine and role behaviors?

Motor Control Model
- What is Kinu's current ability to control her movements (especially those involving her upper extremity) while performing self-care and other occupational tasks?

- What factors are most affecting any difficulties with controlling movements?

Model of Human Occupation
- What is Kinu's knowledge of her current capacities?
- What is her sense of efficacy in being able to do what is important to her?
- What are the most important things, in Kinu's view, that she wants to achieve and that should be the emphasis of her rehabilitation?
- How has Kinu made occupational choices throughout her life and how is she likely to approach choices for her life now, given the changes that she faces?
- What are her roles and which roles are important to her to maintain even while she is in rehabilitation?
- How has her routine changed as a result of the CVA and what aspects of her routine are most important for her to reinstate?
- What is the nature of her social environment and how will it influence her recovery and future occupational functioning?

Intentional Relationship Model
- What are Kinu's interpersonal characteristics (especially her need for control, capacity for trust, communication style, orientation toward relating, and expression of emotion) and their implications for the therapeutic modes that would likely be most helpful for her?
- Is Kinu able to access social support to help her cope with her condition?

Gathering Information On, From, and With Kinu

Hiroyuki ordinarily begins his contact with elderly clients like Kinu with a brief interview. He then continues the interview in a progressive fashion over several sessions. This allows him to build trust as he asks increasingly detailed and more personal questions about the client's life. He also makes it a practice to listen carefully to everything his clients say to get cues about their perceptions of their current situation and needs.

In their first session, Kinu greeted Hiroyuki politely and with a smile. Hiroyuki had the feeling that she would be a forthcoming client with whom he could easily collaborate. He began by asking Kinu about what had happened to her and what she saw as her current needs.

Hiroyuki followed this interview with a range of testing and observation of Kinu in some self-care tasks to get an idea of her movement capacities and limitations. He asked her for more details about her experience of pain. He planned to continue the evaluation of her motor control as they worked on various tasks in therapy that would require her to use her affected arm.

Hiroyuki's Explanation of Kinu's Occupational Situation

Volition (Personal Causation, Interests, and Values)

Kinu's volition appeared intact. She had a strong sense of her priorities and was eager to engage in therapy. She was aware of her impairments and how they were affecting her performance, but she had hope that she would make some recovery. All in all, Kinu appeared to feel in control of her situation. Kinu was able to clearly state that her priority was to reacquire her left hand movements and alleviate the severe pain of her left shoulder and wrist. She was very aware of the nature of her condition and was eager to begin rehabilitation of her upper extremity.

Habituation

Although Kinu expressed no immediate concerns about her occupational life, her roles and habits were interrupted by her current impairments. She was eager to minimize the pain and movement difficulties so that she could return to these aspects of her life.

Motor Skills

Kinu's shoulder pain was severe and she still had minimal movement in her affected hand. Her shoulder passive range of motion was limited (flexion = 120 degrees; abduction = 85 degrees; external rotation = 20 degrees). These limitations were caused by her left shoulder dislocation and increased tone of her pectoralis major and biceps muscles. Her wrist passive range of motion was limited by her ulnar fracture and shoulder-hand syndrome (wrist palmar flexion = 30 degrees; dorsiflexion = 45 degrees; radial deviation = 5 degrees; ulnar deviation = 5 degrees). Finally, her finger passive range of motion was limited by shoulder-hand syndrome (mostly edema).

Finger flexion (for index through little fingers) was 40 degrees at the metacarpophalangeal joints, 40 to 60 degrees at the proximal interphalangeal joints, and 40 degrees at the distal interphalangeal joints.

Kinu's active range of motion was severely limited; she could flex her shoulder and elbow with effort but no other movements were found. Kinu could maintain standing while leaning her upper trunk against a wall or handrail. She used this position when she pulled up her pants. She could do all of her self-care activities using her right hand except for bathing, as she was not able to step into the bath.

Interpersonal Characteristics

Hiroyuki noted that Kinu had a pleasant and direct interpersonal style and could relate her needs clearly. She did not appear to express strong emotion and was able to recognize and trust Hiroyuki as a professional with whom she wanted to collaborate in achieving her rehabilitation goals.

Hiroyuki summarized all this information by completing an initial MOHOST rating, which is show in Figure 19.3.

Therapy Goals and Plans

Based on Kinu's interpersonal characteristics and her clearly stated goals, Hiroyuki planned to use the collaborating mode supplemented with the instructing and problem-solving modes. Because Kinu demonstrated no volitional problems and her major impediments to reinstating roles and habits were her pain and movement difficulties, Hiroyuki decided to emphasize the following goals:

- Improve function of her dislocated shoulder joint and decrease pain by gaining control of Kinu's shoulder girdle muscles, especially those affecting the stability of the shoulder joint
- Decrease excessive tone of her pectoralis major and biceps muscles
- Increase Kinu's shoulder range of motion
- Decrease her edema in order to increase her finger range of motion
- Regain sufficient finger movements for Kinu to execute a total grasp

Motivation for Occupation				Pattern of Occupation				Communication & Interaction skills				Process skills				Motor skills				Environment: Inpatient Hospital			
Appraisal of ability	Expectation of success	Interest	Choices	Routine	Adaptability	Roles	Responsibility	Non-verbal skills	Conversation	Vocal expression	Relationships	Knowledge	Timing	Organization	Problem-solving	Posture & Mobility	Coordination	Strength & Effort	Energy	Physical space	Physical resources	Social groups	Occupational demands
F	F	F	F	F	F	F	F	**F**	**F**	**F**	**F**	**F**	F	**F**	F	F	F	F	F	F	**F**	F	F
A	**A**	**A**	**A**	**A**	**A**	**A**	A	A	A	A	A	A	**A**	A	**A**	**A**	**A**	**A**	**A**	**A**	A	**A**	**A**
I	I	I	I	I	I	I	**I**	I	I	I	I	I	I	I	I	I	I	I	I	I	I	I	I
R	R	R	R	R	R	R	R	R	R	R	R	R	R	R	R	R	R	R	R	R	R	R	R

FIGURE 19.3 Kinu's MOHOST ratings upon admission.

Hiroyuki also planned that, if these goals were achieved, he would work with Kinu to re-learn left upper extremity movements required for self-care. To address the treatment goals, Hiroyuki planned the following strategies:

- Using neurodevelopmental treatment (NDT) for increasing stability of Kinu's left upper trunk; this involved eliciting the sitting balance reaction, which is connected with the stability of the left shoulder muscles
- Using NDT strategies for relearning the sensation of shoulder flexion and abduction movements of the left side of her upper extremity
- Using NDT strategies for facilitating total grasp and release movement of left fingers

- Passive stretching of her pectoralis major and biceps muscles
- Passive range of motion exercise of Kinu's left upper extremity joints
- Using a hot pack for Kinu's left shoulder and icing her wrist and fingers

Implementing and Monitoring Therapy

Kinu often complained during the implementation of the aforementioned strategies that her left hand would have functioned better had it not been for the accident during her initial rehabilitation. With tears, she sometimes recalled her physician's prognosis that she would never walk again. Hiroyuki listened to these narratives carefully using the empathizing

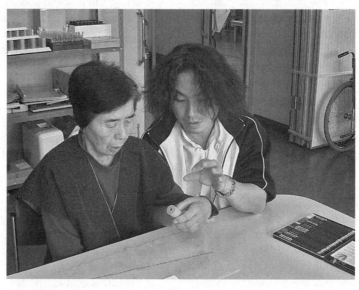

Hiroyuki helps Kinu practice her grasp and release using a soft sponge.

mode. His listening helped to solidify their therapeutic relationship.

One day about two weeks into therapy, Kinu revealed to Hiroyuki that she had begun to practice haiku (a Japanese art of writing brief poems that are represented on a background with a watercolor painting) in her eighties. She proudly stated that it was never too late to learn something new. She talked about how her grandchildren had collected her haiku and had made them into a book. When Hiroyuki showed interest in this story, Kinu lit up and showed Hiroyuki the book, which she had kept with her in the rehabilitation center. It was clear that Kinu was passionate about writing haiku and drawing the pictures used in the haiku. However, she had not continued this occupation since her cerebral infarction.

Hiroyuki considered this intimate self-disclosure to be very important. Creating haiku was clearly a very meaningful activity for Kinu. It was related to her lifelong desire to develop her intellect and it was a way for her to be connected to her family. It also allowed Kinu an important form of emotional expression. Hiroyuki knew that it was important to respond therapeutically to this significant interpersonal event. Moreover, the information she had given provided new insight into her volition. Kinu had a strong interest in writing haiku and drawing pictures. She

attached a high value to this creative process. However, she had a greatly decreased sense of capacity and efficacy as her motor dysfunction prevented her from doing this meaningful occupation.

Therefore, in the next session Hiroyuki used the instructing mode, recommending that Kinu draw pictures and write haiku poems as part of her occupational therapy. Kinu agreed to this recommendation with delight. She began to compose haiku on her own time in the ward. Kinu felt unable at that time to draw the backgrounds for the poems. So Hiroyuki found an occupational therapy fieldwork student who volunteered to help with these drawings. When Kinu's granddaughter saw that her grandmother had resumed haiku, she also volunteered to draw pictures. As a result of their collaboration, Hiroyuki and Kinu decided to modify the contents of every occupational therapy session to include time writing haiku to facilitate her hand function.

After five weeks of this new program, Kinu had progressed to drawing some haiku pictures. At this point, she was able to independently complete most of her self-care. She had acquired total grasp and release movement of her left fingers. She was able to walk with a cane. Despite these gains, the severe pain of her left shoulder had increased.

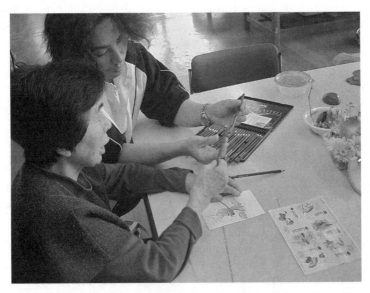

Hiroyuki and Kinu select colored pencils for her to use while working on her haiku.

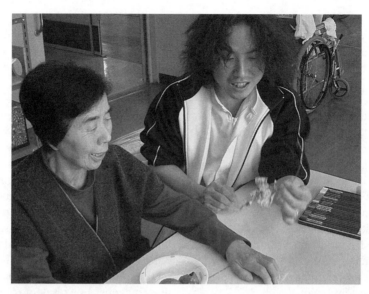

Hiroyuki shows Kinu some plants he has gathered for her to serve as inspiration for her haiku illustrations.

Kinu asked for more time with heat therapy to help with the pain, so Hiroyuki and Kinu decided together to cease the haiku as part of therapy. One of the last two haiku poems she wrote read: 泣きぬれて 夜毎眠れぬ はかなさよ. The Japanese reading of this haiku is "naki nurete yogoto nemurenu hakanasa yo" (In vain, Crying over crying, Under nights).

The other haiku read, 振り向けば 我が人生に 悔いはなし 天命を待つばかり. Hiroyuki translated this haiku to "furimukeba waga jinnsei ni kui wanashi tennmei wo matsu bakari" (Never looking back my way, It's the Providence, Only crying, Only waiting).

One day during therapy, Kinu commented tearfully that that she was resigned to not recovering as she had already lived a good life. Hiroyuki knew that this expression of strong emotion required a careful therapeutic response. He began with the empathizing mode, attempting to understand her experience more fully. Kinu explained that the loss of her most meaningful occupation was a sign to her that her life was basically over. Hiroyuki then used the collaborating mode, indicating to Kinu that she had a choice to resume her haiku again as part of therapy. They decided together that it was important for her to resume working on her haiku as part of therapy since her feelings

of efficacy and meaning were at least as important as the level of pain she experienced.

Therapy Outcomes

Four weeks later Kinu made another intimate self-disclosure. She confided to Hiroyuki that she wanted to live until she was a hundred years old. She confided that working on the haiku had given her confidence that she could go on with life in a meaningful way. Kinu was overheard telling other clients that her best healers were drawing pictures and writing haiku poems.

Just before her discharge, Kinu wrote another haiku: 病葉の 散りて春待つ 桜かな. This haiku read, "wakuraba no chirite haru matsu sakura kana" (Certainly opening up, Hidden cherry buds are there). See Figure 19.4 for Kinu's final haiku.

Kinu said to Hiroyuki that although she felt pain in her shoulder and wrist, she was going to "keep her chin up." Kinu was discharged home with confidence. Her final evaluation with the MOHOST (see Fig. 19.5) reflected the positive changes she had accomplished.

Conclusion

This chapter discussed and illustrated the process of therapeutic reasoning. The use of the

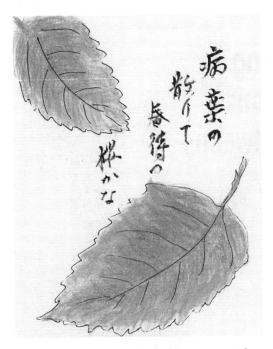

FIGURE 19.4 Kinu wrote this haiku on a postcard painted by her granddaughter.

field's conceptual foundations in understanding and designing intervention for clients is the central work of occupational therapy practice. The quality of occupational therapy will always depend on the extent to which the therapist is able to engage in a thoughtful process of therapeutic reasoning.

The two case examples in this chapter illustrated only two possible ways that therapists may engage in therapeutic reasoning. The reasoning process will vary depending on the conceptual practice models used, the kinds of occupational circumstances and impairments of the client, the length of the therapy process, and the type of context in which the therapy is taking place.

Motivation for Occupation				Pattern of Occupation				Communication & Interaction skills				Process skills				Motor skills				Environment: Inpatient Hospital			
Appraisal of ability	Expectation of success	Interest	Choices	Routine	Adaptability	Roles	Responsibility	Non-verbal skills	Conversation	Vocal expression	Relationships	Knowledge	Timing	Organization	Problem-solving	Posture & Mobility	Coordination	Strength & Effort	Energy	Physical space	Physical resources	Social groups	Occupational demands
F	F	**F**	**F**	F	**F**	**F**	**F**	**F**	**F**	**F**	**F**	**F**	F	**F**	**F**	F	F	F	**F**	F	F	F	**F**
A	**A**	A	A	**A**	A	A	A	A	A	A	A	A	**A**	A	A	**A**	**A**	**A**	A	**A**	**A**	**A**	A
I	I	I	I	I	I	I	I	I	I	I	I	I	I	I	I	I	I	I	I	I	I	I	I
R	R	R	R	R	R	R	R	R	R	R	R	R	R	R	R	R	R	R	R	R	R	R	R

FIGURE 19.5 Kinu's MOHOST ratings upon discharge.

REFERENCE

Parkinson, S., Forsyth, K., & Kielhofner, G. (2006). *Model of human occupation screening tool* (version 2.0). Chicago: Department of Occupational Therapy, University of Illinois at Chicago.

CHAPTER 20

Activity Analysis: Using the Conceptual Foundations to Understand the Fit Between Persons and Occupations

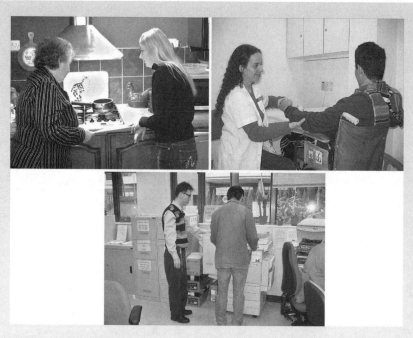

On recently assessing a woman named Roberta with an early diagnosis of Alzheimer's, I learned how she continued to struggle on a daily basis to prepare her disabled husband breakfast in bed. Roberta's priority was to more confidently continue to carry out her breakfast chores as an important part of her role as wife.

Alice Moody

Ah-fai, a client in my vocational rehabilitation setting, wanted to return to his job in the post office. In order to plan interventions, I identified the types of tasks that Ah-fai did on the job and then selected tasks that he could practice in therapy in order to rebuild skills for the job.

Bacon Fung Leung Ng

Benjamin suffered a C5–C6 spinal cord injury. I used different assistive devices to enable him to eat, drink, brush his teeth, shave, read a book/newspaper and operate a computer. Without these aids, Benjamin would have been completely dependent in basic activities of daily living and would not be able to participate in his favorite leisure activities.

Maya Tuchner

While each of these therapists was faced with quite different tasks, they all had to engage in a process referred to as activity analysis. Alice had to consider what was involved in preparing the breakfast that her client wanted to continue making. She had to think about her client's cognitive limitations and examine how this occupation could be modified so the client could continue it safely. Bacon had to consider his client's current abilities and decide what kind of occupational engagement would move the client toward his goal of returning to work. Maya had to carefully examine a number of activities to determine what movements were ordinarily required and decide how she could bridge the gap between the requirements of those movements and what her client could do. By carefully identifying these gaps, she could arrive at decisions about what equipment would bridge them.

In each of these instances, the therapist engaged in activity analysis, a process of finding and/or adjusting an occupation to achieve some therapeutic benefit or allow a person to engage in a former or new occupational role.[1] Activity analysis requires therapists to assess the fit between the characteristics and needs of a client (or client group) and a given activity. As noted in Chapter 19, activity analysis is a necessary component of the therapeutic reasoning process.

Activity analysis always involves asking questions about an activity (Crepeau, 2003). These questions are designed to help the therapist understand:

- What doing the occupation involves
- Whether the client could participate in the activity and what it might be like for the client to do so
- What therapeutic potential the activity might have for the client
- Whether and how the client could perform the activity as part of his/her occupational life

The following are a few examples of the types of questions one might ask about an occupation.

- Is the activity simple or complex?
- Where does the activity ordinarily take place?
- What steps are required for doing the activity?

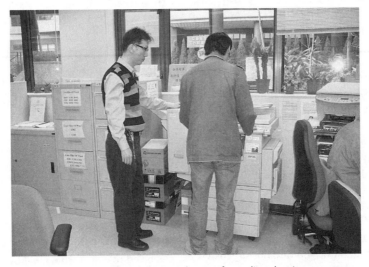

Bacon incorporates office tasks into therapy for a client hoping to return to a job at the post office.

[1]Activity analysis is sometimes taught to students in the absence of considering a particular client or particular client group in order to provide experience in thinking about activities or tasks and what they entail or require of the performer. However, in actual practice activity analysis is undertaken as part of the problem-solving process that matches activities with actual clients.

- What skills are needed to complete the activity?
- Does the activity require more than one performer?
- What sensations, feelings, or meanings might be associated with the activity?

The actual questions that a therapist will ask when analyzing a particular activity should be based on:

- The client or client group that the therapist has in mind when doing the activity analysis
- The conceptual practice models that the therapist uses to guide the activity analysis

Of course, these two factors are interrelated since the therapist's choice of models is related to the needs of the client or client group, as discussed in Chapter 18.

The Role of Conceptual Practice Models in Activity Analysis

While early forms of activity analysis were based on common-sense frameworks, it is now recognized that occupational therapists should use occupational therapy theory as a framework for activity analysis (Crepeau, 2003). Using theory serves to structure the analysis by providing concepts that orient one as to what should be examined about the activity. For instance, the biomechanical model would direct one to ask questions about the strength, range of motion, and endurance needed to do an activity. On the other hand, the sensory integration model would raise questions about the sensations involved in an activity.

> Using theory serves to structure the analysis by providing concepts that orient one as to what should be examined about the activity.

Conceptual practice models also guide the therapists in understanding the extent to which a client has the capacity for doing the activity and/or how the client might experience or react to the activity. Conceptual practice models also provide necessary information for considering how an activity might be modified or organized to achieve a therapeutic benefit and/or to allow the client to do the activity in the future.

The Process of Activity Analysis

Activity analysis consists of the following four steps:

1. Identifying the appropriate practice model(s) to guide the analysis
2. Selecting the occupation to be analyzed
3. Generating questions from the practice model(s) to guide the analysis
4. Identifying ways that the occupation(s) can be adapted and/or graded to accommodate the characteristics and needs of a client or client group

Each of these steps is discussed here.

Step One: Identify the Appropriate Conceptual Practice Model(s) to Guide the Analysis

Before selecting the models, one should reflect on the person or group for which the analysis is being done. These characteristics should determine the choice of conceptual practice models to be used for the activity analysis. The process and principles behind choosing models to guide activity analysis are those outlined in Chapter 18. The aim is to select the models that allow one to center the analysis on the needs of the particular client or client group for whom the activity analysis is being done. Moreover, to achieve a holistic view of the activity in relation to the client, therapists generally will select more than a single model to guide the analysis.

For instance, Alice Moody, in working with the woman with Alzheimer's, would utilize the cognitive model because the client has a cognitive impairment that will likely affect what she can prepare for breakfast and how she will go about it. Alice would also use the model of human occupation to guide considerations of this client's strong motivation for the activity, how it is part of her perceived role as a wife, and how it can be incorporated into her future habit structure. From the perspective of this model, Alice would also consider how her client's values and interests might influence the type of breakfast she wants to prepare. The intentional relationship model would help Alice to consider what emotionally charged events might occur when her client engages in the activity both in therapy and later at home.

Step Two: Select the Activity to be Analyzed

Selection of the activity or activities to be analyzed should be guided by a holistic approach that considers many features of the activity in relation to the client. For instance, one might ask whether the activity would be motivating for the client, whether the activity is relevant to the client's roles and routines, and how the activity's motor, sensory, cognitive, and emotional demands will resonate with the client's capacities and characteristics. Such considerations will help the therapist consider which activities are worth analyzing for the client or group in question.

In the case of the client with Alzheimer's, Alice knew that the general area of activity was preparing breakfast. She had to find out what kind of breakfast the woman was accustomed to preparing in order to choose specifically which activity she would analyze. For instance, the activity could be simply gathering materials for a bowl of cereal or could be more complex, such as preparing toast, eggs, and tea. If it turned out that a more complex form of meal preparation was not feasible for the client, she might need to creatively identify and analyze other activities appropriate for breakfast preparation.

Maya Tuchner had to analyze many self-care activities through her process of therapy with the client who had a spinal cord injury. She considered both what was a priority for her client and what activities could be done most easily with her client's remaining capacities, so that engaging in the activity would lead to success.

Maya knew that it was very important for Benjamin to be independent in activities of daily living. However, a careful activity analysis was necessary in order to determine which specific self-care activities were feasible for Benjamin. It was important to offer him and to discuss with him practicing activities that would lead to success and that were not too complex or tiring. Some important questions included whether Benjamin had the motor capacities (muscle strength and balance) to participate in a chosen activity and whether he wanted to and was willing to make the effort. Maya wanted to know what adaptive equipment might bridge gaps between Benjamin's movement capacities and what was required for desired activities.

> **Selection of the activity or activities to be analyzed should be guided by a holistic approach that considers many features of the activity in relation to the client.**

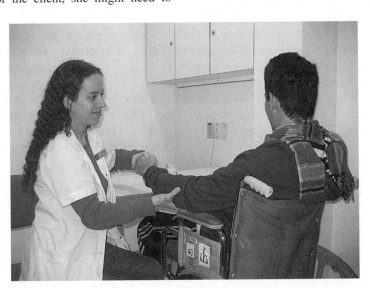

Maya tests out a client's capacities while listening to him prioritize his therapeutic goals.

For example, dressing and bathing by himself were not options for Benjamin but careful analysis showed that he had the potential to eat, drink, brush his teeth, and shave with assistive devices. Indeed, after several treatments in which he practiced these activities, Benjamin gained independence. The second domain of occupation that was extremely important for Benjamin was leisure. Reading books, especially novels, was one of his major hobbies, but at the time he was unable to hold a book and to turn the pages. After examining the steps required for this activity, a special assistive device was adjusted for his hand and a special book holder was added; also, his whole sitting position was adjusted to this activity. This activity required Maya to adapt the environment creatively to enable Benjamin to read a small book but also a larger newspaper.

The same process was completed with another activity: operating a computer. Before his injury, Benjamin used to communicate with some of his friends through the internet and also liked to read and find information online. In this example, an important question was whether he could perform this activity at home. He needed some changes to his room involving accommodations to the physical environment, including the use of special technologies and adaptations. Initially, Benjamin perceived some frustration, but because he had the physical capacities and was highly motivated he had the potential to succeed after several treatment sessions. He gained independence in very intimate and personal activities, which gave him a sense of control. Also, he was able to enjoy his time in favorite activities like reading. He even started writing about his feelings and "telling his story" through the use of the computer and keyboard.

Step Three: Generate Questions to Guide the Analysis

Once an occupation is selected for analysis, the therapist must begin to carefully examine it. This process is guided by the conceptual practice models the therapist is using for the analysis. The aim is to generate a detailed inspection of the occupation, its relationship to the client's characteristics, and the potential for the activity to be used in therapy and/or to be incorporated into the client's life.

This inspection of the activity in relation to the client and the potential of the activity for therapy and/or the client's life are guided by questions that emanate from the conceptual practice models used. Table 20.1 lists the conceptual practice models and questions that would typically be generated from these models for an activity analysis. Thus, the table includes questions about the activity itself, the client's capability for doing the occupation, how the occupation might be used in therapy, and how the activity might be incorporated into the client's life. These questions are not exhaustive, but rather they show how each model can be used to generate questions for an activity analysis.

Since activity analysis is done in reference to a particular individual, not all concepts from each model will be required to generate necessary questions. The specific questions that will be asked for the analysis reflect the specific nature of the client's impairments and occupational circumstances. So, for instance, Maya would derive questions that reflected her knowledge of her client's level of spinal cord injury and of the client's self-care routine in generating the questions to guide her activity analysis.

For the experienced therapist, the process of generating questions to guide an activity analysis is automatic. Students or new therapists might find it helpful to refer to Table 20.1 and to list questions to be considered for an analysis.

Step Four: Identify and Test Ways Occupation(s) Can be Adapted and/or Graded Based on Identified Gaps between the Activity and the Person

The final step in activity analysis involves consideration of the activity's potential for the client. The occupational therapist may consider how the activity can be used as a therapeutic tool and/or how the activity might be considered in the client's life after therapy. In both instances, it may be necessary to adapt or grade the activity.

Table 20.1 **Typical Questions Derived From Conceptual Practice Models for Activity Analysis**

Model	Typical questions about the activity	Typical questions about the client's capacity for the activity	Typical questions to guide adaptation of the activity in therapy	Typical questions used to guide adaptation of the activity for incorporation into the client's life after therapy
Biomechanical Model	What parts of the body are used for this activity (e.g., upper extremity, lower extremity, trunk, head)? What motions must be performed to conduct this activity in the involved parts of the body? How much strength is needed to perform this activity? How much endurance does this activity require?	Does the client have adequate range of motion, strength, and endurance to perform this activity? Does the client's lack of sensation affect safe and effective performance? Will the activity increase pain in the client? Does the activity pose any risks of injury for the client?	Can the activity (including objects used in doing the activity) be modified to gradually increase the range of motion, strength, or endurance requirements? Can the client be taught to compensate for sensory loss in the activity? Can the client be shown how to modify performance of the activity to minimize pain?	What adaptive equipment might bridge gaps between the client's movement capacities and what is required for the activity? What modification of the activity procedure (e.g., rest breaks, ergonomic strategies) might reduce the biomechanical demands of the activity or potential for the activity to cause pain?
Cognitive Model	What are the cognitive demands of the activity? How complex is the activity? How many steps does the activity have? How much judgment is required? What are the consequences of errors in terms of danger?	Does the client have adequate executive functions to do the activity? Does the client have adequate memory, problem-solving, judgment, etc., to do the activity? Is the client aware of limitations that might affect performance? How safe is the client to do this activity?	How can the activity be graded to require increasing demands for cognition to improve capacity? How can the activity be organized to allow the client to explore and find effective cognitive strategies for completing the activity?	How can the activity be simplified or broken down to reduce the cognitive requirements? Can memory aids, cues, or other factors help compensate for the client's cognitive limitations in this activity?

(table continues on page 306)

Table 20.1 **Typical Questions Derived From Conceptual Practice Models for Activity Analysis** continued

Model	Typical questions about the activity	Typical questions about the client's capacity for the activity	Typical questions to guide adaptation of the activity in therapy	Typical questions used to guide adaptation of the activity for incorporation into the client's life after therapy
Functional Group Model	Is this activity best done in a group? If the activity is done in a group, how will the activity demands change?	Does the client have the ability to do this activity in a group?	How would doing this activity as part of a group provide opportunities for the client to improve performance and confidence?	How can the client be incorporated into a group that does this activity?
Intentional Relationship Model	What are the interpersonal requirements of this activity?	What interpersonal events are likely to result from the client doing this activity? Is this an emotionally laden activity for the client? How might the client's interpersonal characteristics affect doing this activity?	What interpersonal strategies (e.g., use of encouragement, empathy, instruction) will likely be needed for the client to be able to engage in this activity? What interpersonal benefits might accrue from this activity?	What interpersonal supports will the client need to continue involvement in this activity?
Model of Human Occupation	To whom does this activity typically appeal? What kind of person is motivated to do this activity? What meanings or values are typically attached to this activity? Is this activity typically associated with a particular role?	What are the client's values and interests? Does the client feel capable of doing this activity? Is this activity related to the client's roles or habits? Does the client have the motor, process, and/or	Can the activity be organized/ modified so the client can enjoy/ find value in it? How can the activity be organized so that the client has adequate confidence to try it and build a sense of efficacy from completing it?	What supports will the client need to continue to do this activity that provides a sense of enjoyment/ value? Can this activity be integrated into this person's roles or habits?

Model	Typical questions about the activity	Typical questions about the client's capacity for the activity	Typical questions to guide adaptation of the activity in therapy	Typical questions used to guide adaptation of the activity for incorporation into the client's life after therapy
	How might this activity be part of a person's routine? What motor, process, and communication/interaction skills are required for this activity?	communication/interaction skills necessary for this activity?	Can this activity be modified so the client can use remaining motor, process, and/or communication/interaction skills to complete it? Would this activity provide good opportunities for the client to learn/relearn motor, process, and/or communication/interaction skills?	
Motor Control Model	What movements are required for this activity? How much postural stability, gross motor, and fine motor abilities are required for this activity?	Does the client have the motor control to engage in this activity? How might the client's movement limitations affect this client's ability to do this activity? What factor is likely to be a control parameter affecting whether/how the client performs the activity?	How can the activity, objects used, and/or context be modified to enhance the client's motor performance in this activity? How can the activity, objects used, and/or context be used to provide opportunity for the client to improve motor control?	What physical supports/activity modification will the client need to do this activity given available motor control capacity?

(table continues on page 308)

Table 20.1   **Typical Questions Derived From Conceptual Practice Models for Activity Analysis** continued

Model	Typical questions about the activity	Typical questions about the client's capacity for the activity	Typical questions to guide adaptation of the activity in therapy	Typical questions used to guide adaptation of the activity for incorporation into the client's life after therapy
Sensory Integration Model	What sensory experiences are associated with this activity? What are the necessary sensations that must be processed to complete this activity?	How is the client likely to react to the sensations associated with this activity? Is the client capable of processing the necessary sensations for this activity?	How can this activity be organized to provide sensations that would benefit this client? How can this activity be organized to present demands for sensory processing that will increase this client's capacity to organize/tolerate the sensations involved?	How can this client learn to manage the sensations involved in this activity? How can this client get his/her sensory needs met through this activity?

Some examples of how activities can be adapted and/or graded are:

- Providing adaptive equipment to allow a client with motor limitations to do necessary tasks within the activity
- Modifying how the occupation is done (e.g., allowing rest between steps to manage pain or fatigue)
- Providing assistance or supervision to ensure safety
- Making environmental alterations to accommodate for motor or cognitive limitations
- Providing different objects to use in the activity that are more suited to the client's capacities
- Breaking the activity down into simple steps and having the client complete only one step at a time

Since step four involves coming up with possible strategies to address identified gaps between the activity and the person or group, it is important that these strategies be tested to determine whether they work. Figure 20.1 illustrates the result of an activity analysis for Roberta, the client with Alzheimer's who wanted to continue preparing breakfast for her disabled husband.

In practice, therapists ordinarily complete an activity analysis as part of the process of clinical reasoning and it is rarely documented in written format as is shown in Figure 20.1. However, for someone who is new at creating an activity analysis it is a useful exercise to commit to writing the analysis.

Conclusion

This chapter presented the process of activity analysis, which is a critical component of therapeutic reasoning. The chapter illustrated how an analysis that is based on theory allows a client-centered and holistic analysis of an activity. Through activity analysis, therapists can use the conceptual foundations of the field to make thoughtful decisions about what activities can be used in therapy and how they will need to be

Activity Analysis for Roberta	
Activity Analyzed	Preparing Breakfast
Models Used	Cognitive Model, Intentional Relationship Model, Model of Human Occupation
Characteristics of the activity relative to Roberta	**Motivation:** Roberta has been preparing breakfast for her husband for 20 years since he had a stroke. It has great meaning for her both because it is part of her current caretaking responsibilities as a spouse of a disabled partner and because it is associated with fond memories of making breakfast in bed for her husband on special occasions. It is one of the key activities that characterize her occupational life. **Routine:** Roberta generally rises early before her husband wakes and has a cup of tea while reading the morning paper. Once her husband is up, she typically prepares him an English breakfast consisting of fried eggs, tomatoes, and toast along with a cup of tea from the pot she has already prepared for herself. **Cognitive challenge of the activity and associated risks:** Preparing breakfast according to her custom requires Roberta to operate a gas stove, handle a hot frying pan, manage boiling water, and transport the breakfast to her husband's room. She currently has no problem with the physical demands of these tasks. However, the breakfast she prepares involves many steps and potential for danger if she makes an error (e.g., fire from the stove, burns from hot water or a skillet). Roberta's dementia is mild at this stage and she is able to engage in multi-step activities that are familiar. The breakfast routine is highly familiar to her at this point and she follows it invariantly. **Emotional nature of the activity for Roberta:** This is a highly valued activity tied to the client's role. If she were not to continue it, Roberta would experience a major loss with strong emotional consequences. Roberta is very open to feedback and would likely deal well with suggestions for modifying the activity to assure safety.
Planned adaptation for therapy	No major modification of how Roberta goes about the activity appears necessary at this time. However, the therapist will observe Roberta preparing breakfast during a home visit. To assure safety, the therapist and Roberta will explore use of a laminated reminder checklist that Roberta can keep in the kitchen with critical steps, such as "turn off gas stove," outlined. Roberta can check off each step on her list with a non-permanent pen as she progresses through the task and then wipe it clean for use the following day. Also, the therapist will review with Roberta the equipment that she uses and consider an electric teapot with an automatic turn-off that does not require her to have two items on the stove at once. They will review safety considerations and further possible modifications to ensure safety such as placement of the phone in the kitchen with a posted phone number to dial in case of an accident.
Planned adaptation for Roberta's daily life	Roberta's son lives nearby and he will be instructed to check in routinely with his mother about how things are going and to observe his mother at least monthly to assure that she is able to safely continue the breakfast procedure. If questions arise about safety, Roberta will be referred by the son back to occupational therapy to consider further activity modification.

FIGURE 20.1 Activity Analysis for Roberta.

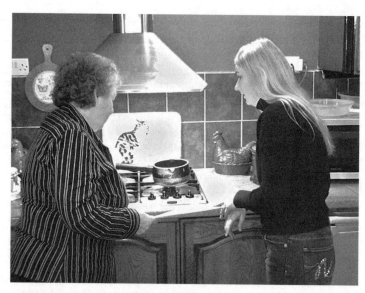

Alice and Roberta try out strategies they have identified to help Roberta with her routine of cooking breakfast.

modified to achieve maximum therapeutic benefit. Moreover, activity analysis can be used to make decisions about activities that clients wish to be part of their occupational lives, so that therapists can assist clients to continue involvement in those activities.

REFERENCES

Crepeau, E.B. (2003). Analyzing occupation and activity: A way of thinking about occupational performance. In E.B. Crepeau, E.S. Cohn, & B.A.B. Schell (Eds.), *Willard & Spackman's occupational therapy* (10th ed., pp. 189–198). Philadelphia: Lippincott Williams & Wilkins.